Cardiac Markers

PATHOLOGY AND LABORATORY MEDICINE

Series Editors: Stewart Sell and Alan Wu

PATHOLOGY AND LABORATORY MEDICINE

Cardiac Markers

Edited by

Alan H. B. Wu

Hartford Hospital, Hartford, CT

Humana Press ✳ **Totowa, New Jersey**

Dedication

This book is dedicated to my parents, for their guidance, my wife, Pamela for her understanding and appreciation, and to our children, Edward, Marcus, and Kimberly.

© 1998 Humana Press Inc.
999 Riverview Drive, Suite 208
Totowa, New Jersey 07512

This publication is printed on acid-free paper. ∞
ANSI Z39.48-1984 (American Standards Institute) Permanence of Paper for Printed Library Materials.

Cover design by Patricia F. Cleary.

For additional copies, pricing for bulk purchases, and/or information about other Humana titles, contact Humana at the above address or at any of the following numbers: Tel.: 973-256-1699; Fax: 973-256-8341; E-mail: humana@humanapr.com; Website: http://humanapress.com

Printed in the United States of America. 10 9 8 7 6 5 4 3 2 1

Library of Congress Cataloging in Publication Data

Cardiac Markers / edited by Alan H. B. Wu.
     p.   cm.—(Pathology and laboratory medicine; 3)
     Includes index.
     ISBN 0-89603-434-8 (alk. paper)
     1. Coronary heart disease—Serodiagnosis. 2. Biochemical markers.
I. Wu, Alan H. B. II. Series.
     [DNLM: 1. Myocardial Infarction—diagnosis. 2. Biological Markers. 3. Angina, Unstable—physiopathology
WG 300 C2668 1998]
    RC685.C6C265 1998
    616.1'23075—dc21
    DNLM/DLC
    for Library of Congress
                                                97-37500
                                                 CIP

Preface

Like most fields of clinical medicine, the practice of cardiology changes at a dramatic rate. New knowledge in the pathophysiology of acute coronary syndromes, coupled with new diagnostic approaches to treat patients with coronary artery diseases (CAD), have placed fresh demands on the clinical laboratory to develop and use more effective markers to answer these clinical needs. This monograph describes the current and future markers for CAD and how they are used in a clinical setting.

As a prelude to treating the markers themselves, the first sections of *Cardiac Markers* defines and classifies coronary artery diseases. An up-to-date review of the underlying pathophysiology of unstable angina and acute myocardial infarction (AMI) are presented. The various therapeutic approaches to the management of patients are described because cardiac markers have an impact on just how such therapies are used. A major use of serum markers lies in the cost-effective triage of patients from the emergency department. Described in this chapter are the conventional and "chest pain center" strategies. The subcellular distribution of the proteins and enzymes used in diagnostic tests provide backround on how they function.

The next two sections describe the cardiac markers in current use. Each chapter begins with a presentation of the biochemistry of the protein marker treated, followed by a discussion of the pertinent analytical methodologies available for its measurement. A description is given of the performance of each test used in cardiac disease, and in selected noncardiac disorders that are important for the proper interpretation of results. The cytoplasmic markers including myoglobin, creatine kinase (CK), CK-MB isoenzymes and isoforms, and lactate dehydrogenase isoenzymes. CK has become recognized as the "gold standard" for diagnosis of AMI. As such, there have been major efforts to develop sensitive and rapid assays for its analysis. Chapters on myoglobin and LD isoenzymes are also important since these are early and late markers for AMI, respectively. The structural proteins represent a new generation of cardiac markers and include cardiac troponin T and I, and myosin light and heavy chains. Assays for cTnT and cTnI are quite specific for cardiac injury. Although assays for myosin are not as specific, they may be important in assessing the severity of AMI.

The final section is devoted to future areas of cardiac marker development and applications. Because of the need to deliver results quickly, point-of-care devices are now being developed that enable testing to be carried out by caregivers at bedside. Discussions of platforms and of the regulatory aspects of point-of-care testing are presented. A look into possible future cardiac markers is also presented. Cardiac troponin will likely become the new gold standard for cardiac injury. Because myoglobin is not specific to cardiac injury, there is a search for earlier and more definitive markers. Whether or not any of these research assays become adopted into routine practice remains to be seen.

Alan H. B. Wu

Contents

Contributors

FRED S. APPLE • *Department of Laboratory Medicine and Pathology, Hennepin County Medical Center, Minneapolis, MN*

EDWARD BESSMAN • *Department of Emergency Medicine, Johns Hopkins Hospital, Baltimore, MD*

ROBERT H. CHRISTENSON • *Department of Pathology, University of Maryland School of Medicine, Baltimore, MD*

ALLEN W. CLARK • *Department of Anatomy, University of Wisconsin Medical School, Madison, WI*

KENNETH J. DEAN • *Boehringer Mannheim Corporation, Indianapolis, IN*

SATYENDRA GIRI • *Department of Internal Medicine, Division of Cardiology, Hartford Hospital, Hartford, CT*

GARY B. GREEN • *Department of Emergency Medicine, Johns Hopkins Hospital, Baltimore, MD*

SOL F. GREEN • *Becton Dickinson Vacutainer Systems, Franklin Lakes, NJ*

ROBERT G. MCCORD • *Department of Pathology and Laboratory Medicine, Chilton Memorial Hospital, Pompton Plains, NJ*

MAURO PANTEGHINI • *First Laboratory of Clinical Chemistry, Spedali Civili, Brescia, Italy*

HEMANT C. VAIDYA • *Dade International, Inc., Newark, DE*

H. KALERVO VAANANEN • *Department of Anatomy, University of Oulu, Oulu, Finland*

DAVID D. WATERS • *Department of Internal Medicine, Division of Cardiology, Hartford Hospital, Hartford, CT*

SHAN S. WONG • *Washington, DC*

ALAN H. B. WU • *Department of Pathology and Laboratory Medicine, Hartford Hospital, Hartford, CT*

Part I
Clinical Aspects

Introduction to Coronary Artery Disease (CAD) and Biochemical Markers

Alan H. B. Wu

INCIDENCE OF CARDIOVASCULAR DISEASES (CVD)*

Cardiovascular disease (CVD) (of which CAD is a subset) is the leading cause of morbidity and mortality in the Western world. In the US, there are approx 70 million people who suffer from one form of this disease or another (Fig. 1) *(1)*. Each year, 500,000 suffer from stroke (cerebrovascular accident, CVA). The annual mortality rate of CVA is about 150,000 and individually ranks third overall behind acute myocardial infarction (AMI) (discussed in Chapter 3) and cancer. Approximately six million Americans are admitted to hospitals with a diagnosis of chest pain. Of those 70 million individuals with CVD, roughly 5% (three million) have silent ischemia. The incidence of AMI from the combination of patients with symptomatic and asymptomatic (silent) CAD is 1.5 million patients/yr. The mortality rate is 500,000/yr. Half of these deaths occur before they reach the hospital for treatment. Unstable angina (discussed in Chapter 2) and congestive heart failure (CHF) account for a large fraction of non-AMI patients who are

admitted to a hospital with chest pain. A large number of chest pain patients are also inappropriately admitted for noncardiac causes. The remainder are discharged to home. From this group, there is roughly 30,000 who are inappropriately discharged from the emergency department. Chapter 4 discusses the impact that cardiac markers have on the discharge of patients from the emergency department.

There are numerous risk factors for CVD, including presence of hypertension (blood pressure ≥ 140/90 on several occasions), smoking, hyperlipidemia (total cholesterol > 200 mg/dL, LDL cholesterol > 130 mg/dL), low HDL cholesterol (≤ 35 mg/dL), family history of premature CAD (definite AMI, AMI, or death at < 55 yr for parent or sibling), presence of the y-chromosome (males) and postmenopausal status (females), diabetes, and a physically inactive lifestyle *(2)*. Some of these factors are discussed further in Chapter 4. Newer risk factors, such as other plasma lipoproteins (apolipoprotein A-I and B, lipoprotein (a), apolipoprotein E genotyping) *(3)*, coagulation factors (fibrinogen, Factor VII, VIII, viscosity) *(4)*, and homocysteine *(5)*, are currently being inves-

---

*See p. 17 for list of abbreviations used in this chapter.

From: Cardiac Markers Edited by: Alan H. B. Wu
© Humana Press Inc., Totowa, NJ

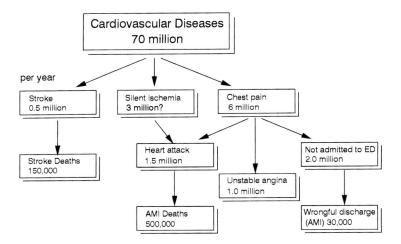

Fig. 1. Estimated annual incidence of cardiovascular diseases.

tigated. A thorough discussion of these and other cardiovascular risk factors are beyond the scope of this book.

CAD DEFINITIONS

CAD and thrombus formation are the underlying pathologies responsible for the majority of patients with AMI. Asymptomatic patients with CAD are classified as silent myocardial ischemia. Symptomatic patients have a clinical presentation of chest pain and are classified as angina pectoris. Those with chest pain at rest may have unstable angina (UA), an acute syndrome associated with plaque rupture, platelet aggregation ("white clot") and thrombus formation ("red clot"). Unstable angina that is associated with a total occlusion of a coronary artery is a prelude to AMI. Unstable angina, non-Q-wave, and Q-wave AMI are collectively termed acute coronary syndromes (6). Detection and treatment of patients with UA are essential in reducing the incidence of AMI, or minimizing its morbidity and mortality. However, medical and surgical therapies are costly and have risks. For example, percutaneous transluminal coronary angioplasty has a morbidity of 0.32%, whereas diagnostic cardiac catheterization has a mortality of 0.1% (7).

AMI incidence is 0.61 and 0.05%, respectively. Therefore, a strategy of diagnosis and risk assessment is appropriate so that patients who are the most likely to suffer acute events in the near future are treated over those who are at low risk. Since sensitive biochemical markers for myocardial injury are now being proposed for diagnosis of minor myocardial injury and risk stratification, a description of these clinical syndromes is warranted to rationalize the need for developing new markers to meet these needs

Silent Myocardial Ischemia

Silent myocardial ischemia can be defined as the presence of transient myocardial injury from coronary artery disease in the absence of chest pain or other typical signs and symptoms (8). Silent ischemia can occur in individuals without a previous history of cardiac disease and presumed to be healthy, or in patients who have had an AMI and are asymptomatic. Some patients with coronary artery disease may have episodes of both silent and symptomatic ischemia. Documentation of silent ischemia is made through evidence by electrocardiogram (ECG) and radionuclide studies. The reason why some ischemic patients are free of pain has been the subject of intense investigations for many years and remains unresolved. It may be possible that some of these patients have an alteration in their sensitivity to pain. This may be manifested by higher plasma concentrations of β-endorphins *(9)*. The precipitation of chest pain in silent ischemia patients following administration of naloxone (opioid antagonist) would support this hypothesis. Unfortunately, results of such experiments have been equivocal *(10)*. Studies in diabetics suggest that there may be some pathological involvement of the autonomic nervous system resulting in raised thresholds to pain. Hyposensitivity to pain, however, cannot alone explain all cases of silent ischemia. It is tempting to postulate that during silent ischemia, less myocardial tissue is at jeopardy for irreversible damage than symptomatic episodes. Radionuclide ventriculography, echocardiography, and myocardial blood flow studies suggest that there is little difference between symptomatic and asymptomatic ischemia for area of necrosis or risks for subsequent events *(11)*.

Determining the prevalence of silent ischemia in patients who are totally asymptomatic is very difficult. One mechanism to determine retrospectively the prevalence of atherosclerotic heart disease in adults is to use autopsy data on individuals who died of noncardiac causes and who had no symptoms or history of coronary artery disease prior to death. In one review, a prevalence of 6.4 and 2.6% was reported for males and females (age range 30–69), respectively *(12)*. Prospective detection of silent ischemia is helpful for clinical management. There are two approaches: exercise (treadmill) testing with electrocardiogram (ECG) monitoring and ambulatory (Holter) electrocardiography, whereby ECG tracings are recorded over a 24-h period. In both cases, the presence of significant ST-segment depression of >1 mm is suggestive of an ischemic event. The confirmation of silent ischemia can be performed by angiography on patients screened positive by these techniques.

Stable Angina Pectoris

Stable angina has been defined by the World Health Organization (WHO) as transient episodes of chest pain precipitated by exercise or other situations, resulting in an increased myocardial oxygen demand *(13)*. The pain usually disappears with rest or with drugs, such as nitroglycerin, that diminish the oxygen demands of the heart. It is divided into three categories:

1. *De novo* effort angina, angina of <1 mo duration;
2. Stable effort angina, <1 mo duration; and
3. Worsening effort angina, sudden worsening in frequency severity, or duration of chest pain caused by the same effort.

Stable angina is caused by years of atherosclerotic deposition of plaque onto coronary arteries. It is one of the entry points for patients with acute coronary syndrome, defined collectively as unstable angina and AMI.

UA Pectoris

UA is principally defined as chest pain occurring at rest. A more thorough definition has been made by the Agency for Health Care Policy and Research *(14)*:

1. Symptoms of angina at rest (usually prolonged >20 min);
2. New-onset (<2 mo) exertional angina of at least Canadian Cardiovascular Society Classification (CCSC) *(15)* class III in severity;
3. Recent (<2 mo) acceleration of angina as reflected by an increase in severity of at least one CCSC class to at least CCSC class III;
4. Variant angina;
5. Non-Q-wave myocardial infarction; and
6. Post-MI (>24 h) angina.

The CCSC for UA is presented in Chapter 3. In addition to the CCSC classification, there are other systems that have been proposed. The one used frequently in the US was proposed by Braunwald *(16)*. This scheme classifies patients with unstable angina in terms of severity (from class I–III) and clinical circumstances surrounding its presence (class A–C). An abbreviated version is shown in Table 1.

Class I is new onset of severe angina (<2 mo) or accelerated angina, and is characterized by the absence of pain at rest. Class II is angina at rest within the prior month, but not within the preceding 48 h. Class III is angina at rest within the preceding 48 h. Class A is UA secondary to the presence of extracoronary clinical conditions that decrease the oxygen supply (e.g., respiratory failure) or increase the oxygen demand (unusual emotional stress) to the heart. Class B is primary UA, where an extrinsic condition cannot be identified. Class C is chest pain developing within 2 wk after AMI. This classification may be further divided according to the intensity of treatment and presence or absence of transient ST-T-wave abnormalities during an anginal episode.

Unlike stable angina, UA is an acute event characterized by rupture of a coronary artery plaque. The pathophysiology of UA is described in Chapter 2. UA is important because it is a prelude to AMI.

Diagnosis of AMI

The pathophysiology of AMI is presented in Chapter 3. The WHO has also defined the criteria for diagnosis of AMI as a triad *(13)*:

1. The history is typical if severe and prolonged chest pain is present;
2. Unequivocal ECG changes are the development of abnormal, persistent Q- or QS-waves, and evolving injury lasting longer than 1 d; and
3. Unequivocal change consists of serial enzyme change, or initial rise and subsequent fall of levels. The change must be properly related to the particular enzyme and

Table 1
Braunwald Classification
of Unstable Angina

Severity	Clinical circumstances		
	Extracardiac cause, 2° UA	No extracardiac cause, 1° UA	After AMI, post-AMI UA
New or accelerated onset	IA	IB	IC
Rest angina (within 1 mo to 48 h)	IIB	IIB	IIC
Rest angina (within 48 h)	IIIA	IIIB	IIIC

to the delay time between onset of symptoms and blood sampling.

When all of these milestones are present, the diagnosis of AMI is unequivocal. The diagnosis is less certain when the chest pain is atypical, if the ECG is equivocal (stationary injury current, symmetrical inversion of the T-wave, pathological Q-wave in a single ECG record, or conduction disturbances), or if enzyme changes are not accompanied by a subsequent fall. The WHO definition is nearly 20 yr old, and is antiquated with the advent of cardiac markers that are not themselves enzymes (such as myoglobin, cardiac troponin T [cTnT] or I [cTnI]). A revision of the WHO AMI diagnostic criteria is now in dire need.

Assessment of Coronary Artery Perfusion Status

Patients with AMI can be emergently treated with thrombolytic agents, such as intravenous (iv) streptokinase or tissue plasminogen activator (tPA) *(17–19)* (Chapter 4). The goal of iv therapy is to recanalize previously occluded coronary arteries. Successful salvage of jeopardized myocardium requires treatment of AMI patients within the first 6 h of chest pain *(20)*. Because some patients present after this time interval and thrombolytic agents have the potential to cause serious bleeding, not all patients are candidates for this therapy. Fortunately, in some patients, spontaneous reperfusion can occur without the aid of clot-dissolving agents. The assessment of coronary artery perfusion status is important in the management of AMI patients. In cases where iv thrombolytic therapy has failed, emergency ("rescue") percutaneous transluminal coronary angioplasty (PTCA) has been used. The effectiveness of rescue PTCA is being studied in clinical trials. Although rescue PTCA has been successful in a majority of cases, the mortality rate for unsuccessful cases is unacceptably high *(21–23)*.

Successful or spontaneous reperfusion is indicated by the secession of chest pain or the presence of reperfusion arrhythmias *(24)*. Since these indicators are highly subjective, definitive assessment of coronary artery patency is performed by cardiac angiography. The Thrombolysis in Myocardial Infarction (TIMI) Study Group has established a grading scale for the extent of patency *(17)*:

1. Grade 0: No antegrade flow beyond the point of occlusion;
2. Grade 1 (penetration without perfusion): Contrast media pass beyond the area of obstruction, but fail to opacify the entire coronary bed distal to the obstruction for the duration of the filming;
3. Grade 2 (partial perfusion): Contrast media pass across the obstruction and opacify the coronary bed distal to the obstruction. However, the rate of entry into the vessel distal to the obstruction or its rate of clearance from the distal bed (or both) is perceptibly slower than its entry into or clearance from comparable areas not perfused by the previously occluded vessel (i.e., the opposite

coronary artery or coronary bed proximal to the obstruction); and
4. Grade 3 (complete perfusion): Antegrade flow into the bed distal to the obstruction occurs as promptly as antegrade flow into the bed proximal to the obstruction, and clearance of contrast material from the involved bed is as rapid as clearance from an uninvolved bed in the same vessel or the opposite artery.

The TIMI grading scale is used as the "gold standard" in characterizing the success of biochemical markers and other indicators of coronary artery reperfusion status.

Congestive Heart Failure (CHF)

Heart failure is a condition whereby the heart is unable to generate a sufficient cardiac output to meet the needs of metabolizing tissues *(25)*. It is characterized by intravascular and interstitial volume overload, which can lead to shortness of breath, rales, and edema, or inadequate tissue perfusion, which can produce fatigue or exercise intolerance *(26)*. Heart failure can be precipitated by a variety of causes, including pulmonary embolism, infection, anemia, thyrotoxicosis, arrhythmias, rheumatic fever, infective endocarditis, systemic hypertension, and myocardial infarction. The manifestations of heart failure include dyspnea, orthopnea, parosysmal (nocturnal) dyspnea, Cheyne-Stokes respiration, fatigue and weakness, lower extremity edema, and abdominal symptoms associated with ascites and/or hepatic engorgement *(25)*. The National Heart, Lung, and Blood Institute has estimated that there are two million Americans with CHF, with about 400,000 new cases each year. Total costs for treating patients exceeds $10 billion/yr. The 5-yr mortality rate is 50% *(26)*. Because of this high mortality rate, early detection and appropriate treatment would be helpful. Unfortunately, many patients with CHF present with no symptoms, and diagnosis in these patients is very difficult *(27)*.

There are several classifications for CHF. The New York Heart Association classification is based on functional capacity and objective assessment *(28)*:

Functional capacity

Class I: Patients with cardiac disease, but without resulting limitation of physical activity. Ordinary physical activity does not cause undue fatigue, palpitation, dyspnea, or anginal pain;

Class II: cardiac disease resulting in slight limitation of physical activity. They are comfortable at rest. Ordinary physical activity results in fatigue, palpitation, dyspnea, or anginal pain;

Class III: marked limitation of physical activity. They are comfortable at rest. Less than ordinary activity causes fatigue, palpitation, dyspnea, or anginal pain; and

Class IV: cardiac disease resulting in inability to carry on any physical activity without discomfort. Symptoms of heart failure or of the anginal syndrome may be present even at rest. If any physical activity is undertaken, discomfort is increased

Objective assessment

1. No objective evidence of cardiovascular disease;
2. Objective evidence of minimal cardiovascular disease;
3. Objective evidence of moderately severe cardiovascular disease; and
4. Objective evidence of severe cardiovascular disease

Since the criteria for minimal, moderately severe, and severe disease cannot be precisely defined, this classification scheme, is in fact, highly subjective. The Killip Classification is also a frequently used system for CHF *(29)*. Patients with suspected CHF should undergo echocardiography to assess left ventricular function *(26)*. The majority of patients with moderate to severe CHF will have ejection fractions of < 35–40%. New biomarkers for heart failure are being developed and are discussed in Chapter 17.

BIOCHEMICAL MARKERS

Historical Perspective

A brief history of cardiac markers in CAD is outlined in Fig. 2. The first biochemcial marker used in AMI was aspartate aminotransferase described in 1954 *(30)*. This was gradually replaced by use of creatine kinase (CK) described in 1965 *(31)*. With the development of electrophoresis methods, CK and lactate dehydrogenase (LD) isoenzymes were recognized as markers with higher specificity than CK *(32)*. In 1975, the immunoinhibition was developed for CK-MB *(33)*, whereas radioimmunoassay was developed for myoglobin *(34)*. Shortly thereafter, the WHO criteria for AMI was established in 1979 *(13)*. The WHO criteria includes enzymes as part of the triad of for AMI diagnosis. In 1985, the first mass assays from two different manufacturers were simultaneously evaluated on AMI patients *(35,36)*. This led to the development of the first antibody to CK-MB, which is used in nearly all commercial CK-MB immunoassays today *(37)*. Although antibodies to the M- and B-subunit existed, many thought that MB did not have any unique antigenicity. cTnT as a marker for AMI was first demonstrated in 1989 *(38)*, while cTnI appeared in 1992 *(39)*. The use of CK-MB isoform for triaging patients from the emergency department was described in 1994 *(40)*. The use of cTnT for unstable angina was first described in 1992 *(41)*. Both have been validated for risk stratification in large clinical trials published in 1996 *(42,43)*.

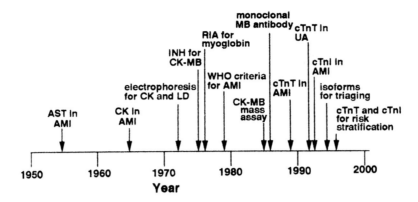

Fig. 2. History of the development of cardiac markers.

Today, cardiac markers are a multibillion dollar industry. In the Western world, multiple determinations of cardiac markers are performed on every patient who is seen with chest pain. The interest in markers continues to grow at a tremendous rate. There have been many review articles *(44–47)* and monographs *(48,49)* published within the last four years. The next generation of markers have already been developed (Chapter 17). It remains to be seen which will survive the test of time.

Criteria for Assay Performance in Clinical Studies

Like other tests in the clinical laboratory, the clinical performance of cardiac markers is evaluated in patient populations diagnosed with and without the disease in question. Equations for clinical sensitivity, specificity, predictive value, and efficiency are given in the Appendix. These terms are used throughout the volume.

Requirements for an Ideal Cardiac Marker

Owing to the changes in the practice of cardiology, new biochemical markers for ischemia and necrosis are needed and are being developed and studied. There are several characteristics of an ideal cardiac marker *(47,50,51)*. Some of them are listed below.

Substantial Distribution Within Cardiac Tissue

A basic premise for the success of a biochemical marker is that it is present in relatively high concentration in the tissue of interest. Because cardiac tissue has an essential contractile function, structural proteins of the contractile apparatus are logical candidates for use as a cardiac marker. Also, proteins and enzymes that are required in energy production and utilization are also potential markers, since energy is needed to fuel contractions. Logically, proteins that are not present in substantial concentrations within the heart would not be useful markers. The size and subcellular distribution of proteins and enzymes will dictate how quickly the proteins arrive into the general circulation. Small proteins and those located predominately in the cytoplasm will appear first. Proteins and those located in the nucleus or mitochondria will appear later, since they must cross through another set of membranes. Structural proteins will appear last, since they are released only after degradation of the matrix has been initiated, such as by macrophages and lysosomal enzymes.

High Cardiac Specificity

The marker should have no significant tissue sources other than the target organ (the heart). Although CK-MB is the most widely used cardiac marker, it is not ideal, because skeletal muscles contain a significant amount of CK-MB that contributes to the baseline concentration of this isoenzyme in the serum of healthy individuals. Abnormal pathologic concentrations of CK-MB must exceed this baseline level.

High Analytical Specificity

Most cardiac markers make use of immunoassays with monoclonal antibodies (MAbs) and polyclonal antibodies. The ideal assay for a cardiac marker must use antibodies that do not crossreact with other structurally related proteins. Even if there is no direct avidity of the interferent protein with the antibody, nonspecific binding of the protein can occur when the interferrent is present at very high concentrations *(52)*. For monoclonal (murine-based) assays, the antibodies should not react in the presence of heterophile or human anti-mouse antibodies (HAMAs) *(53)*. Significant titers of HAMA can be present in individuals who handle domestic animals or patients undergoing MAb anticancer drug therapy and falsely positive results can occur in "sandwich"-type immunoassays *(54)*.

High Assay Sensitivity and Precision

The reference range for cardiac markers in blood is dictated by the normal turnover of tissues containing significant amount of the protein in question. The upper limit of normal ranges from 100 pg/mL for specific assays, such as cardiac troponin, to 100 ng/mL for myoglobin (since it is also found in skeletal muscles). An assay with poor sensitivity cannot be used to detect minor myocardial injury, such as that seen in unstable angina. Because analytical sensitivity is defined as the noise level in the absence of analyte, highly sensitive assays must also necessarily be highly precise (CVs of <5%).

Early Appearance in Blood After Myocardial Injury

This facilitate the early diagnosis of injury or infarction, and can be useful for triaging patients from the emergency department to the appropriate beds within the hospital or discharged to home (Chapter 4). Chapter 17 discusses a strategy for development of new early cardiac markers based on the pathophysiology of acute coronary syndromes. A serum marker for early AMI diagnosis requires development of an assay with a short turnaround time (TAT) to take full diagnostic advantage of the earlier marker.

Prolonged Elevation After Injury

A marker that remains abnormal beyond 2–3 d after the onset of chest pain is useful for diagnosing the few patients who present to the hospital late, i.e., after results of early markers, such as CK-MB and myoglobin have returned to normal. Although acute iv therapy is not indicated, a full cardiac workup is warranted on these late-presenting AMI patients. Procedures, such as PTCA and coronary artery bypass graft surgery, may be considered on an elective basis.

Validated by Clinical Studies

Cardiac markers must be evaluated against appropriate standards in clinical studies *(55,56)*. For AMI markers, the criteria for diagnosis must be carefully established (such as the WHO criteria) and consistently applied. For UA and detection of minor injury, diagnostic criteria are not as well established. In either case, results of the marker in question cannot be used as part of the diagnostic criteria. The cutoff concentration must be rigorously established, since the clinical sensitivity and specificity are interrelated. Assignment of the cutoff concentration can be established by receiver operating characteristic (ROC) curves. A standardized method for performing ROC plots and statistically comparing the performance of multiple markers has recently been proposed *(57)*. For determination of

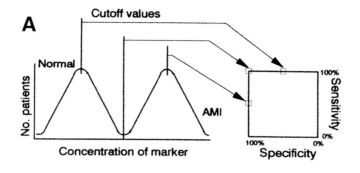

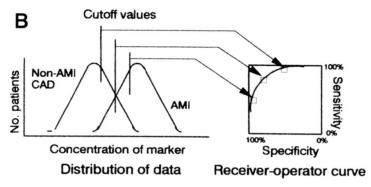

Fig. 3. Use of ROC plots for optimum assessment of cutoff concentrations. **(A)** Use of normal individuals as the non-AMI-rule out group produces results with very high clinical sensitivity and specificity. **(B)** Use of non-AMI cardiac patients produces lower clinical sensitivities and specificities, but is more realistic to actual clinical practice.

clinical specificity, it is important to include patients who have similar clinical presentations as the disease in question. For a test that detects AMI, this would include non-AMI patients with CAD. When normal subjects are used as the rule-out group, a falsely inflated clinical specificity might be obtained. Figure 3 illustrates the effect of inappropriate and appropriate populations for an AMI marker using ROC plots.

Assay Available on Automated Analyzer

The most effective cardiac marker used for acute coronary artery diseases will be one that is available at all hours and has a short TAT for results (<15 min). This requires use of either totally automated analyzers or a point-of-care (POC) platform. Cardiac marker assays are available on random-

access immunoassay analyzers that enable stat testing at all hours for most of the analytes discussed in Chapter 9. It has recently been demonstrated that when all testing is performed on a stat basis, hospital length of stay for cardiac diagnosis-related groups (DRG) is significantly reduced over testing performed once or twice per day *(58,59)*. POC devices are an emerging area for testing and are discussed in Chapter 16. They offer the advantage that no instruments are needed, and the sample does not need to be delivered to the laboratory for testing. Many devices make use of whole blood, which further facilitates a rapid TAT for results.

Summary of Release vs Time Curves

By the nature of its pathophysiology, AMI is inherently a very dynamic process. The

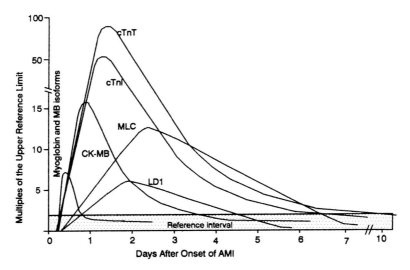

Fig. 4. Release of cardiac markers into blood following AMI.

release of cardiac markers from ischemic areas to the peripheral circulation where it can be measured is a function of its subcellular location (as described in Chapter 5), vascular access from the point of injury, and size of the protein. Figure 4 summarizes the general release pattern of the cardiac markers after AMI. Time zero is defined from the moment of onset of symptoms, and not from the presentation of patient to the emergency department. It should be recognized that the onset of chest pain is not always known, particularly in elderly patients in whom a reliable clinical history is not always available. The ordinate reflects the blood concentration of the marker as expressed in relative units of multiples of the upper reference limit (URL). Myoglobin (Chapter 6) and CK-MB isoforms (Chapter 10) are released within the first 6 h after onset, and return to normal within 24 h. Total CK (Chapter 7) and CK-MB (Chapters 8 and 9) are released within 12 h after chest pain, and return to normal after 48–72 h. Lactate dehydrogenase isoenzyme 1 (Chapter 11), cTnT (Chapter 13) and cTnI (Chapter 14), and myosin light chains (Chapter 15) are released within 12–24 h after chest pain, and remain abnormal for

5 d or more. The release of experimental cardiac markers (Chapter 17) into blood should be compared to results of these markers where the concentration vs time after onset of AMI is well established. Comparative studies of new markers against established markers, such as CK-MB or troponin, should be conducted on the same patient populations.

The kinetics of enzyme release is accelerated when an AMI patient is treated with thrombolytic agents or angioplasty successfully (Fig. 5), which is defined as the reperfusion of previously occluded coronary arteries. Various cardiac markers are being used to identify the reperfusion status of AMI patients. The use of markers to determine coronary artery patency is discussed under the corresponding marker chapter.

Infarct Sizing

One of the earliest applications of cardiac markers was for the estimation of the size or severity of AMI *(60–62)*. Infarct sizing can be calculated by plotting the release of a cardiac marker vs time after the onset of chest pain, and measuring the resulting "area under the curve" or AUC (Fig. 6). Calcula-

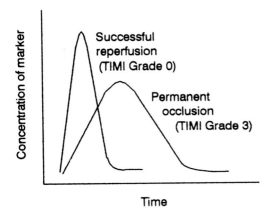

Fig. 5. The effect of successful reperfusion on blood concentrations of cardiac markers relative to permanent occlusion.

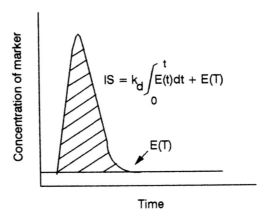

Fig. 6. Use of total enzymes and proteins for infarct sizing (IS). The area under the activity vs time curve is integrated. k_d is the disappearance rate constant, and E is the plasma CK activity at time t. E(T) is the enzyme activity at time T, i.e., when results have returned to baseline concentrations.

tion of infarct size has correlated fairly well with estimates of necrotic zones made on cardiac tissue at autopsy *(62)*, and postinfarction ejection fraction *(63)*. A noninvasive calculation of infarct size may be useful in the future management of patients suffering AMI. The calculation of infarct sizing by biochemical markers resumes a particular shape to the enzyme activity (or concentration) vs time after AMI curve, and that the amount of enzyme or protein that appears in blood is a fixed fraction of the total among released from the necrotic zone. The calculations are summarized below:

$$IS = \frac{\int_0^t f(t)dt \times \text{body wt} \times K_w}{E_d \times K_r} \quad (1)$$

where f(t) is the enzyme appearance function, body wt is the body weight, K_w is the proportion of body wt in which released enzyme is distributed, E_d is the amount of enzyme depleted per gram of infarcted heart, and K_r is the ratio of total enzyme appearance in blood to total enzyme disappearance from the infarcted myocardium. This equation can be simplified by combining the constants to form K_d and defining f(t) as dE/dt + K_dE:

$$K_d \int_0^t E(t)dt + E(T) \quad (2)$$

where E(T) is the enzyme activity when results have returned to baseline concentrations.

The interest in infarct sizing has waned with the development and use of thrombolytic therapy and percutaneous transluminal coronary angioplasty. Because of the "wash-out phenomenon" observed with successful treatment, estimates of infarct sizing are not altered because the enzyme–time curve is altered with reperfusion, and a greater (and unpredictable) fraction of enzymes released from the necrotic zone appear in blood *(64,65)*. Thus, although CK and CK-MB have been successfully used in early infarct sizing studies, markers, such as myosin light and heavy chains, may be more accurate, because they do not respond differently in the presence of reperfusion therapy *(see* Chapter 15). The accuracy of infarct sizing is also affected by the presence of myocardial infarct extension. In experimental dogs, myocardial extension that was produced within 12 h of an initial infarct resulted in a reduction in regional myocardial blood flow, producing a delay in the appearance of cardiac markers into blood *(66)*. Radionuclide ventriculography may provide a more accurate measurement of infarct size *(67,68)*. Although tomography is considered technically difficult and expensive, it is becoming more and more available in hospitals and medical centers.

CARDIAC MARKERS IN ISCHEMIC DISEASES

Silent Ischemia

Little is known concerning the release of cardiac markers in patients with spontaneous episodes of silent ischemia, because in the absence of pain, it is difficult to identify these patients at a time when blood sampling will be meaningful. In patients undergoing stress testing, traditional biochemical markers, such as total CK, CK-MB isoenzyme, and lactate dehydrogenase isoenzymes, are not sufficiently sensitive to be useful for detection of minor injury. With the availability of cTnT and cTnI, and myosin light chains, new studies are warranted to determine if these sensitive markers can be used to monitor minor injury that can occur during stress testing. A disadvantage of serum testing, however, is that there may be a delay of a few hours in the release of proteins from ischemic areas. Therefore, results immediately after testing might remain in the normal range. Collection of blood 3–6 h after a treadmill will not be as convenient as Holter ECG monitoring.

Angina

In symptomatic patients with stable angina and UA, detection of ischemia in blood requires use of a cardiac marker with high analytical sensitivity and specificity because the extent of the injury in these patients is minute compared to that of patients with AMI. Therefore, blood concentrations of cardiac enzymes and proteins may only marginally exceed the upper limit

Table 2
Results of Health Subjects for CK-MB and cTnT[a]

ID	CK-MB	cTnT
1	0.00	0.00
2	0.50	0.00
3	0.00	0.00
4	1.30	0.00
5	0.00	0.00
6	0.00	0.00
7	0.00	0.00
8	3.00	0.00
9	0.00	0.10
10	0.60	0.00
11	0.60	0.00
12	0.00	0.01
13	0.00	0.00
14	1.20	0.00
15	0.00	0.00
16	0.00	0.01
17	0.00	0.00
18	0.20	0.00
19	1.60	0.00
20	0.00	0.00

[a]$x = 0.42, 0.77$ ng/mL; SD $= 0.001, 0.004$ ng/mL.

of a reference population, and be well below that used as a cutoff for AMI. It is obvious that if the cardiac marker does not have high analytical sensitivity, it will be unable to differentiate blood concentrations of normal individuals from those with minor myocardial injury. For example, early generations of thyroid-stimulating hormone (TSH) had limited sensitivity, and results of patients with hyperthyroidism were within the measurement range for normal individuals. When high sensitivity (third-generation) TSH assays became available, they were more useful for hyperthyroid diseases *(69)*.

A cardiac marker with high analytical sensitivity, however, is not enough. High analytical specificity is also important. Table 2 shows results of CK-MB from a group of normal individuals using an automated mass

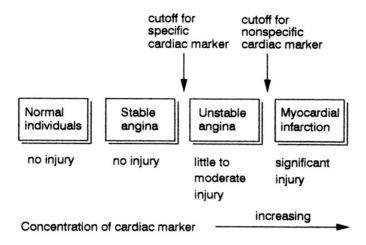

Fig. 7. Selection of cutoff limits for determination of minor myocardial injury with a specific cardiac marker, and AMI with a nonspecific myocardial marker.

assay with a sensitivity of under 0.10 ng/mL. Although the majority of values are within the normal range, there are four subjects in this group that have CK-MB values exceeding 1.0 ng/mL, and might be significant for minor myocardial injury. The normal range from this data, using the central 95% range of values, would be 0.0–1.60 ng/mL. Table 2 also shows results of this same population for cTnT. The normal range from this data calculates to 0.0–0.01 ng/mL. If it is assumed that cTnT has high specificity for myocardial injury, results for CK-MB on subjects 4, 8, 14, and 19 were owing to non-specific release from skeletal muscles.

The impact of nonspecificity on the marker's ability to detect minor myocardial injury is illustrated in Fig. 7. A relatively high cutoff concentration for CK-MB may be necessary (e.g., 5.0 ng/mL) because of the significant residual baseline content of CK-MB present in normal sera (e.g., patient 8). Although new onset of myocardial injury adds to this baseline content, it may still be below the assay's preselected cutoff concentration (Fig. 8A). Because cTnT has high specificity, the residual baseline content in normal sera is very low, and a much lower

cutoff concentration can be selected to detect minor injury (Fig. 8B). With this assay, the same increment of myocardial injury shown in Fig. 8A will produce a positive result for cTnT in Fig. 8B.

AMI

As discussed in Chapter 3, patients with AMI will release very high concentrations of enzymes and proteins. Cutoff concentrations have traditionally been established to differentiate non-AMI conditions, such as congestive heart failure and stable angina and UA from AMI. One is tempted to postulate that irreversible injury only occurs during AMI, following a threshold amount of time after permanent occlusion (Fig. 9A). Under these conditions, the establishment of an AMI cutoff is not difficult (Fig. 9A). The development of highly sensitive biochemical markers has shown, however, that irreversible injury does occur during preinfarction ischemic events, such as UA and that the pathophysiology of AMI progresses along a "continuum" rather than in a "stepwise" fashion (Fig. 9B). The establishment of an AMI cutoff concentration under this concept is vague. Because the differentia-

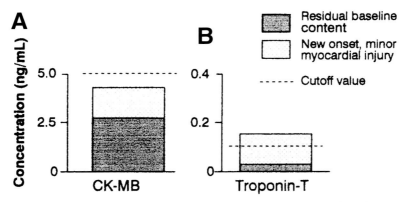

Fig. 8. The effect of specificity on sensitivity of biochemical markers for minor myocardial injury. (From ref. *70*, with permission from the American Association for Clinical Chemistry.)

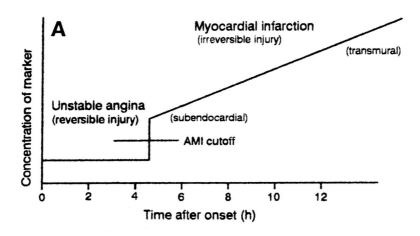

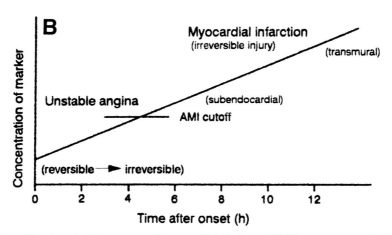

Fig. 9. (A) The threshold concept of irreversible injury. **(B)** The continuous injury concept of irreversible injury.

tion between UA and AMI is important, it may be more meaningful to establish two cutoff concentrations for markers with high specificity (such as cTnT or cTnI): one for minor injury and the other for AMI (Fig. 7) *(70)*. For nonspecific markers, such as total CK, CK-MB, or myoglobin, only a single relatively high cutoff to differentiate UA from AMI may be applicable.

ABBREVIATIONS

AMI, Acute myocardial infarction; AUC, area under the curve; body wt, body weight; CAD, coronary artery diseases; CCSC, Canadian Cardiovascular Society Classification; CHF, congestive heart failure; CK, creatine kinase; cTnI, T, cardiac troponins I and T; CV, coefficient of variation; CVA, cerebrovascular accident; CVD, cardiovascular disease; DRG, diagnosis-related groups; ECG, electrocardiogram; HAMA, human antimouse antibodies; IS, infarct size; IV, intravenous; POC, point-of-care; PTCA, percutaneous transluminal coronary angioplasty ROC, receiver operating characteristic; TAT, turnaround time; TIMI, Thrombolysis in Myocardial Infarction; tPA, tissue plasminogen activator; UA, unstable angina; URL, upper reference limit; WHO, World Health Organization.

APPENDIX

*Equations for Diagnostic Performance of Laboratory Tests***

$$\text{Sensitivity:} \quad \frac{TP}{TP+FN} \times 100$$

$$\text{Specificity:} \quad \frac{TN}{FP + TN} \times 100$$

$$\text{Positive predictive value:} \quad \frac{TP}{TP + FP} \times 100$$

$$\text{Negative predictive value:} \quad \frac{TN}{TN + FN} \times 100$$

$$\text{Efficiency:} \quad \frac{TP}{TP + FP + FN + TN} \times 100$$

___

**TP = true positives; TN = true negatives; FP = false positives; FN = false negatives.

REFERENCES

1. Heart attack and stroke: signals and action. Am. Heart Assoc., Dallas, TX (1992).
2. Expert Panel on Detection, Evaluation, and Treatment of High Blood Cholesterol in Adults (1993) Summary of the second report of the National Cholesterol Education Program (NCEP) Expert Panel on Detection, Evaluation, and Treatment of High Blood Cholesterol in Adults (Adult Treatment Panel II). JAMA 269:3015–3023.
3. Rader DJ, Hoeg JM, and Brewer HB (1994) Quantitation of plasma apolipoproteins in the primary and secondary prevention of coronary artery disease. Ann. Intern. Med. 120:1012–1025.
4. (1992) Ischaemic heart disease: risk stratification and intervention. Risk of progression of coronary artery disease. Eur. Heart J. 13(Suppl. C):3–13.
5. Mayer EL, Jacobsen DW, and Robinson K (1996) Homocysteine and coronary atherosclerosis. J. Am. Coll. Cardiol. 27:517–527.
6. Giri S and Waters DD (1996) Pathophysiology and initial management of the acute coronary syndromes. Curr. Opin. Cardiol. 11, 351–360.
7. Noto TJ, Johnson LW, Krone R, Weaver WF, Clark DA, Kramer JR, and Vetrovec GW (1991) Cardiac catheterization 1990: a report of the registry of the Society for Cardiac Angiography and Interventions (SCA&I). Cathet. Cardiovasc. Diagn. 24, 75–83.
8. Cohn PF (1989) Silent myocardial ischemia and infarction, 2nd ed., New York, Dekker.
9. Heller GV, Garber CE, Connolly MJ, Allen-Rowlands CF, Siconolfi SF, Gann DS, and Carleton RA (1987) Plasma beta-endorphin levels in silent myocardial ischemia induced by exercise. Am. J. Cardiol. 59: 735–739.
10. Ellestad MH and Kuan P (1984) Naloxone and asymptomatic ischemia. Failure to induce angina during exercise testing. Am. J. Cardiol. 54:928–934.

11. Cohn PF (1989) Left ventricular dysfunction and myocardial blood flow disturbances during episodes of silent myocardial ischemia. In: Silent myocardial ischemia and infarction, 2nd ed., New York, Dekker.

12. Diamond GA and Forrester JS (1979) Analysis of probability as an aid in the clinical diagnosis of coronary artery disease. N. Engl. J. Med. 300:1350–1358.

13. World Health Organization (1979) Report of the Joint International Society and Federation of Cardiology/World Health Organization Task Force on Standardization of Clinical Nomenclature. Nomenclature and criteria for diagnosis of ischemic heart disease. Circulation 59:607–609.

14. Braunwald E, Mark DB, Jones RH, Cheitlin MD, Fuster V, McCanley KM, et al. (1994) Unstable angina: diagnosing and management, Clinical Practice Guideline, No. 10 (amended). US Department of Health and Human Services Public Health Service, Rockville, MD, May.

15. Campeau L (1976) Grading of angina pectoris. [letter] Circulation 54:522–523.

16. Braunwald E (1989) Unstable angina. A classification. Circulation 80:410–414.

17. The Thrombolysis in Myocardial Infarction (TIMI) Study Group (1985) The thrombolysis in myocardial infarction (TIMI) trial. N. Engl. J. Med. 312:932–936.

18. Gruppo Italiano per lo Studio della Streptochinasi nell "Infarcto Microcardico (GISSI) (1986) Effective of intravenous thrombolytic treatment in acute myocardial infarction. Lancet 1:397–401.

19. Williams DO, Borerk J, Braunwald E, Chesebro JH, Cohen LS, Dalen J, Dodge HT, Francis CK, Knatterud G, Ludbrook P, Markis JE, Mueller H, Desvigne-Nickens P, Passamani ER, Powers ER, Rao AK, Roberts R, Ross A, Ryan TJ, Sobel BE, Winniford M, and Zaret B (1986) Intravenous recombinant tissue-type plasminogen activator in patients with acute myocardial infarction: a report from the NHLBI thrombolysis in myocardial infarction trial. Circulation 73:338–346.

20. The I.S.A.M. Study Group. (1986) A prospective trial of intravenous streptokinase in acute myocardial infarction (I.S.A.M.). N. Engl. J. Med. 314:1465–1471.

21. Ellis SG, Riveiro da Silva E, Heyndrickx G, Talley D, Cernigliaro C, Steg G, Spaulding C, Nobuyoshi M, Erbel R, Vassanelli C, and Topol EJ (1994) Randomized comparison of rescue angioplasty with conservative management of patients with early failure of thrombolysis for acute anterior myocardial infarction. Circulation 90:2280–2284.

22. Cohort of Rescue Angioplasty in Myocardial Infarction (CORAMI) Study group. (1994) Outcome of attempted rescue coronary angiography after failed thrombolysis for acute myocardial infarction. Am. J. Cardiol. 74:172–174.

23. McKendall, GR, Forman S, Sopko G, Braunwald E, Williams DO, and the TIMI investigators. (1995) Value of rescue percutaneous transluminal coronary angioplasty following unsuccessful thrombolytic therapy in patients with acute myocardial infarction. Am. J. Cardiol. 76:1108–1111.

24. Goldberg S, Greenspon AJ, Urban PL, Muza B, Berger B, Walinsky P, and Maroko PR (1983) Reperfusion arrhythmia: a marker of restoration of antegrade flow during intracoronary thrombolysis for acute myocardial infarction. Am. Heart. J. 105:26–32.

25. Braunwald E (1994) Heart Failure. In: Harrison's principles of internal medicine, 13th ed., Isselbacher KJ, Braunwald E, Wilson JD, Martin JB, Fauci AS, and Kasper OL, eds., New York, McGraw Hill, pp. 998–1008.

26. Konstam MA, Dracup K, Baker DW, Bottorff MB, Brooks NH, Dacey RA, et al. (1994) Heart Failure: evaluation and care of patients with left-ventriculay systolic dysfunction. Clinical Practice Guideline, No. 11. US Department of Health and Human Services Public Health Service, June.

27. Marantz PR, Tobin JN, Wassertheil-Smoller S, Steingart RM, Wexler JP, Budner N, Lense L, and Wachspress J. (1988) The relationship between left-ventricular systolic function and congestive heart failure diagnosed by clinical criteria. Circulation 77:607–612.

28. Dolgin M, ed. (1994) Functional capacity and objective assessment. In: Nomenclature and criteria for diagnosis of diseases of the heart and great vessels, 9th ed. New York, Little, Brown and Co., pp. 253–255.

29. Killip T and Kimball J (1967) Treatment of myocardial infarction in a coronary care unit. A two-year experience with 250 patients, Am. J. Cardiol. 20:457–464.

30. Karmen A, Wroblewski F, and LaDue JS (1954) Transaminase activity in human blood. J. Clin. Invest. 34:126–133.

31. Duma RJ and Seigel AL (1965) Serum creatine phosphokinase in acute myocardial infarction. Arch. Intern. Med. 115:443–451.

32. Roe CR, Limbird LE, Wagner GS, and Nerenberg ST (1972) Combined isoenzyme analysis in the diagnosis of myocardial injury: application of electrophoretic methods for the detection and quantitation of creatine kinase phosphokinase MB isoenzyme. J. Lab. Clin. Med. 80:577–590.

33. Jockers-Wretou E and Pfleiderer G (1975) Quantitation of creatine kinase isoenzymes in human tissues an sera by an immunological method. Clin. Chim. Acta 58:223–232.

34. Gilkeson G, Stone MJ, Waterman M, Ting R, Gomez-Sanchez CE, Hull A, and Willerson JT (1978) Detection of myoglobin by radioimmunoassay in human sera: its usefulness and limitations as an emergency room screening test for acute myocardial infarction. Am. Heart J. 95:70–77.

35. Chan DW, Taylor E, Frye T, and Blitzer RL (1985) Immunoenzymetric assay for creatine kinase MB with subunit-specific monoclonal antibobides compared with an immunochemical method and electrophoresis. Clin. Chem. 31:465–469.

36. Wu AHB, Gornet TG, Bretaudiere JP, and Panfili PR (1985) Comparison of enzyme immunoassay and immunoinhibition for creatine kinase MB in diagnosis of acute myocardial infarction. Clin. Chem. 31:470–474.

37. Vaidya HC, Maynard Y, Dietzler DN, and Ladenson JH (1986) Direct measurement of creatine kinase-MB activity in serum after extraction with a monoclonal antibody specific to the MB isoenzyme. Clin. Chem. 32:657–663.

38. Katus HA, Remppis A, Looser S, Hallermeier K, Scheffold T, and Kubler W (1989) Enzyme linked immuno assay of cardiac troponin T for the detection of acute myocardial infarction in patients. J Mol Cell Cardiol 21:1349–1353.

39. Bodor GS, Porter S, Landt Y, and Ladenson JH (1992) Development of monoclonal antibodies for the assay of cardiac troponin I and preliminary results in suspected cases of myocardial infarction. Clin. Chem. 38:2203–2214.

40. Puleo PR, Meyer D, Wathen C, Tawa CB, Wheelers, Hamburg RJ, Ali N, Obermueller SD, Triana JF, Zimmerman JL, Perryman MB, and Roberts R (1994) Use of a rapid assay of subforms of creatine kinase-MB to diagnose or rule out acute myocardial infarction, N. Engl. J. Med. 331:561–566.

41. Hamm CW, Ravkilde J, Gerhardt W, Jorgensen P, Peheim E, and Ljungdahl L (1992) The prognostic value of serum troponin T in unstable angina. N. Engl. J. Med. 327:146–150.

42. Ohman EM, Armstrong PW, Christenson RH, Granger CB, Katus HA, Hamm CW, O'Hanesian MA, Wagner GS, Kleiman NS, Harrell FE, Califf RM, and Topol EJ (1996) Risk stratification with admission cardiac troponin T levels in acute myocardial ischemia. N. Engl. J. Med. 335:1333–1341.

43. Antman EM, Tanasijevic MJ, Thompson B, Schactman M, McCabe CH, Cannon CP, Fischer GA, Fung AY, Thompson C, Wybenga D, and Braunwald E (1996) Cardiac-specific troponin I levels to predict the risk of mortality in patients with acute coronary syndromes. N. Engl. J. Med. 335:1342–1349.

44. Apple FS (1992) Acute myocardial infarction and coronary reperfusion. Serum cardiac markers for the 1990s. Am. J. Clin. Pathol. 97:217–226.

45. Keffer JH (1996) Myocardial markers of injury. Am. J. Clin. Pathol. 105:305–320.

46. Bhayana V and Henderson AR (1995) Biochemical markers of myocardial damage. Clin. Biochem. 28:1–29.

47. Adams JE, Abendschein DR, and Jaffe AS (1993) Biochemical markers of myocardial injury. Circulation 88:750–763.

48. Apple FS, Wu AHB, Vaidya HC, Katus HA, Scheffold T, Remppis A, Zehlein J, and Panteghini M (1992) Myocardial markers. Lab. Med. 23:297–322.

49. Apple FS, Preese LM, Panteghini M, Vaidya HC, Bodor GS, and Wu AHB (1994) Markers for myocardial injury. Clin. Immunoassay 17:6–48.

50. Statland BE (1996) Signals from the injured heart: the role of cardiac markers in managing patients with acute coronary syndrome. Med. Lab. Observer 28(7):42–44.

51. Wu AHB (1996) Analytical and clinical evaluation of new diagnostic tests for myocardial damage. Clin. Chim. Acta, in press.

52. Katus HA, Simon M, Zorn M, Scheffold T, Remppis A, Zehelein J, Grvenig E, and Fiehn W (1993) Cardiac troponin T measurements are highly specific for myocardial damage [Abstract]. J. Am. Coll. Cardiol. 21:88A.

53. Kricka LJ, Schmerfeld-Pruss D, Senior M, Goodman DBP, and Kaladas P (1990) Interference by human anti-mouse antibody in two-site immunoassays. Clin. Chem. 36:892–894.

54. Dillman RO and Royston I (1984) Applications of monoclonal antibodies in cancer therapy. Br. Med. Bull. 40:240–246.

55. Jaeschke R, Guyatt G, and Sackett DL (1994) User's guides to the medical literature. III. How to use an article about a diagnostic test. A. Are the results of the study valid? JAMA 271:389–391.

56. Werner M, Brooks SH, Mohrbacher RJ, and Wasserman AG (1982) Diagnostic performance of enzymes in the discrimination of myocardial infarction. Clin. Chem. 28: 1297–1302.

57. Henderson AR and Bhayana V (1995) A modest proposal for the consistent presentation of ROC plots in clinical chemistry. Clin. Chem. 41:1205–1206.

58. Anderson FP, Jesse RL, Nicholson CS, and Miller WG (1996) The costs and effectiveness of a rapid diagnostic and treatment protocol for myocardial infarction. In: Assessing clinical outcomes. Utilizing appropriate laboratory testing to decrease healthcare costs and improve patient outcomes, Bowie LJ, ed., Washington DC, AACC Leadership Series, pp. 20–24.

59. Wu AHB and Clive J (1997) Impact of CK-MB testing policies on hospital length of stay and laboratory costs for myocardial infarction and chest pain patients. Clin. Chem. 42:326–332.

60. Grande P, Hansen BF, Christiansen C, and Naestoft J (1982) Estimation of acute myocardial infarct size in many by serum CK-MB measurements. Circulation 65:756–764.

61. Sobel BE, Markham J, and Roberts R (1977) Factors influencing enzymatic estimates of infarct size. Am. J. Cardiol. 39:130–132.

62. Grande P, Christiansen C, and Alstrup K (1983) Comparison of ASAT, CK, CK-MB, and LD for the estimation of acute myocardial infarct size in man. Clin. Chim. Acta 128:329–335.

63. Vollmer RT, Christenson RH, Reimer K, and Ohman EM (1993) Temporal creatine kinase curves in acute myocardial infarction. Implications of a good empiric fit with the log-normal function. Am. J. Clin. Pathol. 100: 293–298.

64. Vatner SF, Baig H, Manders WT, and Maroko PR (1977) Effects of coronary artery reperfusion on myocardial infarct size calculated from creatine kinase. J. Clin. Invest. 61:1048–1056.

65. Horie M, Yasue H, Omote S, Takizawa A, Nagao M, Nishida S, and Kubota J (1984) The effects of reperfusion of infarct-related coronary artery on serum creatine phosphokinase and left ventricular function. Jpn. Circulation J. 46:539–945.

66. Cobb FR, Irvin RG, Hagerty RC, and Roe CR (1979) Effect of extension of infarction on serial CK activity. Circulation 60:145–154.

67. Antunes ML, Seldin DW, Wall RM, and Johnson LL (1989) Measuremen of acute Q-wave myocardial infarct size with single photon emission computed tomograph imaging of indium-111 antimyosin. Am. J. Cardiol. 63:777–783.

68. O'Connor MK, Gibbons RJ, Juni JE, O'Keefe J, and Ali A (1995) Quantitative myocardial SPEC for infarct sizing: feasibility of a multicenter trial evaluated using a cardiac phantom. J. Nucleic Med. 36:1130–1136.

69. Spencer CA, Takeuchi M, Kazarosyan M, MacKenzie F, Beckett GJ, and Wilkinson E (1995) Interlaboratory/intermethod differences in functional sensitivity of immunometric assays of thyrotropin (TSH) and impact on reliability of measurement of subnormal concentrations of TSH. Clin. Chem. 41:367–374.

70. Wu AHB, Valdes R Jr, Apple FS, Gornet T, Stone MA, Mayfield-Stokes S, Ingersoll-Stroubos AM, and Wiler B (1994) Cardiac troponin-T immunoassay for diagnosis of acute myocardial infarction and detection of minor myocardial injury. Clin. Chem. 40:900–907.

2

Pathophysiology of Acute Coronary Syndromes

Satyendra Giri, David D. Waters, and Alan H. B. Wu

INTRODUCTION

Definition

Acute coronary syndromes encompass a spectrum of symptomatic manifestations of ischemic heart disease, including unstable angina (UA)*, and non-Q-wave and Q-wave acute myocardial infarction (AMI). The syndrome of warning chest pain preceding the event was first described in 1912 by Herrick *(1)*. His suspicion of acute coronary occlusion resulting from evolving coronary thrombus as a cause of this chest pain syndrome was further substantiated in 1930s *(2)*. Subsequently, the now near universally accepted term "unstable angina" was coined in 1971 *(3)*. Since then, descriptive classifications of UA have been proposed, and their prognostic value in managing acute coronary syndromes has been substantiated *(4–6)*.

The treating physician, when confronted with a presentation of chest pain at rest and accompanying electrocardiograph (ECG) abnormalities, cannot distinguish between the diagnosis of UA, non-Q-wave AMI, or an infarct in evolution until the ECG patterns evolve or the cardiac enzymes become available. Where uncertainty exists regarding diagnosis, the immediate management of patients does not depend on differentia-

tion of UA and non-Q-wave AMI *(7,8)*. Diagnosis of UA does not require the presence of ECG changes, although its presence increases the diagnosis specificity and indicates a worse prognosis *(7–10)*.

Clinical Spectrum

In its broader definition, acute coronary syndrome should include all patients with the initial occurrence of increasing severity of angina. Although the Framingham study showed that UA was the first manifestation of coronary artery disease (CAD) in only about 10% of cases, retrospectively excluding AMI patients *(11)*, the majority of patients experience a cyclic, changing pattern of chest pain. Only a minority seek medical attention and fewer are hospitalized.

INITIATION AND PROGRESSION OF ATHEROSCLEROSIS: LIPID VS THROMBIN HYPOTHESIS

The pathophysiology of acute coronary syndromes is still imperfectly understood, but can be considered in terms of complementing hypotheses that were first formulated in this century. The thrombogenic hypothesis was postulated by vok Rokitansky in 1844, who after observing the process of intimal thick-

---

*See p. 36 for list of abbreviations used in this chapter.

From: Cardiac Markers   Edited by: Alan H. B. Wu
© Humana Press Inc., Totowa, NJ

ening from fibrin deposition followed by subsequent fibroblast organization and lipid accumulation, deduced the idea of "dyscrasia,"
since the deposit was derived from abnormal
blood *(12)*. The lipid hypothesis was propa-
gated by vok Virchow in 1856, who described
the location of intimal thickening to be in the
subendothelial layer, hence questioning the
derivation from surface deposits as proposed
by the thrombogenic hypothesis *(13)*.

In the ensuing period, a single multifac-
torial theory that integrates both initial con-
templation has evolved and recognizes
endothelial dysfunction as a response to
injury as the common step *(14)*. Many risk
factors acting singly or in unison (hyperlipidemia, smoking, hypertension, diabetes)
along with the local factors (shear stress,
endothelin, abnormal vasomotion) contribute to the development and progression of
endothelial atherosclerotic lesions.

The altered endothelial barrier allows
circulating monocytes and plasma lipids
into the vessel wall, and simultaneous
aggregation and adherence of platelets to
the endothelial cells. Release of platelet-
derived growth factor (PDGF) and other
mitogenic factors potentiate the migration
and proliferation of vascular smooth
muscle cells. Together with lipid accumulation and enhanced connective tissue synthesis, these processes lead to the typical
atheroma *(15)*.

NATURAL HISTORY
OF CORONARY HEART DISEASE
(CHD)

The natural history of CHD involves two
distinct stages. The first stage consists of
an initial asymptomatic period during which
nonobstructive atherosclerotic plaque is
formed with further progression depending
on its associated risk factors (Fig. 1A). The
second stage consists of rapid thrombogenesis due to plaque rupture exposing thrombogenic contents, such as collagen and

tissue thromboplastin, which promotes
platelet aggregation, fibrin formation, and
development of occlusive or near occlusive
thrombus. *(16)*. The final result of a plaque
rupture will essentially depend on the
"hemostatic balance," a concept introduced
in 1956 *(17)*. The hemostatic balance is a
complex interaction between the dynamics
of blood flow, components of the vessel
wall, platelets, and plasma proteins, as well
as numerous regulatory factors within the
platelets, coagulation system, and the fibrinolytic system (Fig. 2) *(18)*. Prospective
epidemiological studies have demonstrated
association between disturbance of the
hemostatic balance and the occurrence of
coronary events *(19,20)*. Figure 3 illustrates
rupture of an atherosclerotic vessel with a
nonocclusive thrombus.

MECHANISMS' CONTRIBUTION
TO PROGRESSION
OF ATHEROSCLEROSIS
AND INTRACORONARY
THROMBOGENESIS

The occurrence of thrombosis in atherosclerotic heart disease is potentiated by several factors (Fig. 1B) *(7)*. Some of the
important causes are discussed below.

Vascular Endothelium Dysfunction

The vascular endothelium plays an important role not only in the control of vascular
tone, but also as a barrier against plasma proteins and cells. Figure 2 illustrates the cellular and biochemical events that take place.
It regulates lipid transport, and contributes to
inflammatory responses, platelet aggregation, cell proliferation, and angiogenesis.
Formation of an atherosclerotic lesion in the
vascular endothelium increases permeability
to fibrinogen, albumin, monocytes, and
lipoprotein (a) [Lp(a)] *(15,16)*. Circulating
monocytes are converted into activated
macrophages, which oxidize low-density
lipoproteins (LDL) and augment the pro-

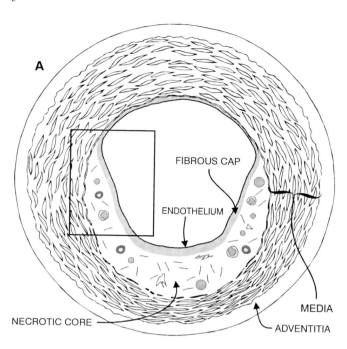

Fig. 1. (A) Schematic picture representing the cross-section of a coronary artery with an atherosclerotic plaque. **(B)** Inset of (A): Amplified image of shoulder region of the atherosclerotic plaque displaying mechanisms contributing to the progression of atherosclerosis and intracoronary thrombogenesis. **(C)** Inset of (A): Amplified image displaying mechanisms contributing to the progression of thrombus following plaque rupture and exposure of core components.

duction of growth factors, which further damage the endothelium *(21,22)*. Endothelial cells release thrombogenic factors, such as von Willebrand factor (vWF), factor V, and plasminogen activator inhibitors (PAI) 1 and 2, chemotactic agents for monocytes called tissue factor (TF), which are activated by interleukin-1 (IL-1), interferon (IFN-γ) and tumor necrosis factor (TNF), and surface proteins for monocyte adhesion, such as endothelium-leukocyte adhesion molecule-1 (ELAM-1), intracellular adhesion molecule-1 (ICAM-1), and endothelin-1 (ET-1). ET-1 is a powerful vasoconstrictor and proaggregator *(23,24)*. Endothelial cells also release antithrombotic agents, such as tissue-plasminogen activator (t-PA), prostacyclin (PGI-2), thrombomodulin, heparin, protein S, tissue factor pathway inhibitor (TFPI), and endothelial-derived relaxing factor (EDRF). EDRF, which is identical to nitric oxide (NO), is a powerful antiplatelet agent and vasodilator *(25)*. Growth factors, such as transforming growth factor-β (TGF-β), fibroblast growth factor (FGF), TNF, interleukin 1 (IL-1), PDGF, and so forth, are released *(26)*. Any injury to the endothelium would result in platelet-thrombus formation owing to the exposure of subendothelial substances and increased shear stress *(27)*. The normal endothelium helps modulate the vasomotor response of the vascular smooth muscle cells. Atherosclerosis impairs the normal vasodilator capability of the endothelium, and in the absence of normal endothelium, the smooth muscle cells will be constricted by thrombin, thromboxane A_2 (TxA_2), serotonin, and other agents. Thus far, a relationship between many of these factors and CHD remains hypothetical.

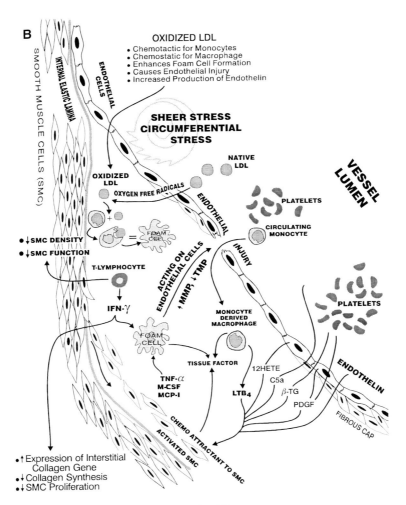

Fig. 1B.

Platelet Hyperactivity

Patients with CHD demonstrate exaggerated platelet reactivity causing platelet aggregation and adherence to the vessel wall stimulating local thrombus formation *(25)*. Platelet adhesion is mediated by membrane receptors with high affinity for fibronectin, thrombospondin, collagen, vWF, and other factors that are synthesized by endothelial cells *(28)*. The exposure of platelet glycoprotein IIb/IIIa receptors is the final common pathway in platelet aggregation, resulting in binding of fibrinogen and fibronectin. These receptors are found only on activated platelets and are mediated by TxA_2, thrombin, Adenosine diphosphate (ADP), and collagen. At this point, glycoprotein IIb/IIIa exposure can occur despite a complete inhibition of arachidonic acid pathway by acetylsalicylic acid (ASA), whereas by blocking the glycoprotein IIb/IIIa receptors, a total inhibition of platelet aggregation can be achieved *(29)*.

Activated platelets are responsible for the release of biologically active compounds, which stimulate aggregation, vasoconstric-

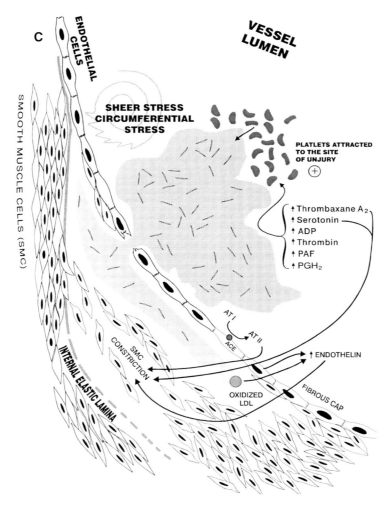

Fig. 1C.

tion, and smooth muscle cell migration and proliferation. In addition, the activated platelet surface catalyzes the coagulation process and generates thrombin. This thrombin plays a pivotal role in the hemostatic process by causing fibrinogenesis, platelet stimulation, and factor V and XIII activation *(30)*.

Patients presenting with CHD and arrhythmias have thrombocytosis, which persists in AMI or sudden death survivors even 7 yr after the event *(30)*. Also, even in healthy subjects, high platelet count correlates with higher CHD mortality *(20)*. Fur-

thermore, an increased platelet aggregability can be demonstrated in patients with unstable angina and predicts future coronary events in patients with a history of an AMI *(31,32)*. Since platelets have β-2- as well as α-2-adrenoceptors, the catecholamines released from the ischemic myocardium can cause platelet activation. This is in agreement with the inhibition of platelet function by selective β-1 blockers. Calcium seems to play a major role in platelet activation and calcium antagonists may inhibit the formation of TxA_2 *(32)*.

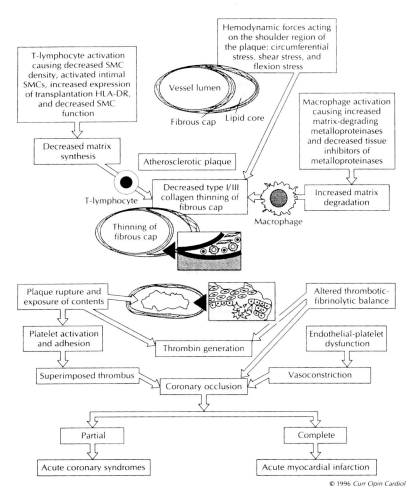

Fig. 2. Sequence of events in the pathophysiology of acute coronary syndromes. SMC–smooth muscle cell. (Used with permission from ref. *7.*)

An increase in the number of platelet α-receptors has been shown during ischemia *(33)*. The role of platelet-activating factor (PAF) is unsettled, but may cause arrhythmia during ischemic insult *(34)*. Similarly, platelets have 5-hydroxytryptamine receptors and release of serotonin also may lead to arrhythmias. The exposure of the glyco-protein IIb/IIIa receptors binding fibrinogen during platelet activation with TxA_2, thrombin, collagen, ADP, and other agents is critical for platelet aggregation. Thus platelets

play a central role in the development of arterial thrombi. Consistent association of increased volume and activity of platelets with acute coronary syndrome have been shown, which may contribute to necrosis and arrhythmogenesis.

Enhanced Procoagulant Activity

Fibrin deposition is present in the arterial walls of developing atherosclerotic lesions, and has been shown to bind LDL *(33)*. This

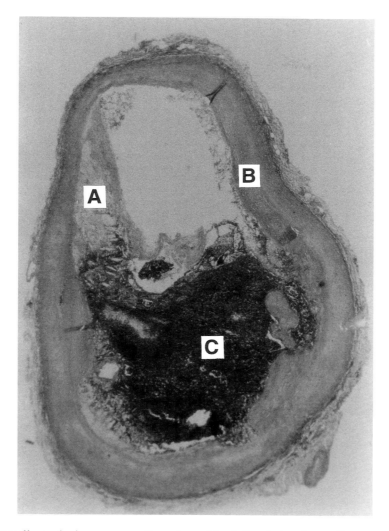

Fig. 3. Nontotally occlusive coronary thrombus of the left anterior descending coronary artery following rupture of an atherosclerotic plaque (UA). Trichrome stain magnification, ×10. (**A**) Ruptured area. (**B**) Intact atherosclerotic plaque. (**C**) Thrombi. (Slide courtesy of Krzysztof Podjaski, MD, Department of Pathology, Hartford Hospital, Hartford, CT.)

process of fibrin deposition followed by the growth of the atherosclerotic plaque has been suggested to be the main pathogenetic component behind atherosclerosis *(35,36)*. The oxidized LDL present in the lipid core of the atherosclerotic plaque induces positive chemotactic response for macrophages, which synthesize TF and may stimulate smooth muscle cells to do the same *(37,38)*.

Also, ischemic injury of the atherosclerotic plaque induces synthesis of tissue thromboplastin in the adventitia of the arterial wall *(39)*. Tissue factor is a membrane-associated lipoprotein expressed in the atherosclerotic lesions by macrophages and possibly smooth muscle cells, and acts as the procoagulant for tissue thromboplastin. On exposure to blood, tissue factor forms a calcium-dependent complex with factor VIIa on phospholipid membranes, and this complex is regulated by TFPI released from endothelial cells *(40)*. Formation of a prothrombin activator complex on a lipid membrane, such as platelet or smooth muscle cell surface, can accelerate thrombin generation by 278,000 times *(39)*. A significant proportion of thrombin remains fibrin-bound, augmenting thrombogenicity of the thrombus. The heparin therapy cannot completely inhibit action of thrombin, since the receptors for antithrombin III (ATIII) and heparin cofactor II on thrombin are concealed when thrombin is fibrin-bound. Also, heparin is neutralized by the platelet factor IV released from the activated platelets *(39,41)*.

Several other coagulation proteins are related to the risk of CHD. Plasma fibrinogen is elevated in healthy persons with a high risk of CHD *(19,36)* and is associated with progression to AMI *(42)*. Further elucidation regarding the role of fibrinogen is needed because it is possible that raised plasma fibrinogen levels merely represent inflammation-induced acute-phase reaction *(43)*. Factor VII activity has been shown to be independently associated with the risk of future CHD in middle-aged men *(19)*. Also, several cross-sectional studies show increased factor VII mass and activity in patients with or at risk for CHD *(43,44)*. A relationship between the dietary influence on plasma triglyceride concentration and phospholipid–factor VII complex has been postulated *(45)*. The Northwick Park Heart (NPH) Study found an association between factor VIII activity and the incidence of CHD *(46)*, and among hemophiliacs, there is a low incidence of CHD *(47)*. The vWF has an important role to play in atherogenesis, since it is responsible for platelet adhesion to endothelial cells. Several studies demonstrate an association between a high vWF level and CHD *(48,49)*. Endogenous anticoagulants (proteins C and S, ATIII, heparin cofactor II,

and TFPI) are also activated with the activation of the coagulation system *(36)*. Thrombin inhibition by heparin cofactor II is also ATIII-dependent *(50)*, and induction of TFPI release from endothelial cells by heparin inhibits the prothrombinase complex *(41)*.

Although logically low concentrations of these endogenous anticoagulants should be associated with an increased risk of CHD, study results have been controversial *(36)*. In the NPH Study, both low and high ATIII levels were associated with an increased risk of CHD *(51)*, and similar conflicting results are reported for ATIII and protein C *(36)*. This could be owing to the inconsistency in methodology involved in measuring antigen level and functional activity of the endogenous anticoagulants between studies. In addition, the previously unrecognized activated protein C resistance may also explain some of these conflicting results *(52)*.

Impaired Fibrinolytic Capacity

Endothelial cells release t-PA, which mediates clot lysis by cleaving fibrin-bound plasminogen to plasmin. The extent of clot lysis is regulated by inhibitors of t-PA and plasmin *(53)*. Plasminogen activator inhibitor-1 (PAI-1) released from endothelial cells is the primary inhibitor of t-PA *(54)*. An increase in circulating PAI-1 can attenuate physiological fibrinolytic activity and the rate of clot lysis *(54)*.

Low fibrinolytic activity has been shown to be a major determinant of CHD in younger men (40–54 yr) even after adjusting for plasma fibrinogen *(19)*. In recent years, specific and sensitive methods to determine the different components of the fibrinolytic system (PAI-1, t-PA antigen, t-PA activity, and so forth) have been developed, and several cross-sectional studies examining levels of these markers in patients with acute coronary syndrome have been performed *(55,56)*. Measurement of PAI-1 has produced conflicting results possibly because its concentration varies depending on age, sex, risk factors, and the degree of atherosclerosis in an individual *(36)*. Furthermore, the plasma levels of t-PA and PAI-1 are subject to circadian variations *(57)*. The plasma PAI-1 activity peaks in the early morning and may show wide intraindividual variation. PAI-1, like other serine-protease inhibitors *(53)*, is synthesized by many cells, but it is suggested that the vascular endothelial cells of various tissues are primarily responsible for plasma levels of PAI-1. Another important source of PAI-1 is platelets, which release their pool from the α-granules along with procoagulant factors *(58,59)*. In an in vitro model of a platelet-fibrin thrombus, presence of platelet PAI-1, which is bound to fibrin after clot lysis, have been shown to correlate with the amount of residual clot *(51)*. This may explain the inefficacy of thrombolysis in UA, as thrombolytic agents without antithrombotic agents stimulate platelets. PAI-1 is an acute-phase reactant and increases after AMI *(56,60)*, surgery, endotoxemia, and septicemia *(61)*. It also appears to be important in angiogenesis, wound healing, and in affecting the composition of extracellular matrix *(62)*.

Apolipoprotein B-containing particles (very low density lipoprotein [VLDL] and oxidized LDL particles) stimulate the production of PAI-1 in cultured human endothelial cells *(63,64)*. Serum triglycerides are strongly associated with PAI-1 levels in plasma, and lipid-lowering intervention is accompanied by improvement in the fibrinolytic capacity *(65,66)*. Factor XII-dependent fibrinolytic activity is significantly decreased in the survivors of an acute coronary event *(67)*. Also, a significant increase in the frequency of reinfarction and recurrent thromboembolism in patients with a factor XII deficiency have been documented *(68,69)*. Furthermore, factor XII-dependent fibrinolytic activity decreases during t-PA infusion if >40% of the circulating pool of plasminogen is converted to plasmin *(70)*. This underscores the significance of optimum dosing regimens that generate minimal systemic plasmin and ensure adequate levels of plasminogen.

PATHOPHYSIOLOGY BEHIND TRIGGERING OF ACUTE CORONARY SYNDROMES

In the majority of cases, the mechanism accountable for abrupt conversion of coronary disease is rupture of the surface of an atherosclerotic plaque in a focal segment of an epicardial coronary artery exposing thrombogenic plaque components to flowing blood with formation of superimposed thrombus at the site of pre-existing stenosis *(16,71,72)*. The clinical consequence following this event depends on the resultant obstruction, duration of compromised perfusion, and the oxygen demand of the myocardial substrate in jeopardy. If there is extensive local thrombosis, a flow-limiting coronary stenosis would result in myocardial ischemia associated with UA or with the necrosis that characterizes non-Q-wave AMI. When plaque rupture and thrombosis are extensive enough to occlude the coronary artery completely, it may result in an acute Q-wave infarction. Likewise, superimposed enhanced and abnormal vasomotion resulting in constriction and degree of collateral circulation also influence the clinical outcome.

Mechanisms behind the induction of plaque rupture and thrombus formation are still an area of active research. The spontaneous episodes of ischemia in patients with UA predominantly result from episodic reductions in coronary blood flow. This reduction, in turn, is caused by the combined effects of fixed (atherosclerotic plaque) and dynamic (thrombosis and vasoconstriction) forces. Current research has tried to understand the interaction between the hemostatic system and components of atherosclerotic plaque, which act as triggers of thrombotic cascade.

Evidence of Thrombus Involved in Acute Coronary Syndromes

The active atherosclerotic plaque seems to be fissured in 50–90% of cases of acute coronary syndromes. Disruption of a plaque exposes its thrombotic components, including collagen, lipids, macrophages, and tissue factor *(37,38)*. This leads to platelet aggregation and activation of the coagulation system, which results in the formation of a platelet-rich thrombus (white thrombus). Secondary to this thrombotic response and as a result of stasis in the affected coronary vessel, a thrombus rich in fibrin and erythrocytes (red thrombus) may evolve and extend upstream or downstream. In addition, other factors, such as the local blood flow disturbances (high shear rates within severe stenosis) and the systemic or local equilibrium, may influence the magnitude of the thrombotic response *(73)*.

This "thrombinocentric" hypothesis explaining the initiation of acute coronary syndromes is supported by many observations. For example, thrombotic occlusion in acute coronary syndrome-related deaths is shown to be 21–91% *(74–76)*. Using coronary angiography to evaluate patients within 4 h of symptoms, an 87% incidence of total coronary occlusion has been reported *(77)*. Similarly, pathological studies of patients who died suddenly or soon after the acute coronary syndrome show ruptured plaque with superimposed thrombus as the underlying mechanism in the development of acute coronary syndromes *(72,78)*. The recent angiographic and angioscopic studies *(79,80)* demonstrate thrombotic occlusion in up to 90% of patients during the early hours of myocardial infarction. In the Thrombolysis In Myocardial Infarction (TIMI) 3A trial, thrombus was definitely present in 35% of primary culprit lesions and possibly present in an additional 40% *(81)*. Likewise, an 80% incidence of plaque rupture has been demonstrated with layered thrombus in patients with UA *(78)*. Total coronary occlusion was the most common finding in UA patients who died *(82)*.

Plaque Morphology and Its Components

The committee of Vascular lesions of the council of Atherosclerosis, American Heart Association, have proposed classification of atherosclerotic lesions. The atherosclerotic plaque progresses through stages of evolution, and is differentiated by its proportion of lipids (intra- or extracellular), macrophages, and smooth muscle cells *(16)*. Plaques with a predominance of extracellular lipids are called Type IV lesions. Accumulation of extracellular lipids occupying within the intima separated from the vascular lumen by a thin fibrous cap constitutes Type Va lesions. This extracellular lipid accumulation is called the lipid core *(83)*. This lipid core is associated with erosion and destruction of adjacent tissue. The thinning of fibrous cap overlying the lipid core makes it vulnerable to tearing or disruption. The fibrous cap may rupture if the strain on the cap components exceeds their deformability *(84)*, leading to exposure of the thrombogenic lipid core components to flowing blood (Type VI or complicated lesion) *(85)*.

Effect of Hemodynamic Forces

In a susceptible plaque weakened by various causes, hemodynamic forces (including circumferential stress, shear stress, and flexion stress) seems to cause further disruption *(86)*. Acute changes in coronary pressure, fluctuations in shear stress, and arching of the artery during each cardiac cycle contribute to plaque rupture. Circumferential stress is directly related to a vessel's luminal diameter and intraluminal pressure, and is inversely related to its wall thickness. However, plaque rupture does not always occur at high stress regions, probably because of the local variations in plaque material properties *(87)*. It seems that plaques containing strands of collagen are resistant to disruption, because the collagen anchors the fibrous cap. Compared with intact caps, ruptured ones are deficient of collagen bundles, and their tensile stress is reduced *(88)*. In addition, when the lipid core is situated eccentrically in the plaque, it is more likely to fissure *(81)*. According to computer models, circumferential stress is localized at the shoulder region of the plaques with soft lipid-rich cores, which are the most common sites of disruption. The level of circumferential stress seems to be higher in plaques that cause mild or moderate obstruction than in those that lead to severe stenosis *(85,89)*. Computer model analysis shows increased tensile stress at the ends of plaque caps, particularly when the extracellular lipid pool exceeds >45% of the vessel wall circumference *(89)*. This may be the reason why 60–70% of all acute coronary syndromes evolve from obstructive plaques that produce <50% stenosis. It is possible that not only do these plaques have high lipid content and thinner fibrous cap, but also that such plaques are subject to high levels of circumferential stress and thus are more likely to become disrupted.

Role of Inflammation

In recent times, the role of inflammation as the principal underlying pathophysiological process in acute coronary syndromes has been proposed *(90–92)*. All atherosclerotic plaques contain monocytes, macrophages, and T-lymphocytes. However, as demonstrated by cell-specific monoclonal antibodies (MAbs), these cell types are much more abundant in unstable compared with stable coronary plaques, suggesting that an acute inflammatory process may be present. At the local level of disrupted plaques, macrophages are plentiful, particularly near the shoulder regions, and they have the unique ability to produce metalloproteinases in vitro and in vivo *(93–96)*. These metalloproteinases can cause degradation of virtually all components of the fibrous cap of an atherosclerotic plaque, which supports the hypothesis of a role in plaque instability and disruption *(93,97,98)*. There is also increased accumulation of T-lymphocytes and activated degranulated mast cells. Significant mononuclear infiltrate in the culprit lesion has been demonstrated in patients dying within 1 mo of UA *(99)* and also in the atherectomy specimens *(98)* obtained from patients with UA. Not only are there more inflammatory cells in patients with stable angina, but they are also more likely to be activated, and the activated macrophages and lymphocytes appear to be contiguous with the site of disruption of the coronary plaque. van der Wall and his colleagues *(98)* demonstrated scarcity of smooth muscle cells in the culprit lesions of patients dying soon after the onset of AMI. These lesions showed a large number of macrophages and lymphocytes expressing the HLA-DR antigens, indicating their activated state.

The macrophage-derived foam cells release free radicals, lipid oxidation products, and proteolytic enzymes, degrading the connective tissue matrix and thinning the fibrous cap *(89,101)*. Metalloproteinases, which are derived from macrophages (interstitial collagenase, gelatinase, and stromelysin), are also abundant in the shoulders and base regions of the plaque *(97,102)*. Experiments demonstrating an increased gelatinolytic and caseinolytic activity at the sites of macrophage accumulations *(102)*, and an increase in collagen breakdown when monocyte-derived macrophages are incubated with human aortic plaques, clearly insinuate macrophages as being responsible for plaque disruption. There is also a 50-fold increase in the number of activated mast cells at the shoulder region of the plaques when compared to normal coronary intima. These mast cells, through their release of tryptase and chymase, can activate metalloproteinases produced by plaque macrophages and smooth muscle cells. This could be the mechanism for triggering matrix degradation, fibrous cap digestion, and rupture of coronary plaques *(103)*. Finally, significantly large macrophage-rich areas are detected in atherectomy specimens obtained from patients with unstable coronary syndromes as compared to stable angina *(104)*. This further supports the crucial role of macrophages in the triggering of the acute coronary syndromes.

Potentiation of Thrombosis by Inflammation

In patients with UA, monocytes, after exposure to immunogenic or other stimuli, express a procoagulant-inducing factor on their surfaces, a lymphokine that stimulates clotting *(105)*. Monocyte procoagulant activity is comparatively low in patients with stable angina, noncardiac chest pain, dilated cardiomyopathy with ventricular thrombus, and from normal control patients *(106)*. The hypercoagulability induced by monocytes in the acute coronary syndromes has been investigated in two recent studies *(90,107)*.

Evidence of Systemic Inflammation in Acute Coronary Syndrome

Systemic evidence of acute inflammation is present in UA and is an independent predictor of outcome. C-reactive protein alone *(108)* or both C-reactive protein and serum amyloid A protein *(91)* have been found to be elevated in patients with UA compared with those who have stable angina. Patients with UA who had elevated levels of these inflammatory markers were more likely to experience recurrent chest pain, have more ischemia on Holter monitoring, and have significantly higher rates of revascularization compared with patients with UA without elevated levels of these markers. Interleukin-6 (IL-6) levels were also found to be significantly elevated in 59% of patients with UA compared with 21% of patients with stable angina, and the elevation correlated with short-term events *(81)*.

Thrombogenicity of Atherosclerotic Plaques

The degree of plaque disruption and the different level of thrombogenicity of different core components exposed appear to determine the amount of thrombus formation *(109,110)*. Superficial plaque injury with exposure of collagen-rich matrix present in small plaque fissures is associated with less platelet deposition compared to that seen after deep injuries with exposure of the lipid-rich core. The lipid core is much more thrombogenic than the collagen-rich component *(110)*. Therefore, plaques containing lipid-rich "gruel" are not only more prone to rupture, but they are also the most thrombogenic when their content is exposed to flowing blood. The atheromatous gruel is derived from core lipids, disintegrated cells, macrophages, and extracellular matrix. It contains cholesteryl esters, Lp(a), phospholipids, cellular debris and collagen degradation products. The components responsible for the high thrombogenicity, in the gruel is unknown. However, two recent studies indicate that tissue factor may play a role in activating the coagulation cascade after plaque rupture *(37,38)*. Tissue factor antigen, which is present in the atheromatous gruel, is upregulated in circulating and endothelium-adhered monocytes, and is also increased in coronary tissue from patient with UA *(106,111–113)*. The macrophages and possibly the smooth muscle cells are responsible for tissue factor content of the plaque in patients with acute coronary syndrome. Tissue factor is also associated with macrophages and its membranous debris *(114)*. However, it is likely that other components of the gruel, such as lipids, might also induce platelet aggregation and activation of the coagulation system *(37,38)*.

At present, it is quite apparent that atherosclerotic plaques occupying <50% of the diameter of a coronary artery can develop fissure and become a nidus for thrombosis. Even though coronary arteriography can diagnose the severity of coronary disease *(115)*, it cannot predict the site of future coronary occlusion. Probably, the reason why severe coronary disease at angiography is able to predict high coronary morbidity and mortality is because there is higher likelihood of the presence of small plaques prone to rupture *(116)*. This underscores the need for a practical method to identify the vulnerable lesions that are subject to an abrupt disruption with subsequent thrombus formation.

CORONARY ARTERY THROMBOSIS

The sequence of events in the acute coronary syndromes, which consist of plaque disruption, thrombus formation, abnormal vasomotion, platelet activation, and aggregation, are all highly interrelated, since they share common mediators.

Mechanisms Contributing to the Progression of Thrombus (Fig. 3C)

Born and colleagues *(117)* have proposed the possibility of the plaque fissuring being a random event, analogous to the appearance of cracks in the wings of an airplane, the result of a natural wear and tear phenomena on a vulnerable composition. Probably, plaques rupture frequently, but are resealed by a small mural thrombus, which organizes and contributes to an episodic, yet clinically silent growth *(86)*. This may be the reason for the benefit of β-blocker therapy in patients with CHD. However, if the thrombus is extensive, it can impair coronary blood flow leading to ischemia *(16,86)*. Many variables determine whether a ruptured plaque proceeds rapidly to an occlusive thrombus and an acute ischemic events,

or persists at an intermediate stage as a nonocclusive clinically silent thrombus.

Plaque Injury and Resulting Exposure of Core Components

It is uncertain why a particular disruption of a plaque would lead to occlusive thrombus in some cases but not others. The depth of injury may be important, since the deeper injuries expose a greater amount of thrombogenic core components. When subendothelial layers are exposed to flowing blood at a high shear rate, platelet adhesion and aggregation are induced. However, the thrombus is labile and can be partially dislodged by the blood flow leaving a smaller residual mural thrombus *(118,119)*. On the other hand, exposure of deeper vascular layers to blood flow results in a dense platelet thrombus formation, which is not easily dislodged. In patients presenting with acute coronary syndromes, a large and complex plaque rupture exposing highly thrombogenic components leads to extensive coronary thrombus formation and, if persistent and occluding, may lead to acute Q-wave myocardial infarction.

Resulting Stenosis and Shear Rates

The degree of occlusion resulting from plaque disruption causes sudden geometric changes resulting in high shear rates *(86)*. Higher shear rates resulting from stenosis increase platelet and fibrinogen deposition at the site of plaque rupture *(86,118,120)*. Therefore, the larger the geometric change, the more persistent the thrombotic occlusion causing prolonged ischemia. Similarly, surface roughness and irregularities at the site of plaque rupture also influence thrombogenicity *(121)*.

Residual Intracoronary Thrombus

Residual intracoronary thrombus can contribute to recurrent thrombotic vessel occlusion in several ways *(121–123)*. First, by increasing stenosis and shear rate, it may facilitate the activation and deposition of platelets and fibrinogen *(119,123,124)*. Second, recent studies demonstrate thrombus itself being very thrombogenic, and it continues to grow despite heparin therapy *(125,126)*. It is possible that the enhancement of platelet and thrombin activity by thrombolytic agents themselves may contribute to rethrombosis by exposing the fibrin-bound thrombin to the circulating blood *(127,128)*.

Vasoconstriction

Atherosclerosis and its related risk factors are associated with impaired vasodilation and enhanced vasoconstriction *(129)*. Coronary vasospasm has been established in patients with UA *(130)*. Both abnormal vasodilation and enhanced vasoconstriction have been studied and attributed to being owing to dysfunction in endothelial-dependent dilation mechanisms *(131,132)*, which primarily results in the increased inactivation of nitric oxide (NO) (EDRF). In addition, altered platelet function resulting in platelet-dependent vasoconstriction mediated by serotonin and TxA_2, *(133,134)*. Thrombin-dependent vasoconstriction *(135)* at the site of plaque disruption, and increased production of the peptide endothelin (vasoconstrictor) *(16)* suggest a direct interaction of these substances with smooth muscle cells. This is in agreement with the recent observation that transient vasoconstriction accompanies plaque disruption and thrombosis in the acute coronary syndromes *(136)*.

Sympathetic Nervous System Activation

Catecholamines have been shown to induce a hypercoagulable state and also cause vasoconstriction. Circulating catecholamines also enhance platelet activation and thrombin generation *(137,138)*. States of sympathetic hyperactivity, like emotional stress, unaccustomed exercise, morning awakening, and smoking, may contribute to the development of arterial thrombosis. It is possible that plaque disruptions that occur at the time of sympathetic hyperactivity are more prone to develop an acute coronary syndrome *(136)*.

Hypercholesterolemia and Lipoprotein (a)

High cholesterol levels are associated with hypercoagulability and platelet hyperactivity at the site of experimentally induced acute vascular injury *(139,140)*. High-density lipoprotein (HDL)-associated Apo A-1 is reduced in patients presenting with UA and AMI. This suggests that HDL may also influence intracoronary thrombus formation, in addition to mobilizing free cholesterol from tissues and macrophages. Furthermore, HDL may also stabilize PGI-2 through Apo A-1, which is present on the surface of HDL particles and has been identified as a PGI-2-stabilizing factor *(141)*.

Lp(a) has been proposed to be a link between atherogenesis and thrombogenesis. Lp(a) has been shown to be associated with coronary heart disease, especially in subjects with familial hypercholesterolemia or a family history of premature coronary heart disease *(142)*. Glycoprotein Apo (a) present in Lp(a) is structurally homologous to plasminogen *(143)*, with both genes linked on the long arm of chromosome 6 *(144)*. This close homology may result in competitive inhibition of the binding of plasminogen to fibrin monomer and to the plasminogen receptor of the endothelial cell, thus inhibiting the action of t-PA *(145)*, and cause acute thrombotic complications. However, the direct thrombogenic effect of high Lp(a) results has not been confirmed in unfractionated plasma, and the clinical importance of the association between Lp(a) and plasminogen is still uncertain.

in vascular disease patients. Principal results. Arteriosclerosis Thrombosis 12:1063–1070.

50. Eisenberg PR (1994) Thrombosis and fibrinolysis in acute myocardial infarction. Alcohol Clin. Exp. Res. 18:97–104.

51. Meade TW, Cooper J, Miller GJ, Howarth D, and Stirling Y (1991) Antithombin III and arterial disease. Lancet 337:850–851.

52. Svensson PJ and Dahlback B (1992) Resistance to activated protein C as a basis for venous thrombosis. N. Engl. J. Med. 33:517–522.

53. Dawson S and Henney A (1992) The status of PAI-1 as a risk factor for arterial and thrombotic disease. A review. Atherosclerosis 95:105–117.

54. Knapp RM, Chiu AT, and Reilly TM (1990) Effects of recombinant plasminogen activator inhibitor type 1 on fibrinolysis *in vitro* and *in vivo*. Thrombosis Res. 59:309–317.

55. Ridker PM, Vaughan DE, Stampfer MJ, Manson JE, and Hennekens CH (1993) Endogenous tissue-type plasminogen activator and risk of myocardial infarction. Lancet 341:1165–1168.

56. Gurfunkel E, Altman R, Scazziota A, Rouvier J, and Mauntner B (1994) Importance of thrombosis and thrombolysis in silent ischemia: comparison of patients with acute myocardial infarction and unstable angina. Br. Heart J. 71:151–155.

57. Andreotti F, Davies GJ, Hackett DR, Khan MI, DeBart AC, Aber VR, Maseri A, and Kluff C (1988) Major circadian fluctuations in fibrinolytic factors and possible relevance to time of onset of myocardial infarction, sudden cardiac death and stoke. Am. J. Cardiol. 62:635–637.

58. Booth NA, Simpson AJ, Croll A, Bennett B and MacGregor IR (1988) Plasminogen activator inhibitor-1 in plasma and platelets. Br. J. Haemotol. 70:327–333.

59. Hantgan RR, Handt S, Kirkpatrick CJ, and Lewis JC (1991) Role of platelet-released Plasminogen activator inhibitor-1 in regulation of fibrinolysis. Thrombosis Haemostas. 65:718.

60. ECAT Angina Pectoris Study Group. (1993) ECAT angina pectoris study: baseline associations of haemostatic factors with extent of coronary arteriosclerosis and other coronary risk factors in 3,000 patients with angina pectoris undergoing coronary angiography. Eur. Heart J. 14:8–17.

61. Colucci M, Paramo JA, and Collen D (1985) Generation in plasma of a fast-acting inhibitor of plasminogen activator in response to endotoxin stimulation. J. Clin. Invest. 75:818–824.

62. Suffredini AF, Harpel PC, and Parrillo JE (1989) Promotion and subsequent inhibition of plasminogen activation after administration of intravenous endotoxin to normal subjects. N. Engl. J. Med. 320:1165–1172.

63. Stiko-Rahm A, Wiman B, Hamsten A, and Nilsson J (1990) Secretion of plasminogen activator inhibitor-1 from cultured human umbilical vein endothelial cells is induced by very low density lipoprotein. Arteriosclerosis 10:1067–1073.

64. Witxtum JL and Steinberg D (1991) Role of oxidized low density lipoprotein in atherosclerosis. J. Clin. Invest. 88:1785–1792.

65. Anderson P, Nielson DWT, Lyberg Beckman S, Holme I, and Hjermann I (1988) Increased fibrinolytic potential after diet intervention in healthy coronary high-risk individuals. Acta. Med. Scand. 223:499–506.

66. Anderson P, Smith P, Seljeflot I, Brataker S, and Arnesen H (1990) Effect of gemfibrozil on lipids and haemostasis after myocardial infarction. Thrombosis Haemostas. 63:174–177.

67. Lodi S, Isa L, Pollini E, Bravo AF, and Scalvini A (1984) Defective intrinsic fibrinolytic activity in a patient with severe factor XII deficiency and myocardial infarction. Scand J. Haemotol. 33:80–82.

68. Halbmayer W-M, Mannhalter C, Feichtinger C, Rubi K, and Fischer M (1992) The prevalence of factor XII deficiency in 103 orally anticoagulated outpatients suffering from recurrent venous and/or arterial thromboembolism. Thrombosis Haemostas. 68:285–290.

69. Goodnought LT, Saito H, and Ratnoff OD (1983) Thrombosis or myocardial infarction in congenital clotting factor abnormalities and chronic thrombocytopenias: A report of 21 patients and a review of 50 previously reported cases. Medicine 62:248–255.

70. Munkvad S, Jesperson J, Gram J, and Kuft C (1992) Association between systemic generation of plasmin and activation of the

factor XII dependent fibrinolytic proactivator system in coronary thrombosis. Fibrinolysis 6:57–62.

71. Falk E, Shah PK, and Fuster V (1995) Coronary plaque disruption. Circulation 92: 657–671.

72. Davies MJ and Thomas AC (1985) Plaque fissuring: the cause of acute myocardial infarction, sudden ischemic death, and crescendo angina. Br. Heart J. 53:363–373.

73. Falk E, Shah PK, and Fuster V (1995) Coronary plaque disruption. Circulation 92: 657–671.

74. Roberts WC and Buja LM (1972) The frequency and significance of coronary arterial thrombi and other observations in fatal acute myocardial infarction: a study of 107 necropsy patients. Am. J. Med. 52:425–443.

75. Erhardt LR, Lundman T, and Mellstedt H (1973) Incorporation of ^{125}I-labelled fibrinogen into coronary arterial thrombi in acute myocardial infarction in man. Lancet 1:387–390.

76. Baroldi G, Radice F, Schmid G, and Leone A (1974) Morphology of acute myocardial infarction in relation to coronary thrombosis. Am. Heart J. 87:65–75.

77. DeWood MA, Spores J, Notske R, Mouser LT, Burroughs R, Golden MS, and Lang HT (1980) Prevalence of total coronary occlusion during the early hours of transmural myocardial infarction. N. Engl. J. Med. 303:897–902.

78. Falk E (1985) Unstable angina with fatal outcome: dynamic coronary thrombosis leading to infarction and/or sudden death: autopsy evidence of recurrent mural thrombosis with peripheral embolization culminating in total vascular occlusion. Circulation 71:699–708.

79. Forrestor JS, Litvack F, Grundfest W, and Hickey A (1987) A perspective of coronary disease seen through the arteries of living man. Circulation 75:505–513.

80. Mizuno K, Satomura K, Miyamoto A, Mouser LT, Burroughs R, Golden MS, and and Lang HT (1992) Angioscopic evaluation of the character of coronary thrombus in acute coronary syndromes. N. Engl. J. Med. 326:287–291.

81. The TIMI 3A Investigators: (1993) Early effects of tissue-type plasminogen activator added to conventional therapy on the culprit lesion in patients presenting with ischemic cardiac pain at rest: result of the Thrombolysis in Myocardial Infarction (TIMI 3A) trial. Circulation 87:38.

82. Kragel AH, Gertz SD, and Roberts WC (1991) Morphologic comparison of frequency and types of acute lesions in the major epicardial coronary arteries in unstable angina pectoris, sudden coronary death and acute myocardial infarction. J. Am. Coll. Cardiol. 18:801–808.

83. Starg HC, Chandler AB, Dinsmore RE, Fuster V, Glagov S, Insull W Jr., Rosenfeld ME, Schwartz CJ, Wagner WD, Wissler RW. (1995) Definitions of advanced types of atherosclerotic lesions and a historical classification of atherosclerosis. Circulation 92:1355–1374.

84. MacIsaac AI, Thomas JD, and Topol EJ (1993) Toward the quiescent coronary plaque. J. Am. Coll. Cardiol. 87:1179–1187.

85. Fuster V (1994) Lewis A Conner Memorial Lecture. Mechanisms leading to myocardial infarction: Insights from studies of vascular biology. Circulation 90:2126–2146.

86. Gertz SD and Roberts WC (1990) Hemodynamic shear force of coronary arterial atherosclerotic plaques. Am. J. Cardiol. 66: 1368–1372.

87. Cheng GC, Loree HM, Kamm RD, Fishbein MC, and Lee RT (1993) Distribution of circumferential stress in ruptured and stable atherosclerotic lesions. A structural analysis with histopathological correlation. Circulation 87:1179–1187.

88. Kragel AH, Reddy SG, Wittes JT, and Roberts WC (1989) Morphometric analysis of the composition of atherosclerotic plaques in the four major epicardial coronaries in acute myocardial infarction and sudden coronary death. Circulation 80:1747–1756.

89. Richardson RD, Davies MJ, and Born GVR (1989) Influence of plaque configuration and stress distribution on fissuring of coronary atherosclerotic plaques. Lancet 2:941–944.

90. Jude B, Agraou B, McFadden EP, Susen S, Bauters B, Lepelley P, Vanhaesbroucke C, Devos P, Cosson A, and Asseman P (1994) Evidence for time-dependent activation of monocytes in the systemic circulation in

unstable angina but not in acute myocardial infarction or in stable angina. Circulation 90:1662–1668.

91. Liuzzo G, Biasucci LM, Gallimore JR, Grillo RL, Rebuzzi AG, Pepys MB, and Maseri A (1994) the prognostic value of C-reactive protein and serum amyloid A protein in severe unstable angina. N. Engl. J. Med. 331:417–424.

92. Biasucci LM, Cliberto G, Liuzzo G, Altamura S, Monaco C, Quaranta G, Caliguri G, Vitelli A, and Maseri A (1995) Elevated serum concentration of interleukin-6 in unstable angina [abstract]. Circulation (suppl I):I664.

93. Shah PK, Falk E, Badimon JJ, Fernandez-Ortiz A, Mailhac A, Villareal-Levy G, Fallon JT, Regnstrom J, and Fuster V (1995) Human monocyte-derived macrophages induce collagen breakdown in fibrous caps of atherosclerotic plaques: potential role of matrix-degrading metalloproteinases and implications for plaque rupture. Circulation 92:1565–1569.

94. Hansson GK (1993) Immune and inflammatory mechanisms in the development of atherosclerosis. Br. Heart J. 69(suppl I):S38–S41.

95. Buja LM and Willerson JT (1994) Role of inflammation on coronary plaque disruption. Circulation 89:503–505.

96. Lendon CL, Davies MJ, Born GVR, and Richardson PD (1991) Atherosclerotic plaque caps are locally weakened when macrophage density is increased. Atherosclerosis 87:87–90.

97. Henney AM, Wakeley PR, Davies MJ, Foster K, Hembry R, Murphy, G, and Humphries S (1991) Localization of stromelysin gene expression in the atherosclerotic plaques by in situ hybridization. Proc. Natl. Acad. Sci. USA 88:8154–8158.

98. van der Wall AC, Becker AE, van der Loos CM, and Das PK (1994) Site of intimal rupture or erosion of thrombosed coronary atherosclerotic plaques is characterized by an inflammatory process irrespective of the dominant plaque morphology. Circulation 89:36–44.

99. Sato T, Takebayashi S, and Khochi K (1987) Increased subendothelial infiltration of the coronary arteries with mono cytes/macrophages in patients with unstable angina. Atherosclerosis 68:191–197.

100. Moreno PR, Falk E, Palacios IF, Newell JB, Fuster V, and Fallon JT (1994) Macrophage infiltration in acute coronary syndromes: implications for plaque rupture. Circulation 90:775–778.

101. Mitchinson MT and Ball RY (1987) Macrophages and atherogenesis. Lancet 2:146–149.

102. Galis ZS, Sukhova GK, Lark MW, and Libby P (1994) Increased expression of matrix metalloproteinases and matrix degrading activity in vulnerable regions of human atherosclerotic plaques. J. Clin. Invest. 94:2493–2503.

103. Kaartinen M, Penttil A, and Kovanen PT (1994) Accumulation of activated mast cells in the shoulder region of human coronary atheroma, the predilection site of atheromatous rupture. Circulation 90:1669–1678.

104. Moreno P, Falk E, Palacios IF, Newell JB, Fuster V, and Fallon JT (1994) Macrophage infiltration in acute coronary syndromes: implications for plaque rupture. Circulation 90:775–778.

105. Gregory SA, Kornbluth RS, Helin H, Remold HG, and Edington TS (1986) Monocyte procoagulant inducing factor: a lymphokine involved in the T-cell instructed monocyte procoagulant response to antigen. J. Immunol. 137:3231–3239.

106. Serneri GGN, Abbate R, Gori AN, Attanasio M, Martini F, Giusti B, Dabizzi P, Poggesi L, Modesti A, and Trotta F (1992) Transient intermittent lymphocyte activation is responsible for the instability of angina. Circulation 86:790–797.

107. Leathman EW, Bath PMW, Tooze JA, and Camm AJ (1995) Increased monocyte tissue factor expression in coronary disease. Br. Heart J. 73:10–13.

108. Berk BC, Weintraub WS, and Alexander RW (1990) Elevation of C-reactive protein in active coronary disease. Am. J. Cardiol. 65:168–172.

109. Lam JYT, Chesebro JH, Steel PM, Dewanjee MK, Badimon L, and Fuster V (1986) Deep arterial injury during experimental angioplasty: relation to positive 111In-

labeled platelet scintigram, quantitative platelet deposition and mural thrombosis. J. Am. Coll. Cardiol. 8:1380–1386.

110. Fernandez-Ortiz A, Badimon JJ, Falk E, Fuster R, Meyer B, Marlhac A, Weng D, Shah PK, and Badimon L (1994) Characterization of the relative thrombogenicity of atherosclerotic plaque components: Implications for consequences of plaque rupture. J. Am. Coll. Cardiol. 23:1562–1569.

111. Kovanen PT, Kaartinen M, and Paavonen T (1995) Infiltrates of activated mast cells at the site of coronary atheromatous erosion or rupture in myocardial infarction. Circulation 92:1084–1088.

112. Lo SK, Cheung A, Zheng Q, and Silverstein RL (1995) Induction of tissue factor on monocytes by adhesion to endothelial cells. J. Immunol. 154:4768–4777.

113. Annex BH, Denning SM, Keith MC, Sketch MH, Stack RS, Morrisey JH, and Peters KG (1995) Differential expression of tissue factor protein in directional atherectomy specimens from patients with stable and unstable coronary syndromes. Circulation 91:619–622.

114. Toschi V, Fallon JT, Gallo R, Lettino M, Fernandez-Ortiz A, Badimon L, Chesbro JT, Nemerson Y, Fuster V, and Badimon JJ (1995) Tissue factor predicts thrombogenicity of human atherosclerotic plaque components. Circulation 92(Suppl I): I-112.

115. Moise A, Lesperance J, Theroux P, Taeymans Y, Goulet C, and Bourassa MG (1984) Clinical and angiographic predictors of new total coronary occlusion in coronary artery disease: analysis of 313 nonoperated patients. Am. J. Cardiol. 54:1176–1181.

116. Hangartner JRW, Charleston AJ, Davies MJ, and Thomas AC (1986) Morphological characteristics of clinically significant coronary artery stenosis in stable angina. Br. Heart J. 56:501–508.

117. Born GVR (1979) Unstable angina. In: Cardiology, proceedings of the VIII world congress of cardiology, Tokyo, September 17–23, 1978, Hayase S and Murao S, eds. Amsterdam, Excerpta Medica, pp.81–91.

118. Badimon L, Badimon JJ, Turitto VT, Vallabhajosula S, and Fuster V (1988) Platelet thrombus formation on collagen type I: a model of deep vessel injury: influence of blood rheology, von Willebrand factor, and blood coagulation. Circulation 78: 1432–1442.

119. Badimon L and Badimon JJ (1989) Mechanism of arterial thrombosis in nonparallel streamlines: platelet thrombi grow at the apex of stenotic severely injured vessel wall: experimental study in pig model. J. Clin. Invest. 84:1134–1144.

120. Turitto VT and Baungartner HR (1979) Platelet interaction with subendothelium in flowing rabbit blood: effect of blood shear rate. Microvasc. Res. 17:38–54.

121. Davies SW, Marchart B, Lyons JP, and Timmis AD (1991) Irregular coronary lesion morphology after thrombosis predicts early clinical instability. J. Am. Coll. Cardiol. 18:669–674.

122. Hackett D, Davie G, Ghierchia S, and Maseri A (1987) Intermittent coronary occlusion in acute myocardial infarction: value of combined thrombolytic and vasodilatory therapy. N. Engl. J. Med. 317: 1055–1059.

123. Mailhac A, Badimon JJ, Fallon JT, Fernandez-Ortiz A, Meyer B, Chesbro JH, Fuster V, and Badimon L (1994) Effect of an eccentric severe stenosis on fibrinogen deposition on severely damaged vessel wall in arterial thrombosis. Relative contribution of fibrinogen and platelets. Circulation 90:988–996.

124. Lassila R, Badimon JJ, Vallabhajosula S, and Badimon L (1990) Dynamic monitoring of platelet deposition on severely damaged vessel wall in flowing blood: effect of different stenosis on thrombus growth. Arteriosclerosis 86:385–391.

125. Meyer BJ, Badimon JJ, Mailhac A, Fernandez-Ortiz A, Chesbro JH, Fuster V, and Badimon L (1994) Inhibition of growth of thrombus on fresh mural thrombus. Targeting optimal therapy. Circulation 90: 2432–2438.

126. Weitz JI, Hudoba M, Massel D, Maraganore J, and Hirsh J (1994) Clot bound thrombin is protected from inhibition by heparin-antithrombin III but is susceptible to inactivation by antithrombin III-independent inhibitors. J. Clin. Invest. 86:385–391.

127. Owen J, Friedman KD, Grossman BA, Wilkins C, Berke AD, and Powers ER (1988) Thrombolytic therapy with tissue plasminogen activator or streptokinase induces transient thrombin activity. Blood 72:616–620.

128. Eisenberg PR, Sherman LA, and Jaffe AS (1987) Paradoxic elevation of fibrinopeptide A after streptokinase: evidence for continued thrombosis despite intense fibrinolysis. J. Am. Coll. Cardiol. 10: 527–529.

129. Zeiher AM, Schachinger V, Weitzel SH, Wollschlager H, and Just H (1991) Intracoronary thrombus formation causes focal vasoconstriction of epicardial arteries in patients with coronary artery disease. Circulation 83:1519–1525.

130. Maseri A, L'Abbate A, Baroldi G, Chlerchia S, Marzilli M, Ballestra AM, Severis, Parodi O, Blagini A, Distante A, and Pesola A (1978) Coronary vasospasm as a possible cause of myocardial infarction. A conclusion derived from the study of "preinfarction" angina. N. Engl. J. Med. 299:1271–1277.

131. Zeiher AM, Drexler H, Wollschlager H, and Just H (1991) Modulation of coronary vasomotor tone in humans: progressive endothelial dysfunction with different early stages of coronary atherosclerosis. Circulation 83:391–401.

132. Celermajer DS, Sorenson K, Gooch LM, Spiegelhalter DJ, Miller OI, Sullivan ID, Lloyd JK, and Dearfield JE (1992) Noninvasive detection of endothelial dysfunction in children and adults at risk of atherosclerosis. Lancet 340:1111–1115.

133. Willerson, JT, Golino P, Eidt J, Campbell WB, and Buja LM (1989) Specific platelet mediators and unstable coronary artery lesions: experimental evidence and potential clinical implications. Circulation 80: 198–205.

134. Lam JYT, Chesebro JH, Steele PM, Badimon L, and Fuster V (1987) Is vasospasm related to platelet deposition? Relationship in a porcine preparation of arterial injury in vivo. Circulation 75:243–248

135. Vanhoutte PM and Shimokawa H (1989) Endothelium-derived relaxing factor and coronary vasospasm. Circulation 80:1–9.

136. el-Tamimi H, Davies GL, Hackett D, Sritara P, Bertrand O, Crea F, and Maseri A (1991) Abnormal vasomotor changes early after coronary angioplasty. Circulation 84: 1198–1202.

137. Larson PT, Wallen NH, and Hjemdahl P (1994) Norepinephrine-induced platelet activation in vivo is only partly counteracted by aspirin. Circulation 89: 1951–1957.

138. Kimura S, Nishinaga M, Ozawa T, and Shimada K (1994) Thrombin generation as an acute effect of cigarette smoking. Am. Heart J. 128:7–11.

139. Davies MJ, Bland MJ, Hangartner WR, Angelini A, and Thomas K (1989) Factors influencing the presence or absence of acute coronary thrombi in sudden ischemic death. Eur. Heart J. 10:203–208.

140. Badimon JJ, Badimon L, Turitto VT, and Fuster V (1991) Platelet deposition at higher shear rates is enhanced by high plasma cholesterol levels: in vivo study in a rabbit model. Arteriosclerosis Thrombosis 11:395–402.

141. Kawai C (1994) Pathogenesis of acute myocardial infarction. Novel regulatory systems of bioactive substances in the vessel wall. Circulation 90:1033–1043.

142. Rader DJ, Hoeg JM, and Brewer HB Jr (1994) Quantitation of plasma apolipoproteins in the primary and secondary prevention of coronary artery disease. Ann. Intern. Med. 120:1012–1025.

143. McLean JW, Tomlinson JE, Kuang WJ, Eaton DL, Chen EY, Fless GM, Scanu AM, and Lawn RM (1987) cDNA sequence of human apolipoprotein (a) is homologous to plasminogen. Nature 30:132–137.

144. Frank SL, Klisak I, Sparkes RS, Mohandas T, Tomlinson JE, McLean JW, Lawn RM, and Lusis AJ (1988) The apoprotein (a) gene resides on human chromosome 6q26-27 in close proximity to the homologous gene for the plasminogen. Hum. Genet. 79:352–356.

145. Loscalzo J (1990) Lipoprotein (a): a unique risk factor for athero-embolic disease. Arteriosclerosis 10:672–679.

146. Benoussan D, Levy-Toledano S, Passa P, Caen J, and Caniver J (1975) Platelet hyperaggregation and increased plasma level of

von Willebrand factor in diabetics with retinopathy. Diabetologia 11:307–312.

147. Schwartz CJ, Kelley JL, Valente AJ, Cayatte AJ, Sprague EA, and Rozek MM (1992) Pathogenesis of the atherosclerotic lesion: implications for diabetes mellitus. Diabetes Care 15:1156–1167.

148. The diabetes control and complications trial research group (1993) The effect of intensive treatment of diabetes on the development and progression of long-term complications in insulin-dependent diabetes mellitus. N. Engl. J. Med. 329:977–986.

149. Jacoby RM and Nesto RW (1992) Acute myocardial infarction in the diabetic patient: pathophysiology, clinical course and prognosis. J. Am. Coll. Cardiol. 20: 736–744.

150. Lam JYT, Latour JG, Lesperance J, and Waters D (1994) Platelet aggregation, coronary artery disease progression and future coronary events. Am. J. Cardiol. 73: 333–338.

151. Merlini A, Bauer KA, Oltrona L, Ardissino D, Cattanco M, Belli C, Mannucci PM, and Rosenberg RD (1994) Persistent activation of coagulation mechanism in unstable angina and myocardial infarction. Circulation 90:61–68.

152. Wilhemsen L, Svardsudd K, Korsan-Bengsten K, Larsson B, Welin L, and Tibblin G (1984) Fibrinogen as a risk factor for stroke and myocardial infarction. N. Engl. J. Med. 311:501–505.

153. McGill DA and Ardlie NG (1990) The relationship between blood fibrinogen level and coronary artery disease. Coronary Artery Disease 1:557–566.

154. Rosengren A, Wilhelmsen L, Wellin L, Tsipogianni A, Teger-Nilsson AC, and Wedel H (1990) Social influences and cardiovascular risk factor as determinant of plasma fibrinogen concentration in a general population sample of middle age men. Br. Med. J. 330:634–638.

155. Fuster V, Dyken ML, Vokonas PS, and Hennekens C (1993) Aspirin as a therapeutic agent in cardiovascular disease. Circulation 87:659–675.

156. Cohen M, Adams PC, Parry G, Kiong J, Chamberlain D, Wieczorek I, Fox KA, Chesbro JH, Strain J, Keller C, Kelly A, Lancaster G, Ali J, Kronmal R, and Fuster V (1994) Combination antithrombotic therapy in unstable rest angina and non-Q wave infarction in nonprior aspirin users: primary endpoints analysis from the ATACS trial. Circulation 89:596–603.

3

Pathophysiology and Treatment of Acute Myocardial Ischemia and Infarction

Gary B. Green, Edward S. Bessman, and Sol F. Green

PATHOPHYSIOLOGY OF ATHEROSCLEROTIC CORONARY ARTERY DISEASE (CAD)

Historical

Atherosclerotic vascular disease has been present in humans for thousands of years. Atherosclerotic lesions were identified in Egyptian mummies dating as early as the 15th century B.C. In the 19th century, researchers speculated that arterial wall injury may cause an inflammatory response, resulting in atherosclerotic lesions (1). By the early 1900s investigators had proposed a correlation among the degree of atherosclerotic lesions, acute myocardial infarction (AMI)*, and stroke (2). The prevention and treatment of coronary artery atherogenesis is a major public health concern today (3).

Coronary Artery Atherogenesis

Atherogenesis begins in childhood. Lipid-rich lesions containing macrophages and T-lymphocytes (fatty streaks) are found in the aorta shortly after birth, and increase in number between the second and third decade. Eventually, expanding lesions become elevated and may affect normal laminar blood flow. These lesions contain smooth muscle cells that have migrated into the intimal layer of the arterial wall with accumulation of lipids, forming a fibrous plaque. As migration and proliferation of smooth muscle cells continue, a fibrous cap is formed containing dense connective tissue matrix, macrophages, T-lymphocytes, cell debris, and intracellular and extracellular lipids.

In more advanced lesions, the fibrous plaque can become vascularized, and the lipid-rich core increases in size and becomes calcified. At this stage, the surface of the intima may develop cracks and thrombi, and hemorrhage. If a thrombus is involved, it can lead to occlusive disease by reducing the size of the vascular lumen (4).

Plaque Disruption

Coronary atherosclerotic plaque is composed of connective tissue, calcium phosphates, lipids, inflammatory cells (T-lymphocytes, macrophages), and smooth muscle cells in the residual medial layer. The proportion of each component varies among individuals and is related to lesion age. Older, heavily fibrotic or calcified plaque is

---

*See p. 66 for list of abbreviations used in this chapter.

From: Cardiac Markers   Edited by: Alan H. B. Wu
© Humana Press Inc., Totowa, NJ

hard, whereas younger, soft plaque consists predominantly of lipids and foamy macrophages. Regardless of composition, lesion progression consistently leads to the formation of a fibrous cap.

Rupture of the fibrous cap may occur from smooth muscle spasm, causing the release of plaque contents into the lumen of the blood vessel, and ultimately leading to coronary thrombus and AMI *(5,6)*. The pathogenesis and pathophysiology of myocardial ischemia are complex events involving the interaction of several processes, including vascular spasm and plaque rupture as well as platelet and thrombin system activation. The series of events leading to a specific coronary event may be variable. For example, plaque rupture, caused by vasospasm, can induce thrombosis, or platelet adherence can lead to vasoconstrictive substance release, causing vasospasm and plaque rupture.

Coronary Artery Spasm

The endothelial cells lining the vessel wall play a critical role in maintenance of vascular homeostasis. They are actively involved in plaque formation as well as platelet and inflammatory cell adhesion. Endothelial cells also release mediators controlling vascular relaxation (endothelium-derived relaxing factor [EDRF], nitric oxide [NO]), and spasm (endothelins). Three mechanisms have been proposed for the induction of coronary vasospasm:

1. A decrease in NO release. NO has been shown to be an important endothelial-derived vasodilator. However, immunohistochemical studies of atherosclerotic lesions demonstrate increased, rather than decreased, expression of NO synthetase in diseased arteries, suggesting increased NO production is more characteristic of CAD *(7)*.
2. Increased NO degradation by oxygen via free radicals ($NO + O_2 \rightarrow NO_3$).
3. Increased sensitivity of vascular smooth muscle constrictors. The efficacy of calcium

entry blockers in decreasing vasospasm suggests that there may be abnormal expression of voltage-dependent calcium channels in diseased vessels, which could enhance contractility.

Platelet Activation and Thrombus Formation

Experimental and clinical observations of platelet participation in ischemia indicate that platelets function in the following roles. Once activated, they form aggregates that can restrict coronary perfusion and eventually cause AMI. Alternatively, activated platelets release their granular contents (ADP, thrombin, thromboxane A_2), which are involved in the induction of cell proliferation and thrombosis *(8)*.

Platelets usually circulate freely in blood and rarely adhere to endothelial cells. One possible explanation for this behavior may be that both platelets and endothelium have a negative charge, and thus are mutually repulsive. However, in the event of vessel injury, subendothelial connective tissue is exposed and causes platelets adherence (collagen and fibronectin interact with platelet membrane glycoproteins). This interaction triggers a conformational change in the platelet's shape from disk to stellate forms (activation) *(9–11)*. In the presence of calcium, activated platelets induce intraplatelet regulatory proteins. These proteins activate the actin-myosin system, resulting in platelet contraction, which results in the release of ADP, serotonin, and thromboxane A_2. Once released, these mediators further induce platelet aggregation and also promote thrombin production.

Other changes in platelet structure and function may be observed, but are of unclear significance. For example, studies have shown an increased mean platelet volume (MPV) in patients with sudden death and AMI (both during and after infarction) *(12–14)*. However, it has been suggested that since MPV measurements are derived from automated hematology instruments, an elevated MPV may actually reflect the presence of platelet agglutinates rather than individually enlarged platelets.

Thrombin System Activation

Thrombin is generated on the membrane of activated platelets from circulating prothrombin as an end product of coagulation. The coagulation process converts a number of plasma procoagulants into activated factors via an intrinsic and extrinsic pathway. The intrinsic pathway involves factors within blood that lead to the conversion of prothrombin to thrombin. The extrinsic pathway is initiated by substances outside the blood such as tissue thromboplastin.

Factor X acts as a bridge between the intrinsic and extrinsic pathways, and activates prothrombinase, which converts prothrombin to thrombin. Thrombin also activates platelets on vascular endothelial and smooth muscle cells via a thrombin receptor, leading to the release of factor V and producing a positive feedback mechanism for further pathway activation. Ultimately, thrombin converts fibrinogen to fibrin. Fibrin can form coupled monomers (polymers) that make up the skeleton of a thrombus, trapping platelets as well as red and white blood cells *(15)*.

Risk Factors

Atherosclerotic lesions and their rate of development are highly variable and depend on anatomic site as well as various genetic, physiologic, and environmental risk factors.

Hyperlipidemia

Hyperlipidemia from dietary lipids is the most important environmental cause for atherosclerotic disease. There is a direct association between lowering of plasma cholesterol and a reduced incidence of coronary atherosclerosis *(16,17)*. The National Cholesterol Education Program has established guidelines for normal plasma values of cholesterol and lipoproteins: Cholesterol levels <200 mg/dL are considered "desirable," 200–239 is considered "borderline," and "high blood cholesterol" is defined as a level >240. Low-density lipoproteins (LDLs) levels <130 mg/dL are considered "desirable," 130–159 are "borderline," and those with levels >160 mg/dL are classified as "high-risk" *(18)*.

Oxidized LDL (oxLDL)

Native LDL transports lipids into the intima through the endothelium. During this process, LDL may become oxLDL. Macrophages actively take up oxLDL, leading to an accumulation of lipid and formation of foam cells within the intima. Oxidized lipids are activators of monocytes as well as being cytotoxic and are considered to be a major factor in plaque progression *(19,20)*. Oxidized lipids can injure the endothelium and smooth muscle cell membranes during transport of extracellular cholesterol into the cell. Antioxidants, such as probucol, have been shown to induce lesion regression by preventing membrane damage of free radicals *(21)*.

Hypertension

Hypertension has clearly been established as an independent risk factor for CAD *(22)*, although the mechanism of atherosclerosis induction remains unsubstantiated. Altered flow characteristics may result in injury to the endothelium and development of lesions leading to atherosclerosis *(23)*. The effects of hypertensive agents, such as angiotensin and renin, may also be factors *(23)*.

Cigaret Smoking

A strong correlation has been established between cigaret smoking and CAD. Components of cigaret smoke may be injurious to the arterial wall. However, the exact pathways of the metabolic effect remain an active area of investigation *(24)*.

Gender

The reason for increased male incidence of atherogenesis is not clear. It has been suggested that estrogens may play a role in decreased female incidence, since post-menopausal women have an increased risk of CAD. However, increases in cardiovascular mortality have been documented in men receiving large doses of estrogenic hormones after a myocardial event *(22)*.

Diabetes

Although a specific mechanism has not been elucidated, a correlation between diabetes and hypertension with decreased concentrations of HDL cholesterol has been well established *(22)*.

Other Factors

Other risk factors for the presence of CAD that have been established include family history, age (>45 yr in males, >55 in females), previous myocardial infarction (MI), and sedentary lifestyle *(18)*.

There may also be an association between inflammation caused by *Chlamydia pneumoniae* infections and coronary atherosclerosis. In one study involving 90 patients undergoing coronary arthrectomy, 79% of assayed specimens were positive for the presence of *Chlamydia*, whereas only 4% of patients with normal coronary arteries showed evidence of *Chlamydia (25)*.

PATHOPHYSIOLOGY OF SYNDROMES OF MYOCARDIAL ISCHEMIA (REVERSIBLE INJURY)

Vascular Pathophysiology

Stable Angina Pectoris

Stable angina is a clinical syndrome defined by the occurrence of recurrent ischemic chest pain or other symptoms of myocardial ischemia (angina equivalent) in a pattern that does not change significantly over time. Symptom occurrence remains consistent over a period of several weeks or longer with respect to the level of exertion that triggers an episode, as well as the duration, severity, and frequency of episodes.

Although significant variability in the characteristics of individual ischemic episodes typically does occur, an unchanging pattern can be observed over time *(26)*.

Coronary artery angiography of patients with stable angina patterns typically reveals hemodynamically significant vessel stenosis owing to atherosclerotic plaque without evidence of acute thrombosis *(27,28)*. During periods of low myocardial oxygen demand, blood flow through the stenosed vessel remains adequate and the patient remains asymptomatic. However, during times of increased oxygen demand, flow through the fixed lesion cannot be proportionately increased, and the region of myocardium perfused by the culprit vessel becomes ischemic. The increase in myocardial work and oxygen demand is relatively constant at a given level of exertion, thus explaining the typically reported initiation of symptoms during similar activities on a daily or weekly basis. The finding of a relatively reproducible ischemic threshold on serial exercise testing of stable angina patients further supports this mechanism *(26)*. The variability of reported symptoms is likely owing to various transient alterations in coronary vascular tone, such as those caused by circadian rhythms *(29)*.

Unstable Angina

The clinical diagnosis of unstable angina is given to patients who report a change in pattern of their ischemic symptoms. This includes patients with new onset of anginal symptoms as well as those who have recently experienced an increased frequency, duration, or severity of symptoms. Patients experiencing chest pain at rest are included and are a particularly high-risk subgroup *(30)*. Several systems have been proposed to further categorize patients with unstable angina according to symptom severity. At present, the most widely used grading system was developed by the Canadian Cardiovascular

Table 1
Canadian Classification System
for Unstable Angina[a]

Class	Description
I	Day-to-day activity, such as walking or climbing stairs; angina occurs only with strenuous, rapid, or prolonged exertion
II	Slight limitation of ordinary activity; angina occurs on walking or climbing stairs rapidly, walking uphill, walking or stair climbing after meals, in cold or windy conditions, under emotional stress, or only during the few hours after awakening; angina occurs when walking more than two blocks on a level surface and climbing more than one flight of ordinary stairs at a normal pace and in normal condition
III	Marked limitations of ordinary physical activity; angina occurs on walking one to two blocks on a level surface or climbing one flight of stairs in normal conditions and at a normal pace
IV	Inability to carry on any physical activity without discomfort; angina may be present at rest

[a]Adapted from ref. *36*.

Society (Table 1) *(31)*. The pathophysiology of unstable angina is presented in Chapter 2.

Myocardial Cell Pathophysiology

Although the process of ischemic cell injury and death can be measured using many indicators, observation of energy usage is perhaps the most relevant. In the myocyte, as in all cells, energy is stored and transferred within the high-energy phosphate bonds of ATP. The needs of the many energy-requiring processes of the cell are met through the continuous regeneration of ATP by aerobic metabolism of glucose and fatty acids. However, within minutes of oxygen deprivation to the myocardial cell, the oxygen-dependent synthesis of ATP (oxidative phosphorylation) dramatically decreases *(32)*. In the continued absence of oxygen, a shift to anaerobic metabolism takes place, and this does result in some continued ATP production. However, the metabolism of 1 mol of glucose by anaerobic metabolism results in 2 mol of ATP, compared to the 36 mol of ATP produced by aerobic processes. Further, the byproducts of anaerobic metabolism have deleterious effects on other intracellular processes. The overall result is that soon after oxygen deprivation, ATP demand surpasses production and existing stores of the energy-rich compound are depleted. As ATP becomes scarce, the function of ATP-dependent ion channels in the sarcoplasmic and cell membranes quickly becomes compromised. This results in impairment of the cells' ability to maintain ionic gradients necessary for contractility and cellular integrity *(33,34)*.

If oxygen is restored to the cell rapidly, these changes are reversible. Aerobic metabolism is resumed, ATP levels are restored, and the necessary ionic gradients are maintained. In experimental models of a transient ischemic insult, cell recovery occurs reproducibly when intracellular ATP content is reduced by <40%. These cells do exhibit microscopic changes, such as intermyofibrillar edema and mitochondrial swelling, but do not exhibit the typical changes associated with necrosis *(32)*.

Hemodynamic Affects

Transient myocardial ischemia of even brief duration is associated with predictable hemodynamic abnormalities *(35)*. Several invasive hemodynamic studies of patients with induced or spontaneous episodes of ischemia have demonstrated the rapid onset of left ventricular (LV) dysfunction as indicated by increases in LV and pulmonary artery diastolic pressures and decreased LV ejection fraction *(36–38)*. These findings are consistent with echocardiographic observations of regional akinesis and global ventricular dysfunction associated with transient ischemia induced during coronary artery angioplasty procedures *(39)*.

Impairment of systolic function is observable as early as 1 min following coronary occlusion and corresponds to a sudden decrease in contractile force at the cellular level *(40)*. Several biochemical processes have been implicated in this phenomenon, including intracellular changes in Ca^{2+} transport and concentration gradients, depletion of ATP and inorganic phosphate stores, and intracellular acidosis. Whatever the cause, within 10 min of ischemia, contraction ceases and the ischemic region becomes dyskinetic during systole. Diastolic dysfunction is also observed soon after occlusion and is the result of decreased myocardial compliance *(41)*. Ischemic contracture of myocytes associated with intracellular ATP depletion is postulated to be the cause. In addition to systolic and diastolic dysfunction, transient mitral regurgitation may occur if the hypoperfused region includes the region of the LV overlying the papillary muscles *(42)*.

If coronary flow is restored within 20 min of occlusion, all of the observed metabolic derangements are reversed. Although complete restoration of myocardial function does occur, recovery is a slow process. After an ischemic insult, systolic dysfunction may persist for up to 24 h. Diastolic impairment has an even longer recovery period, requiring up to 2 d for return to normal filling rates *(43)*. The occurrence of this period of recovery is termed "myocardial stunning," and is thought to explain the transient myocardial dysfunction observed after cardiac surgery and cardiopulmonary bypass *(44)*. The recognition of myocardial stunning also has other important clinical implications. For example, after an ischemic event, stunned but viable myocardium may exist adjacent to a region of infarction, making early assessment of residual ventricular function difficult.

In addition to the episodic occurrence of acute ischemia, coronary artery disease may also result in a chronic reduction in coronary flow that is not sufficient to cause infarction. Although myocardial viability may be maintained with as little as 15% of normal perfusion, changes in ventricular function do occur. A persistent state of reduced perfusion results in chronic contractile dysfunction, with the degree of dysfunction being proportional to the decrease in flow. If adequate coronary flow is restored, such as after coronary bypass graft surgery, normal contractile function resumes. This reversible ischemic dysfunction is termed "myocardial hibernation," and its pathophysiology is an active area of research *(45,46)*.

PATHOPHYSIOLOGY OF AMI

Vascular Pathophysiology

Plaque rupture with associated thrombus formation can be demonstrated in most patients with a crescendo pattern of unstable angina as well as those with AMI *(47–49)*. Accordingly, it is presumed that the underlying pathophysiologies of these different clinical entities are identical, and therefore, myocardial infarction must also be considered to be the result of a complex, dynamic vascular process. The defining difference between the two entities is simply whether the thrombus–plaque complex is sufficiently occlusive to lead to identifiable cell death within the hypoperfused region of myocardium.

Analogous to the continuum occurring in the degree of coronary artery thrombosis, it is also apparent that the "downstream" processes in AMI also occur in shades of gray. On one end of the spectrum is the "classic" presentation of acute, uniform, full wall thickness (transmural) necrosis resulting from sudden, total thrombosis of a coronary vessel. However, many variables may ultimately affect the level of myocardial cell death and, subsequently, the patient's clinical manifestations. For example, even in the presence of complete vessel occlusion, if significant collateral flow to the affected region is present, infarction may be reduced or precluded. Another point on the spectrum is the development of a subendocardial infarction. Myocardial oxygen consumption is higher in the subendocardium than in other regions of the heart, and collateral flow is relatively poor. Therefore, this region is the most susceptible to an ischemic insult. If the occlusion is incomplete or transient, or if epicardial collateral flow is adequate, necrosis may be limited to the subendocardial region *(50,51)*. Further, if an intracoronary thrombus is unstable, fragmentation and distal embolization may occur, the result being small, patchy zones of necrosis within a larger region of viable myocardium. In other cases, if the ischemic insult is even less severe, the vast majority of myocardium may remain intact, with only microscopic areas of cell death occurring. Patients with these "microinfarcts" are usually clinically indistinguishable from those with unstable angina and may be detected only by using sensitive serum markers *(52,53)*. Other factors affecting the extent and characteristics of an ischemic lesion include the rapidity of thrombus formation, the presence and timing of antegrade flow restoration, and the condition of the affected myocardium prior to occlusion.

Myocardial Cell Pathophysiology

If oxygen is not restored to the cell within 10–15 min, cell death becomes inevitable. When oxidative phosphorylation is not rapidly resumed, continued dysfunction of ATP-dependent ion channels leads to increased intracellular levels of Na^+. Na^+/Ca^{2+} exchange and dysfunction of ATP-dependent Ca^{2+} transport then contribute to increased intracellular Ca^{2+} levels. The increase of intracellular Ca^{2+} is associated with, and may be the trigger of, a cascade of processes that eventually result in irreversible organelle damage and loss of cell membrane integrity. These events occur reproducibly after a reduction in intracellular ATP content of 80% or more *(32,54)*.

Hemodynamic Affects

Q-Wave vs Non-Q-Wave Infarction

As previously stated, a wide spectrum exists in the degree and pattern of cell death following coronary occlusion. However, clinicians have traditionally classified AMI into two broad categories based on electrocardiographic (ECG) findings. "Q-wave" and "non-Q-wave" infarctions were initially thought to correspond to transmural and subendocardial patterns of necrosis, respectively. Although pathologic studies have since demonstrated that this is not reliably true, the ECG designations are still used because of significant clinical and prognostic differences between the two groups. Presence of Q-waves on the ECG is still thought to represent a more "complete" infarction of the affected area *(50,51)*. Conversely, a non-Q-wave infarct seems to indicate that a significant mass of viable myocardium still exists in the ischemic region. Consistent with this idea are the findings that infarct size is larger in patients with Q-wave infarction and that early mortality is significantly greater in these patients compared to those with non-Q-wave infarcts. Conversely, patients with non-Q-wave infarcts are more likely subsequently to suffer reinfarction in the affected region. The end result is that the two groups have an equivalent 2-yr mortality. The term "myocardium at risk" is often used to describe viable myocardium perfused by the culprit vessel following a non-Q-wave infarct. Angiographic studies show a higher rate of early patency in non-Q-wave patients and have led to the suggestion that non-Q-wave infarction may be the result of

Table 2
Classification of AMI

Subset	Description	Measures	
Clinical exam (Killip classification)			
I	No evidence of heart failure	Rales and S_3 absent	
II	Evidence of CHF	Rales up to 50% of lung fields	
III	Pulmonary Edema	Rales 50% of lung fields	
IV	Cardiogenic shock	Hypotension, hypoperfusion	
Hemodynamic			Pulmonary
measurements (Forrestec classification)		Cardiac index	artery occl.
		L/m²/min	pressure, (mmHg)
I	Normal hemodynamics	2.7 ± 0.5	≤ 12
II	Hyperdynamic state	>3.0	<12
III	Hypovolemia	≤ 2.7	≤ 9
IV	LV failure		
	A. Mild	≤ 2.5	$>18, \leq 2$
	B. Severe	≤ 1.8	≥ 22
V	Cardiogenic shock	≤ 1.8	≤ 18
VI	Shock attributable to RV infarction	≤ 1.8	≤ 18

[a]Adapted from refs. *63* and *64*.

early, spontaneous reperfusion of the occluded vessel. This theory is also supported by data demonstrating an earlier peak in creatine kinase (CK) levels in non-Q-wave MI, thought to represent "early washout" of the enzyme owing to continued perfusion of the infarcted area *(48,51,55,56)*.

Infarct Size

The single most important determinant of the clinical course of an AMI is infarct size. Patients with a larger infarct are more likely to have significant LV dysfunction, and the degree of dysfunction is predictive of infarct survival *(57)*. This was recognized as early as 1967 when Killip and Kimball developed a system of classification of AMI patients based on clinical signs of congestive heart failure (CHF) that was able to predict prognosis (Table 2) *(58)*. Using this system, patients were placed in one of four "Killip classes." Class 1 patients had the lowest mortality (6%) and included those patients without any physical signs of CHF. Class 4

represents patients in cardiogenic shock and was associated with an 80% mortality rate, whereas classes 2 and 3 had intermediate levels of CHF and correspondingly intermediate mortality rates. More recently, more precise classification systems have been devised that categorize patients based on results of invasive hemodynamic measurements (Table 2) *(59)*. Each of these systems also demonstrates that mortality increases according to the degree of LV dysfunction.

Infarct Location

The circulatory system of the human heart is predominantly regional, with each coronary artery branch perfusing a specific region of myocardium. This is most dramatically demonstrated by studies of AMI patients undergoing early angiography, in which 90% of patients exhibit a total occlusion of the coronary vessel that anatomically corresponds to the myocardial region identified by ECG *(60,61)*. However, it is important to note that the myocardial regions perfused by the various coronary vessels are not uniform with respect to either size or function. The implication of this is that myocardial infarction is a regional disease, and the clinical manifestations of AMI can depend on infarct location as well as infarct size.

There are three main coronary trunks that have a relatively constant pattern of regionalization. The left anterior descending coronary artery supplies the anterior wall of the LV near the apex, the adjoining anterior wall of the right ventricle (RV), and the anterior two-thirds of the interventricular septum. The right coronary artery supplies the posterior wall of the LV, the posterior one-third of the septum, and in most people, the remainder of the RV. The left circumflex coronary artery supplies the lateral wall of the LV. Occlusion of the left anterior descending or one of its branches is most common, occurring in 40–50% of AMIs. Right coronary occlusion occurs in 30–40% of cases and left circumflex occlusion in 15–20% of cases *(62)*.

Acute anterior infarction is associated with a relatively higher mortality compared to other regions, primarily attributable to the adverse hemodynamic affects of larger infarct size and greater degree of LV dysfunction *(63)*. Complications, such as acute bundle branch block and high-grade atrioventricular conduction blocks owing to direct conduction system infarct involvement, also contribute to the poorer prognosis *(64,65)*.

Inferior infarctions are generally smaller in size and have a correspondingly lower mortality. Sinus bradycardia, the most common arrhythmia in AMI patients, is observed in 40% of patients with inferior MI and is usually attributed to increased vagal tone *(66)*. Transient low-grade atrio-ventricular conduction blocks are also common. Papillary muscle dysfunction and/or rupture causing acute mitral valve regurgitation is a less common, but more serious complication of inferior MI *(67)*.

Right ventricular infarction occurs uncommonly (3–5%) in isolation, but can be documented in up to 50% of patients with acute inferior MI *(68,69)*. In about half of these patients, the extent of RV involvement will be hemodynamically significant. Although the presence of right-sided infarction is frequently overlooked, these patients may demonstrate dramatic hemodynamic changes in a characteristic pattern. The RV becomes a passive conduit, with increasing RV-filling pressures. Simultaneously, LV-filling pressures remain normal and cardiac output drops, leading to hypotension. The importance of early recognition of RV infarction has led to the recommendation that right-sided ECG leads be recorded in all patients presenting with inferior AMI.

THERAPY OF AMI

Overview

The goal of therapeutic intervention in AMI is to reduce morbidity and mortality by limiting infarct size and preventing or treating complications. The need for early intervention has long been recognized. More than half of AMI deaths occur within 1 h of the onset of symptoms and prior to arrival at a hospital *(70)*. Furthermore, the effectiveness of certain interventions, particularly reperfusion therapies, depends on their early administration *(71,72)*. Consequently, there is increasing pressure to identify patients with AMI rapidly and promptly initiate therapy *(73)*.

Acute myocardial ischemia represents a continuum from unstable angina, through non-Q-wave MI, to Q-wave AMI, collectively referred to as acute coronary syndromes *(74)*. Although specific treatments differ for these entities, distinguishing between them on clinical grounds may be difficult. Accordingly, certain baseline anti-ischemic therapies must be started while diagnostic strategies are being pursued.

Current recommendations from the American College of Cardiology/American Heart Association (ACC/AHA) Task Force on Practice Guidelines emphasize the use of the 12-lead ECG for the purpose of guiding initial decision making *(75)*. Patients with ECG findings of ST-segment elevation or new left bundle branch block (LBBB) are considered for reperfusion therapy. Those without ST-segment elevation, but whose ECGs are strongly suspicious for ischemia (ST-segment depression or T-wave inversion) should be admitted to the hospital for more aggressive anti-ischemic therapy. Patients with normal or nondiagnostic ECGs should receive continued evaluation in the Emergency Department (ED) or an inpatient setting until ischemia/infarction is either ruled in or out.

Routine Measures

The following interventions should be initiated in all patients with possible myocardial ischemia/infarction. If the patient is transported by prehospital personnel capable of providing advanced cardiac life support (ACLS), then certain of these measures may already be in place. If not, they should be started on arrival in the hospital ED.

Intravenous (iv) Access

All patients should have at least one iv line begun. Volume infused must be carefully controlled to avoid precipitating pulmonary congestion. Alternatively, a saline lock may be used.

Oxygen

Oxygen by nasal prongs should be administered to all patients for at least the first 2–3 h. Beyond that time, there is no evidence that oxygen is beneficial for uncomplicated patients. Digital pulse oximetry may be used to guide therapy, with the goal of maintaining an oxygen saturation at >90%.

Continuous Electrocardiographic Monitoring

The primary cause of death in the first 2 h after an AMI is arrhythmia, in particular ventricular fibrillation (VF) *(76)*. ECG monitoring allows for early recognition of conduction abnormalities, and rapid response to life-threatening events. By extension, immediate availability of resuscitation equipment and drugs is necessary.

Nitroglycerin (NTG)

NTG relaxes vascular smooth muscle, thus producing vasodilatation. The mechanism of action appears to be the conversion of nitrate into NO, which is a potent regulator of vascular tone *(77)*. Vasodilatation lowers preload by reducing venous return to the heart and thus reducing cardiac filling. Systemic arterial relaxation reduces afterload, and coronary vasodilatation improves the flow of blood to the heart muscle. Thus, NTG lowers myocardial oxygen demand while simultaneously improving oxygen supply *(78,79)*. In spite of its favorable hemodynamic profile, clinical trials are conflicting regarding the potential for NTG to reduce mortality in AMI *(80,81)*. Nevertheless, current practice dictates that every patient with a possible acute coronary syndrome should receive NTG unless it is contraindicated. NTG can be easily given as a sublingual tablet, but in unstable patients, it is best given iv so its dosing can be titrated to effect.

Most patients given nitrates develop a headache, which generally is mild. Some patients with pulmonary congestion will experience worsening gas exchange because of a redistribution of flow in the pulmonary vasculature leading to ventilation/perfusion mismatch. However, the most clinically significant adverse effect of NTG is hypotension, often accompanied by reflex tachycardia, both of which will aggravate myocardial ischemia. Hypotension can be particularly severe in patients with RV infarcts and/or bradycardia. Thus, NTG should be avoided in patients who are hypotensive, bradycardic, or have RV ischemia.

Analgesics

The pain and anxiety that accompany ischemic-type chest pain lead to stimulation of the sympathetic nervous system. The release of endogenous catecholamines results in heart rate stimulation, increased contractility, and elevation of blood pressure. This causes increased myocardial oxygen demand, which can worsen ischemia and increase myocardial irritability *(82)*. NTG is effective in reducing ischemic-type pain, but may not offer complete relief and does not treat anxiety. Thus, the early use of an analgesic is indicated. Although morphine can produce respiratory depression and hypotension, concerns are often overstated. Furthermore, respiratory depression readily responds to naloxone, and hypotension usually responds to fluid administration or postural changes.

Aspirin

Platelet aggregation plays an important role in the pathogenesis of acute arterial occlusion leading to ischemia. Aggregation is triggered by the prostaglandins thromboxane A2 in platelets and prostacyclin in endothelial cells, both of which are produced by the action of the enzyme cyclo-oxygenase *(83,84)*. Aspirin inhibits platelet aggregation by irreversibly blocking the action of cyclo-oxygenase. Platelets are unable to produce more cyclo-oxygenase and thus are unable to aggregate for the duration of their 10-d lifespan. Endothelial cells are able to generate new cyclo-oxygenase, and thus, are able to recover their ability to induce aggregation.

The use of aspirin in all patients with clinical suspicion of AMI is currently considered to be the standard of care *(75)*. Unequivocal support for the efficacy and safety of aspirin is based on the Second International Study of Infarct Survival (ISIS-2). In that study of 17,187 patients with suspected AMI, the 35-d mortality rate was reduced by 23% *(85)*. The total rate of stroke was also reduced by 42%. The beneficial effect on survival remained significant after a median survival of 15 mo.

Serious complications are rare, and are related to allergic reactions, bleeding, and gastrointestinal irritation *(75)*. There is a small increase in cerebral hemorrhage *(86)*, and there may be increased rate of bleeding from surgical sites *(87,88)*. Gastrointestinal effects are the most common adverse events, and can be minimized by the use of antacids, histamine-2 receptor antagonists, and enteric-coated or buffered aspirin preparations, or suppositories. When allergy to aspirin prevents its use, the clinician can substitute dipyridamole, ticlopidine, or sulfinpyrazone, although these antiplatelet agents have not been as well studied *(89)*. A recent trial reported that clopidogrel, a derivative of ticlopidine, was more effective than aspirin in reducing ischemic events, and was at least as safe *(90)*. Other promising antiplatelet agents are also being studied.

Reperfusion Therapy

Beginning with the work of Herrick over 80 yr ago *(91)*, the usual precipitating event leading to AMI has been shown to be thrombotic occlusion of a coronary artery *(92,93)*. Thrombosis is initiated at the site of a ruptured or fissured atherosclerotic plaque; endothelial injury causes platelets to become activated and trigger the coagulation cascade, whereby fibrinogen is converted to fibrin by the action of thrombin *(94)*. Fibrin deposition results in formation of a clot, or thrombosis. Thrombin, which may be clot-bound or circulating, in turn causes platelet activation (which is not blocked by aspirin), thus reinforcing fibrin deposition. However, simultaneously with thrombosis, a natural fibrinolytic system is activated, converting plasminogen to plasmin, which degrades fibrin and leads to clot lysis. The balance between clot formation and dissolution is complex, but suggests the basis for the current treatment strategy: prevention of platelet activation (aspirin), prevention of clot formation and extension (anticoagulants and antithrombotics), promotion of clot lysis (thrombolytics), and mechanical restoration of coronary blood flow (angioplasty and/or bypass surgery). Each of these therapies will be summarized.

Antithrombotics/Anticoagulants

Heparin acts at multiple sites in the coagulation system to inhibit the formation of fibrin clots. Small amounts of heparin will combine with antithrombin III to inactivate activated factor X and inhibit the conversion of prothrombin to thrombin. Larger amounts of heparin can inactivate thrombin, prevent the conversion of fibrinogen to fibrin, and prevent the activation of fibrin-stabilizing factor.

In spite of its theoretical value, there is little current empiric evidence regarding the value of heparin in AMI other than as an adjunct to the use of thrombolytic agents (*see* the section on thrombolytics). Previous studies have shown a 17% reduction in mortality and a 22% reduction in reinfarction *(95)*. However, these results predate the current routine use of aspirin and other anti-ischemic therapies, so it is unknown whether heparin use has any added benefit. Nevertheless, its use is considered routine in selected circumstances *(75,96)*:

1. Patients undergoing angioplasty or surgical bypass;
2. Patients not treated with a thrombolytic agent; and
3. Patients treated with a nonselective thrombolytic agent who are at high risk for systemic emboli (large or anterior MI, atrial fibrillation, previous embolus, or known LV thrombus).

Furthermore, subcutaneous heparin may be useful to reduce the incidence of deep venous thrombosis in the nonambulatory, post-AMI patient *(97)*.

The major complication of heparin therapy is bleeding, which can be from any site. The risk of bleeding can be minimized by dosing heparin based on weight and by following the activated partial thromboplastin time. Furthermore, heparin causes thrombocytopenia in roughly 3% of treated patients *(98)*. This is because of irreversible platelet aggregation, which can lead, paradoxically, to prothrombotic events (white-clot syndrome) *(99)*. Recent investigations have been made into the use of fractionated, low-mol-wt heparins (e.g., enoxaparin) and the direct antithrombin agent hirudin in AMI *(100,101)*.

Warfarin and other coumarin anticoagulants interfere with the synthesis of vitamin K-dependent clotting factors. Existing thrombus is not affected. Warfarin is given orally, thus providing a mechanism for long-term anticoagulation. Although warfarin anticoagulation of the post-AMI patient makes sense on theoretical grounds, as with heparin, its use is controversial because of the lack of adequate randomized controlled trials. The following indications are suggested by the ACC/AHA *(75)*:

1. For secondary prevention of MI in post-MI patients unable to take daily aspirin;
2. For post-MI patients in persistent (or perhaps paroxysmal) atrial fibrillation; and
3. For patients with LV thrombus or, possibly, with extensive wall motion abnormalities.

Bleeding is the major risk of warfarin therapy and requires close attention to the prothrombin time (international normalized ratio, INR).

Thrombolytic Therapy

Given that acute thrombosis of a coronary vessel is the precipitating event in AMI, clot lysis offers an effective therapy through either intracoronary or iv routes *(102)*. All agents in clinical use are plasminogen activators, i.e., they convert plasminogen into plasmin by enzymatic hydrolysis. Plasmin in turn is a highly efficient fibrinolytic agent, capable of degrading both clot-bound fibrin and circulating fibrinogen.

There are four thrombolytic agents approved by the FDA for iv administration in AMI: streptokinase (SK), anisoylated plasminogen streptokinase activator complex (APSAC or anistreplase), recombinant tissue-type plasminogen activator (alteplase or TPA), and a derivative of alteplase called reteplase (r-PA). There are significant differences between these agents with respect to circulating half-life, systemic fibrinogen depletion, antigenicity, rate of coronary recanalization and reocclusion, risk of intracerebral hemorrhage (ICH), dose, technique of administration, and cost.

SK is an enzyme produced by group C β-hemolytic streptococci. It combines with plasminogen to form an "activator complex" that converts plasminogen to plasmin. SK produces a systemic "lytic state" that persists for several hours. Heparin use increases the risk of bleeding without improving efficacy. Given as a 1.5 million unit dose over 30–60 min, it has a recanalization rate of ~40%, an ICH rate of ~0.3%, and results in ~2.5 lives saved/100 treated *(103)*. Most patients have had previous exposure to streptococci and thus have circulating antibodies to SK. Minor allergic reactions occur in up to 4% of patients; anaphylactic shock is rare. SK costs about $280 for the standard dose.

Anistreplase (APSAC) is a chemically modified complex of plasminogen and SK that is stable until reconstituted. When injected iv, it immediately begins to produce plasmin, both at the site of preformed thrombus and in the general circulation, thus producing a systemic fibrinolytic state. APSAC is given as a 30-mg bolus over 5 min, and heparin anticoagulation is not needed. It has a recanalization rate of ~63%, an ICH rate of ~0.6%, and results in ~2.5 lives saved/100 treated *(103)*. The profile of allergic side effects is similar to that for SK. A dose of APSAC costs about $1700.

Alteplase (TPA) is a tissue-type plasminogen activator that is synthesized by recombinant DNA technology. The DNA sequence used codes for the natural human enzyme. Thus, allergic reactions are very rare (<0.02%). The conversion of plasminogen to plasmin by TPA is enhanced by the presence of fibrin. Accordingly, the activity of TPA is largely clot-specific, with much less systemic depletion of fibrinogen than with SK or APSAC. Consequently, the activity of TPA is enhanced by the addition of heparin, which decreases the rate of reocclusion. Using an accelerated dosing regimen (15-mg bolus, then 0.75 mg/kg to a maximum of 50 mg over 30 min, then 0.50 mg/kg to a maximum of 35 mg over 60 min) *(104)*, TPA has a recanalization rate of ~79%, an ICH rate of ~0.6%, and results in ~3.5 lives saved/100 treated *(103)*. The cost of 100 mg of TPA is about $2200.

Reteplase is the newest thrombolytic to be released for use in AMI. Reteplase is a deletion mutant of wild-type TPA, and shares TPA's lack of antigenicity, clot-specific activity, and enhanced performance in the presence of heparin. Reteplase is given as two 10-U boluses 30 min apart and costs $2200. Clinical trials comparing r-PA to SK and to TPA have shown it to be at least as effective and safe, if not more so *(105,106)*. However, the number of subjects is small (<7000), so further study is warranted. Nevertheless, the ease of administration and promising early results make r-PA an attractive choice.

Indeed, there have been a great many multicenter, international, randomized trials (AIMS, ASSET, GISSI, GUSTO, ISIS, LATE, TIMI, and so forth) comparing various agents and adjuvants at different doses and administration protocols in an attempt to identify the optimum regimen; no doubt there will be more. Furthermore, there are new thrombolytics and adjuvants under investigation. Consequently, specific recommendations for choice of thrombolytic protocol can rapidly become out of date. One principle that is unlikely to change, however, is the repeated observation that the earlier reperfusion is accomplished, the smaller the area of myocardium in jeopardy and the lower the rate of morbidity and mortality.

This has led to the concept of "door-to-needle" time, referring to the interval from when the patient arrives in the ED to when the thrombolytic agent infusion is begun, with the target being <30 min *(107)*. Indeed, making sure to use thrombolytic therapy in every instance where it is appropriate and to initiate treatment early in the course of AMI is more important than the choice of thrombolytic agent actually used *(108)*.

Eligibility criteria relate primarily to stratifying patients in order to maximize potential benefit and minimize complications. The most important risk of thrombolytic therapy is bleeding, but fortunately 70% of bleeding episodes occur at sites of vascular access and can be managed without transfusion *(109)*. However, ICH is a more serious complication with a ~66% mortality *(110)*. The risk of ICH is increased with hypertension, either by history or on presentation. Thus, thrombolytics are relatively contraindicated in hypertensive patients with low-risk AMI (inferior ST elevation or ST depression only) *(110)*. Table 3 summarizes the contraindications and cautions for thrombolytic use in AMI. The AAC/AHA guidelines are *(75)*:

1. Thrombolytic therapy generally beneficial: (a) ST-segment elevation (>0.1 mV in two or more contiguous ECG leads), or (b) LBBB obscuring ST-segment analysis in a history suggestive of AMI with 12 h or less from onset of symptoms, and age <75 yr.
2. Thrombolytic therapy probably beneficial: ST-segment elevation and age >75 yr.
3. Thrombolytic therapy possibly beneficial: (a) ST-segment elevation and time-to-therapy >12–24 h, or (b) presenting blood pressure >180 mmHg systolic or 110 diastolic in high-risk AMI (anterior ST elevation or LBBB)

Table 3
Contraindications and Cautions for Thrombolytic Use in Myocardial Infarction[a]

Contraindications

Previous hemorrhagic stroke at any time; other strokes or cerebrovascular events within 1 yr

Known intracranial neoplasm

Active internal bleeding (does not include menses)

Suspected aortic dissection

Cautions/relative contraindications

Severe uncontrolled hypertension on presentation (blood pressure >180/110 mmHg); especially in low-risk AMI

History of prior cerebrovascular accident or known intracerebral pathology not covered in contraindications

Current use of anticoagulants in therapeutic doses (INR ≥ 2–3); known bleeding diathesis

Recent trauma (within 2–4 wk), including head trauma or traumatic or prolonged (>10 min) CPR or major surgery (<3 wk)

Noncompressible vascular punctures

Recent (within 2–4 wk) internal bleeding

For SK/APSAC: prior exposure (especially within 5 d) or prior allergic reaction

Pregnancy

Active peptic ulcer

History of chronic severe hypertension

[a]Adapted from ref. *80*.

4. Thrombolytic therapy not beneficial—possibly harmful: (a) ST-segment elevation and time-to-therapy >24 h; ischemic pain resolved, or (b) ST-segment depression only.

Currently, accelerated-dose TPA with iv heparin appears to confer the greatest reperfusion rates, but carries a higher risk of ICH and substantially greater cost *(111,112)*. For patients presenting early after onset of symptoms who have a high-risk AMI and are at low risk for ICH, TPA is the agent of choice *(75)*. For patients where the cost–benefit ratio is lower, SK is recommended. Ongoing research is likely to change these recommendations in the near future.

Percutaneous Transluminal Coronary Angioplasty (PTCA)

Angioplasty refers to the mechanical revision of the lumen (fluid path) of an artery in order to relieve an obstruction *(113)*. For AMI, PTCA can either be primary (in place of thrombolysis) or salvage (when thrombolysis has failed). In PTCA, a catheter is inserted percutaneously (through the skin) via needle puncture, into the femoral artery. The catheter is then passed up the aorta and into the opening of the blocked coronary artery. Injection of radiographic contrast media allows delineation of the anatomy via X-ray fluoroscopy. A guidewire with a balloon at its tip is then threaded through the catheter and into the area of blockage within the artery. The balloon is carefully inflated, thus compressing the obstructing clot and/or atherosclerotic plaque against the vessel wall and enlarging the lumen. Other devices, such as a scraper, drill, or laser, can also be used to remove obstructing material. A semirigid tube or stent can be placed into the artery to hold it open. Maintenance of patency of the angioplastied vessel is enhanced by the use of anticoagulants.

Theoretical advantages of PTCA compared to thrombolysis include direct reopening of the infarct-related vessel, avoidance of systemic fibrin depletion, and delineation of coronary anatomy. Disadvantages are cost, need for sophisticated personnel and facilities, and potentially longer time-to-patency. A number of studies have been done to compare PTCA to thrombolysis for primary therapy of AMI, but to date they have been small. A recent meta-analysis pooled 2023 patients from nine trials and showed a borderline statistical benefit of PTCA over thrombolysis when the end point was mortality *(114)*. When both death and rate of AMI were considered, PTCA had a clear advantage over thrombolysis (relative risk = 0.2, $p = 0.001$). However, considering that in excess of 100,000 patients have been enrolled in the various thrombolytic trials, the data for PTCA are quite limited, and the need for further study is apparent.

Complications of PTCA include bleeding at the site of needle puncture, AMI precipitated by balloon inflation, failure to relieve obstruction, reocclusion, and rupture of the coronary artery. The latter event can be catastrophic and requires urgent open heart surgery to repair. Thus, current guidelines recommend that PTCA be performed by experienced personnel *(115)*, and in facilities where emergent access to cardiac surgery is available *(75)*. However, studies are under way to evaluate the safety and efficacy of PTCA in hospitals without cardiac surgery, and broader guidelines may be forthcoming. The current ACC/AHA recommendations for PTCA in AMI are *(75)*:

1. PTCA generally beneficial: as an alternative to thrombolytic therapy only if performed in a timely fashion by skilled practitioners and personnel at a high-volume center.
2. PTCA probably beneficial: (a) for reperfusion candidates who have a risk of bleeding contraindication to thrombolytic therapy, or (b) patients in cardiogenic shock or with persistent hemodynamic instability.
3. PTCA possibly beneficial: (a) for reperfusion candidates who fail to qualify for thrombolytic therapy for reasons other than a risk of bleeding contraindication, or (b) patients with evolving large or anterior infarcts treated with a thrombolytic agent in whom it is believed that the infarct-related artery is not patent.

The role for PTCA in AMI will continue to evolve as experience accumulates and newer techniques and strategies are introduced.

Coronary Artery Bypass Graft (CABG) Surgery

The first coronary bypass surgery was performed in 1964 *(116)*, and within a few years, the surgical technique had been refined and standardized *(117)*. Prior to the advent of thrombolytic therapy and PTCA, CABG was the only revascularization technique available for use in AMI *(118)*. Currently, however, emergency CABG is restricted primarily to circumstances where thrombolysis and/or PTCA have failed or are not appropriate *(119)*. The ACC/AHA guidelines for emergency CABG in AMI that follow presume that the coronary artery anatomy is suitable for bypass.

1. Emergency CABG generally beneficial: (a) patients with persistent pain or hemodynamic instability who have failed or are not candidates for PTCA, or (b) at the time of surgical repair of postinfarction ventricular septal defect or mitral valve insufficiency.
2. Emergency CABG probably beneficial: cardiogenic shock refractory to other therapy.
3. Emergency CABG possibly beneficial: hemodynamically stable patient with small area of myocardium at risk who has failed PTCA.
4. Emergency CABG not beneficial—possibly harmful: when the expected surgical mortality does not exceed the mortality rate for medical management.

With the development of minimally invasive, thoracoscopic techniques, there may be a positive influence on the mortality rate of CABG surgery in the setting of AMI *(120)*. Nevertheless, it is unlikely that CABG will ever again be a first-line reperfusion technique in AMI.

Anti-Ischemic Therapy and Mortality Reduction

There are a number of pharmacologic adjuncts that may be used to treat ongoing ischemia or to reduce mortality in AMI. These therapies are particularly useful in patients who do not meet the criteria for, or who have failed to respond adequately to thrombolysis and/or revascularization. However, this represents a very heterogeneous group of patients that has not been well characterized or studied, so recommendations are subject to revision as experience accumulates.

β-Adrenoreceptor Blocking Agents

β-blockers have several effects on the heart. Primarily they cause a decrease in the force and rate of contraction, and slow the rate of myocardial depolarization. These actions serve to decrease myocardial oxygen demand. In addition, the decrease in heart rate prolongs diastole and can increase myocardial oxygen delivery, particularly to the penumbra of ischemic tissue surrounding an area of infarction. As a result, the use of β-blockers in AMI reduces infarct size and the incidence of complications in patients not given thrombolytics *(121)*, and reduces the rate of reinfarction in patients who are treated with thrombolytics *(122)*. However, these beneficial effects have only been seen in patients given β-blockers early in the course of their infarction (<12 h).

Complications from β-adrenoreceptor blocking agents are common and can be serious. Myocardial depression can lead to hypotension, CHF, and heart block. β-Blockers can produce bronchoconstriction, and thus, worsen asthma or chronic obstructive pulmonary disease. In insulin-requiring diabetics, β-blockers can mask the signs and symptoms of hypoglycemia and delay the recovery of normal blood glucose levels. The contraindications and cautions to the use of β-blockers in AMI are presented in Table 4. Only about 25–50% of AMI patients qualify for β-blocker therapy. The β-adrenoreceptor blocking agents best studied for use in AMI are atenolol *(123)* and metoprolol *(124)*. Either agent is continued indefinitely. The ACC/AHA recommendations for β-adrenoreceptor blockade in AMI include *(75)*:

1. β-Blockers generally beneficial: (a) all patients without contraindications who can be treated within 12 h, (b) continuing or recurrent ischemic-type pain, or (c) patients with tachyarrhythmias, especially atrial in origin.
2. β-Blockers possibly beneficial: non-Q-wave AMI.

Table 4
Contraindications/Cautions to β-Adrenoreceptor Blocking Agents in AMI

Heart rate < 60 bpm
Systolic blood pressure < 100 mmHg
Moderate or severe left ventricular failure
 (Killip Class II or greater)
Signs of peripheral hypoperfusion
First-degree AV block with PR interval
 > 0.255
Second- or third-degree AV block
Severe chronic obstructive pulmonary disease
Wheezing or a history of asthma
Severe peripheral vascular disease
Insulin-dependent diabetes mellitus

ᵃAdapted from ref. 80.

*Angiotensin-Converting Enzyme
(ACE) Inhibitors*

ACE inhibitors have been used for years to control elevated blood pressure. More recently, they have been studied for their cardioprotective effects in AMI. ACE inhibitors have been shown to reduce the incidence of CHF and reinfarction, and to prolong life when given on a long-term basis following AMI *(125)*. The GISSI-3 study followed the effects of oral lisinopril in >19,000 suspected AMI patients *(80)*, and ISIS-4 studied captopril in >58,000 patients *(81)*. A meta-analysis of these two large trials combined with a number of smaller trials (>100,000 patients) reported an absolute reduction of 4.6 deaths/1000 patients treated with ACE inhibitors *(126)*. Subgroup analysis suggests that the benefits are greatest in those patients at highest risk of death (e.g., anterior MI, CHF, previous infarction), but that all patients may benefit from early use of ACE inhibitors in suspected AMI.

ACE inhibitors can precipitate profound hypotension in patients with renal failure, and can produce life-threatening angio-edema of the oropharynx in sensitive individuals. Use should also be avoided when the systolic blood pressure is <100 mmHg or when bilateral renal artery stenosis is present. Furthermore, all agents should be administered orally, since iv ACE inhibitor produces high morbidity *(127)*. There are a variety of ACE inhibitors available for use, including lisinopril (GISSI-3) and captopril therapy (ISIS-4). Other agents should likewise be gradually introduced. The ACC/AHA guidelines for ACE inhibitors to mortality reduction are *(75)*:

1. ACE inhibitors generally beneficial: (a) within the first 24 h of suspected AMI with anterior ischemia or CHF and without hypotension, or (b) patients with AMI and LV ejection fraction of <40%.
2. ACE inhibitors probably beneficial: (a) all other patients within 24 h of suspected AMI, without hypotension, not included in 1(a) above, or (b) asymptomatic patients with old MI and LV ejection fraction of 40–50%.
3. ACE inhibitors possibly beneficial: asymptomatic patients with recent MI and normal or near-normal LV function.

Magnesium

There is considerable experimental evidence that magnesium may be beneficial in cardiovascular disease *(128)*. Nevertheless, the role of magnesium for cardioprotection in AMI has been controversial. Several small studies, when taken independently and after meta-analysis, suggested a decrease in both short- and long-term mortality *(129)*. However, the ISIS-4 trial, which at 58,050 subjects was 20 times the size of the largest of the smaller trials (LIMIT-2), did not reveal any benefit to magnesium therapy *(79)*. Nevertheless, further analysis suggests that magnesium may be beneficial if given early *(130)*, especially to the sickest patients *(131)* and to those who do not qualify for thrombolysis *(132)*. Until there is more clarification, the ACC/AHA recommends the following usage (75):

1. Magnesium probably beneficial: (a) correction of documented magnesium and/or

potassium deficits, or (b) for treating poly-morphic VT (torsades de pointes).

2. Magnesium possibly beneficial: for high-risk patients and those not candidates for thrombolytic therapy.

Calcium Entry Blockers

There are three commonly used calcium entry blocking agents: nifedipine, verapamil and diltiazem. The calcium entry blockers are used extensively to treat hypertension, and angina, and there was hope that these drugs would reduce mortality in the setting of AMI. However, after a number of studies, there is no evidence that these agents reduce mortality in AMI or decrease the rate of rein-farction when used routinely (133). Further-more, several studies have suggested increased mortality when these agents are used, particularly immediate-release nifedip-ine, and especially when LV dysfunction is present (134,135).

The consensus of the ACC/AHA is that calcium entry blockers are overused in the setting of AMI and that β-blockers represent a better choice (75). Calcium antagonists may be considered in the following circumstances:

1. Calcium entry blockers probably beneficial: iv use for relief of ongoing ischemia, or control of rapid atrial fibrillation when β-blockers are ineffective or contraindicated.
2. Calcium entry blockers possibly beneficial: diltiazem may be given in non-ST-segment elevation MI when LV dysfunction is absent, beginning at 24 h and continued for 1 yr.
3. Calcium entry blockers not beneficial, possi-bly harmful: (a) immediate-release nifedipine should be avoided in the setting of suspected AMI, or (b) all of these agents are con-traindicated in AMI with LV dysfunction.

Treatment of Complications

Arrhythmias

As noted previously, VF is the most important cause of death early in the course of AMI (76). In response to ischemia, the myocardium becomes electrically irritable. This is worsened by the release of endoge-nous catecholamines associated with the pain and anxiety of an MI, and further exac-erbated by a number of metabolic derange-ments, including acidosis, hypomagnesemia, and hypokalemia (136). VF is usually, but not always, preceded by VT. The mechanism of VT/VF is thought to be micro-reentry where an irritable focus of myocardium depolarizes repeatedly in a short-circuit effect (137). This spreads a wave front of depolarization throughout the myocardium, precipitating VT and/or VF. VT may be brief (<5 beats), nonsustained (<30 s), or sus-tained in duration, and may be regular (monomorphic) or irregular (polymorphic) in appearance. VF is a nonperfusing rhythm, whereas pulse and blood pressure may be maintained during VT.

Treatment is directed toward abolishing the re-entrant electrical activity, and then aggressively searching for and correcting any aggravating factors. Unstable patients should be treated with an electrical counter-shock. If a regular, monomorphic VT is pre-sent, then the countershock must be synchronized to the ECG to prevent the dis-charge from precipitating VF. Otherwise, the countershock should be unsynchronized. Stable patients should be treated with the appropriate medication. More detailed infor-mation is available (137). The ACC/AHA guidelines are (75):

1. Treatment of VT/VF that is generally beneficial:
   a. for VF: unsynchronized countershock of 200 J, followed by 300 and 360 J if needed.
   b. For sustained polymorphic VT: treat as VF.
   c. For unstable monomorphic VT: synchro-nized countershock(s) beginning at 100 J.
   d. For stable monomorphic VT: (i) lido-caine, procainamide, or amiodarone, and (iv) synchronized countershock(s) start-ing at 50 J, after appropriate analgesia/sedation.
2. Treatment for VT/VF that is probably bene-ficial: (a) after an episode of VT/VF, antiar-

13. Martin JF, Plumb J, Kilbey RS, and Kishk YT (1983) Changes in volume and density of platelets in myocardial infarction. Br. Med. J. 287:456–459.

14. Towbridge WE, Slater DN, Kishk YT, Woodcock BW, and Martin JF (1984) Platelet production in myocardial infarction and sudden cardiac death. Thromb. Hamostasis. 52:167–171.

15. Davies MJ (1994) Mechanisms of thrombosis in atherosclerosis. In *Hemostasis and Thrombosis: Basic Principles and Clinical Practice*, Coleman RW, Hirsh J, Marder VJ, and Salzman EW, eds. Philadelphia, J.B. Lippincott.

16. Lipid Research Program, Lipid Metabolism-Atherogenesis Branch, National, Heart, Lung, and Blood Institute. The Lipid Research Clinics Coronary Primary Prevention Trial Results. (1984) Reduction in incidence of coronary heart disease. JAMA 251: 351–364.

17. Lipid Research Program, Lipid Metabolism-Atherogenesis Branch, National, Heart, Lung, and Blood Institute. The Lipid Research Clinics Coronary Primary Prevention Trial Results. II (1984) The relationship of reduction in incidence of coronary heart disease to cholesterol lowering. JAMA 251: 365–374.

18. National Heart, Lung and Blood Institute (1993) Second report of the expert panel on detection, evaluation and treatment of high blood cholesterol in adults. NIH Publication 93-3096.

19. Steinberg D, Parthasarathy S, Carew TE, Khoo JC, and Witztum JL (1989) Beyond cholesterol. Modifications of low density lipoprotein that increase its atherogenicity. N. Engl. J. Med. 320:915–921.

20. Steinberg D and Witztum JL (1990) Lipoproteins and atherogenesis. JAMA 264: 3047–3052.

21. Steinberg D (1991) Antioxidants and atherosclerosis: a current Assessment. Circulation 84:1420–1425.

22. McGill HC Jr (1978) Risk factors for atherosclerosis. Adv. Exp. Med. Biol. 104:273–280.

23. Fry DL (1976) Hemodynamic forces in atherogenesis. In *Cerebro Vascular Diseases*, Scheinberg P, ed., 10th Princeton Conference. New York, Taven, pp. 77–95.

24. Becker CG, Dubin T, and Wiedemann HP (1976) Hypersensitivity to Tobacco Antigen. Proc. Natl. Acad. Sci. USA 73:1712–1716.

25. Muhlestein JB, Hammond EH, Carlquist JF, Radicke E, Thomson MJ, Karagounis LA, Woods ML, and Anderson JL (1996) Increased incidence of *Chlamydia* species within the coronary arteries of patients with symptomatic atherosclerotic versus other forms of cardiovascular disease. J. Am. Coll. Cardiol. 27:1555-1561.

26. Deanfield JE, Maseri A, Selwyn AP, Riveiro P, Chierchia S, Krikler S, and Morgan M (1983) Myocardial ischemia during daily life in patients with stable angina: its relation to symptoms and heart rate changes. Lancet 2:753–758.

27. Hangartner J, Charleston A, Davies M, and Thomas A (1986) Morphological characteristics of clinically significant coronary artery stenosis in stable angina. Br. Heart J. 56: 501–508.

28. Roberts W (1976) The coronary arteries and left ventricle in clinically isolated angina pectoris. Circulation 54:388–390.

29. Maseri A, L'abbate A, Baroldi G, Chierchia S, Marxilli M, Ballestra AM, Severi S, Parodi O, Biagini A, Distante A, and Pesola A (1978) Coronary vasospasm as a possible cause of myocardial infarction. A conclusion derived from the study of "preinfarction" angina. N. Engl. J. Med. 299:1271–1277.

30. Braunwald E, Mark DB, Jones RH, Cheitlin MD, Fuster V, McCauley KM, et al. (1984) Unstable angina: diagnosing and management, Clinical Practice Guideline, No. 10 (amended). US Department of Health and Human Services Public Health Service, Rockville, MD.

31. Campeau L (1976) Grading of angina pectoris [letter]. Circulation 54:522–523.

32. Jennings RB, Reimer KA, Hill ML, and Mayer SE (1981) Total ischemia in dog hearts in vitro. I. Comparison of high energy phosphate production, utilization and depletion, and of adenine nucleotide catabolism in total ischemia in vitro vs. severe ischmia in vivo. Circ. Res. 49:892–900.

33. Neely JF and Grotyohann LW (1984) Role of lycotic products in damage to ischemic myocardium: dissociation of adenosine triphosphate levels and recovery of function

of reperfused ischemic hearts. Circ. Res. 55:816–824.

34. Heyndrickx GR, Millard RW, MeRitchie RJ, Maroko PR, and Vatner SF (1975) Regional myocardial function and electrophysiological alterations after brief coronary artery occlusion in conscious dogs. J. Clin. Invest. 56:978–985.

35. Swan HJC (1993) Left ventricular systolic and diastolic dysfunction in the acute phases of myocardial ischaemia and infarction, and in the later phases of recovery: function follows morphology. Euro. Heart J. 14(Suppl. A):48–56.

36. Bourdillon PD, Lorell BH, Mirsky I, Paulus WJ, Wynne J, and Grossman W (1983) Increased regional myocardial stiffness of the left ventricle during pacing-induced angina in man. Circulation 67:316–323.

37. Levy RD, Shapiro LM, Wright C, Mockus L, and Fox K (1986) The haemodynamic signifcnace of asymptomatic ST segment depression assessed by ambulatory pulmonary artery pressure monitoring. Br. Heart J. 56:526–530.

38. Hirzel H, Leutwyler R, and Krayenbuehl HP (1985) Silent myocardial ischemia: hemodynamic changes during dynamic exercise in patients with proven coronary artery disease despite absence of angina pectoris. J. Am. Coll. Cardiol. 6:275–284.

39. Wohgelernter D, Jaffe CC, Cabin HS, Yeatman LA, and Cleman M (1987) Silent ischemia during coronary occlusion produced by balloon inflation: relation to regional myocardial dysfunction. J. Am. Coll. Cardiol. 10:491–498.

40. Schott FJ and Schaper W (1989) Effects of transient coronary occlusion: experience with myocardial stunning and precondition. Isr. J. Med. Sci. 25:479–482.

41. Castello R and Pearson AC (1990) Diastolic function in patients undergoing coronary angioplasty: influence of degree of revascularization. J. Am. Coll. Cardiol. 15:1564–1569.

42. Kono T, Sabbah HN, Rosman H, Alam M, Jafri S, Stein PD, and Goldstein S (1992) Mechanism of functional mitral regurgitation during acute myocardial ischemia. J. Am. Coll. Cardiol. 19:1101–1105.

43. Braunwald E and Kloner RA (1982) The stunned myocardium: prolonged, post-ischemic ventricular dysfunction. Circulation 66:1146–1149.

44. Braunwald E (1990) The stunned myocardium: newer insights into mechanisms and clinical implications. J. Thorac. Cardiovasc. Surg. 100:310–311.

45. Rahimtoola SH (1989) The hibernating myocardium. Am. Heart J. 117:211–221.

46. Braunwald E and Rutherford JD (1986) Reversible ischemic left ventricular dysfunction: evidence for "hibernating myocardium." J. Am. Coll. Cardiol. 8:1467–1470.

47. Mizuno K, Satomura K, Miyaamoto A, Arakawa K, Shibuya T, Arai T, Kurita A, Nakamura H, and Ambrose JA (1992) Angioscopic evaluation of coronary-artery thrombi in acute coronary syndromes. N. Engl. J. Med. 326:287–291.

48. Ambrose J, Hjemdahl-Monsen C, Borrico S, Gorlin R, and Fuster V (1988) Angiographic demonstration of a common link between unstable angina pectorisis and non q-wave acute myocardial infarction. Am. Coll. Cardiol. 12:244–247.

49. Sherman C, Litvack F, and Grundfest W (1986) Coronary angioscopy in patients with unstable pectoris. N. Engl. J. Med. 315:913–919.

50. Spodick DH (1983) Q-wave infarction versus ST infarction: non-specificity of electrocardiographic criteria for differentiating transmural and nontransmural lesions. Am. J. Cardiol. 51:913–915.

51. Gibson RS (1988) Non-q-wave myocardial infarction diagnosis, prognosis and management. Curr. Probl. Cardiol. 13:9–72.

52. Heller GV, Blaustein AS, and Wei JY (1983) Implications of increased myocardial isoenzyme level in the presence of normal serum creatine kinase activity. Am. J. Cardiol. 51: 24–27.

53. Ahmed SM, Williamson JR, Roberts R, Clark RE, and Sobel BE (1976) The association of increased plasma MB CPK activity and irreversible ischemic myocardial injury in the dog. Circulation 54:187–193.

54. Marban E, Koretsune Y, Corretti M, Chacko VP, and Kusoaka H (1989) Calcium and its role in myocardial cell injury during ischemia and reperfusion. Circulation 80 (Suppl. IV):80.

55. Marmor A, Geltman EM, Schechtman K, Sobel BE, and Roverts R (1982) Recurrent

myocardial infarction: clinical predictors and prognostic implications. Circulation 66:415–421.

56. Gibson RS, Boden WE, Theroux P, Strauss HD, Pratt CM, Gheorghiade M, Capone RJ, Crawford MH, Schlant RC, Kleiger RE, Young PM, Schechtman K, Perryman MB, and Roberts R (1986) Diltiazem and reinfarction in patients with non-Q-wave myocardial infarction. Results of a double-blind, randomized, multicenter trail. N. Engl. J. Med. 315:423–429.

57. Sobel BE, Bresnahan GF, Shell WE, and Yoder RD (1972) Estimation of infarct size in man and its relation to prognosis. Circulation 46:640–648.

58. Killip T and Kimball J (1967) Treatment of myocardial infarction in a coronary care unit. A two year experience with 250 patients. Am. Cardiol. 20:457–464.

59. Forrester JS, Diamond G, Chatterjee K, and Swan HJ (1976) Medical therapy of acute myocardial infarction by the application hemodynamic subsets. N. Engl. J. Med. 295:1356–1362.

60. DeWood MA, Spores J, Notske RN, Muser LT, Burroughs R, Golden MS, and Lang HT (1980) Prevalence of total coronary artery occlusion during the early hours of transmural myocardial infarction. N. Engl. J. Med. 303:897–902.

61. Ong L, Reiser P, Coromilas J, Scherr L, and Morrison J (1983) Left ventricular function and rapid release of creatine kinase MB in acute myocardial infarction: evidence for spontaneous reperfusion. N. Engl. J. Med. 309:1–6.

62. Falk J and O'Brien JF (1996) Chest pain. In: Emergency Medicine: A Comprehensive Review, 4th ed., Tintinalli JE, Ruiz E, and Krome RL, eds. New York, McGraw-Hill.

63. Wellens H (1993) Right ventricular infarction [editorial]. N. Engl. J. Med. 328: 1036–1038.

64. Meltzer LE and Cohen HE (1972) The incidence of arrhythmias associated with acute myocardial infarction. In Textbook of Coronary Care, Meltzer LE, and Dunning AJ, eds. Philadelphia, Charles.

65. Hindman MC, Wagner GS, JaRo M, Arkins JM, Scheinman MM, DeSanctis RW, Hutter AH Jr, Yeatman L, Rubenfire M, Pujara C, Rubin M, and Morris JJ (1978) The clinical significance of bundle branch block complicating acute myocardial infarction: clinical characteristics, hospital mortality, and one-year follow-up. Circulation 58:679-688.

66. Grauer LE, Gershen BJ, Orlando MM, and Epstein SE (1973) Bradycardia and its complications in the prehospital phase of acute myocardial infarction. Am. J. Cardiol. 32: 607–611.

67. Manning WJ, Waksmonski CA, and Boyle NG (1995) Papillary muscle rupture complicating inferior myocardial infarction: identification with transesophageal echocardiography. Am. Heart J. 129:191–193.

68. O'Rourke RA and Dell'Italia LJ Right ventricular myocardial infarction, in Atherosclerosis and Coronary Artery Disease, Fuster V, Ross R, and Topol EJ (eds), Philadelphia, Lippincott-Raven, pp. 1079–1096.

69. Forman MB, Goodin J, Phelan B, Kopelman H, and Virmani R (1984) Electrocardiographic changes associated with isolated right ventricular infarction. J. Am. Coll. Cardiol. 4:640–643.

70. National Heart, Lung, and Blood Institute (1992) Morbidity and Mortality: Chartbook on Cardiovascular, Lung, and Blood Diseases, Bethesda, Md, US Department of Health and Human Services, Public Health Service, National Institutes of Health.

71. Koren G, Weiss AT, Hasin Y, Applebaum D, Welber S, Rozenman Y, Lotan C, Mosseri M, Sapoznikov D, Laria MH, and Gotsman MS (1985) Prevention of myocardial damage in acute myocardial ischemia by early treatment with intravenous streptokinase. N. Engl. J. Med. 313:1384–1389.

72. Hermens WT, Willems GM, Nijssen KM, and Simoons ML (1992) Effect of thrombolytic treatment delay on myocardial infarct size. Lancet 340:1297.

73. National Heart, Lung, and Blood Institute. 9-1-1: Rapid Identification and Treatment of Acute Myocardial Infarction, Bethesda, MD US Department of Health and Human Services, Public Health Service, National Institutes of Health; May 1994, NIH Publication 94-3302.

74. Antman EM and Braunwald ED (1996) Acute myocardial infarction, in Heart Dis-

ease: A Textbook of Cardiovascular Medicine, Braunwald, E. D., ed. Philadelphia, PA, WB Saunders, pp. 1184–1266.

75. Ryan TJ, Anderson JL, Antman EM, Braniff BA, Brooks NH, Califf RM, Hillis D, Hiratzka LF, Rapaport E, Riegel BJ, Russell RO, Smith EE, and Weaver WD (1986) ACC/AHA guidelines for the management of patients with acute myocardial infarction: a report of the American College of Cardiology/American Heart Association Task Force on Practice Guidelines (Committee on Management of Acute Myocardial Infarction). J. Am. Coll. Cardiol. 28:1328–1419.

76. Gunby P (1992) Cardiovascular disease remains nation's leading cause of death. JAMA 267:335–336.

77. Fung HL, Chung SJ, Bauer JA, Chong S, and Kowaluk EA (1992) Biochemical Mechanism of Organic Nitrate Action. Am. J. Cardiol. 70(Suppl. 5):4B–10B.

78. Abrams J (1985) Hemodynamic effects of nigroglycerin and long-acting nitrates. Am. Heart J. 1410:216–224.

79. Abrams J (1995) The role of nitrates in coronary heart disease. Arch. Intern. Med. 155:357–364.

80. GISSI-3: Effects of lisinopril and transdermal Glyceryl Trinitrate singly and together on 6-week mortality and ventricular function after acute myocardial infarction: Gruppo Italiano per Studio della Sopravvivenza nell'infarto Miocardico. Lancet 343:1115–1122.

81. ISIS-4: A randomized factorial trial assessing early oral captopril, oral mononitrate, and intravenous magnesium sulphate in 58,050 patients with suspected acute myocardial infarction. 1995. Lancet 345:669–685.

82. Antman EM. General hospital management, in Management of Acute Myocardial Infarction, London, Saunders, 1004, pp. 42–44.

83. Burch JW, Stanford N, and Majerus PW (1978) Inhibition of platelet prostaglandin synthetase by oral aspirin. J. Clin. Invest. 61:314–319.

84. Moncada S and Vane JR (1979) The role of prostacyclin in vascular tissue. Fed. Proc. 38:66–71.

85. ISIS-2 (Second International Study of Infarct Survival) Colloabaartive Group. (1988) Randomized trial of intravenous streptokinase, oral aspirin, both, or neither among 17,187 cases of suspected acute myocardial infarction: ISIS-2. Lancet 2:349–360.

86. Hennekens CH, Peto R, Hutchison GB, and Doll R (1988) An overview of the british and American aspirin studies. N. Engl. J. Med. 318:923–924.

87. Goldman S, Copeland J, Moritz T, Henderson W, Zadina K, Ovitt T, et al. (1988) Improvement in early saphenous vein graft patency after coronary artery bypass surgery with antiplatelet therapy: results of a veterans administration cooperative study. Circulation 77:1324–1332.

88. Sanz G, Pajaron A, Alegria E, Coello I, Cardona M, Fournier JA, Gomez-Recio M, Ruano J, Hidalgo R, Medina A, Oller G, Colman T, Mulpartida F, and Bosch Y (1990) Prevention of early aortocoronary bypass occlusion by low-dose aspirin and dipyridamole: grupo espanol para el seguimiento del injerto coronario (GESIC). Circulation 82:765–773.

89. Collaborative Overview of Randomized Trials of Antiplatelet Therapy, II: Maintenance of vascular graft or arterial patency by antiplatelet therapy. 1994. Br. Med. J. 308: 159–168.

90. CAPRIE Steering Committee: A randomized, blinded, trial of clopidogrel versus aspirin in patients at risk of ischaemic events (CAPRIE). 1996. Lancet 348:1329–1339.

91. Herrick JB (1912) Clinical features of sudden obstruction of the coronary arteries. JAMA 59:2015.

92. DeWood MA, Spores J, Notske R, Mouser LT, Burroughs R, Golden MS, and Lang HT (1980) Prevalence of total coronary occlusion during the early hours of transmural myocardial infarction. N. Engl. J. Med. 303:897–902.

93. Mizuno K, Satomura K, Miyamoto A, Arakawa K, Shibuya T, Arai T, Kurita A, Nakamura H, and Ambrose JA (1992) Angioscopic evaluation of coronary-artery thrombi in acute coronary syndromes. N. Engl. J. Med. 326:287–291.

94. Eberst, M. E. (1996) Evaluation of the bleeding patient, in: Emergency Medicine: A Comprehensive Study Guide, Tintinalli JE, Ruiz E, and Frome RL, eds. New York, McGraw-Hill, pp. 973–976.

95. MacMahon S, Collins R, Knight C, Yusuf S, and Peto R (1988) Reduction in major morbidity and mortality by heparin in acute myocardial infarction. Circulation 78(Suppl. II)II:98.

96. The SCATI Group (1989) Randomized controlled trial of subcutaneous calcium-heparin in acute myocardial infarction: The SCATI (Studio sulla Calciparina nell-Angina e nella Thrombosi ventricolare nell'Infarto) Group. Lancet 2:182–186.

97. Chesebro JH and Fuster V (1986) Antithrombotic therapy for acute myocardial infarction: mechanisms and prevention of deep venous, left ventricular, and coronary artery thromboembolism. Circulation 74(Suppl. III):III-1–III-10.

98. Warkentin TE, Levine MN, Hirsh J, Horsewood P, Roberts RS, Gent M, and Kelton JG (1995) Heparin-induced thrombocytopenia in patients treated with low-molecular-weight heparin or unfractionated heparin. N. Engl. J. Med. 332:1330–1335.

99. Harrington RA, Sane DC, Califf RM, Sigmon KN, Abbottsmith CW, Candela RJ, Lee KL, and Topel EJ (1994) Clinical importance of thrombocytopenia occurring in the hospital phase after administration of thrombolytic therapy for acute myocardial infarction: The thrombolysis and angioplasty in myocardial infarction study group. J. Am. Coll. Cardiol. 23:891–898.

100. Gurfinkel EP, Manos EJ, Mejail RI, Cerda MA, Duronto EA, Garcia CN, Daroca AM, and Mautner B (1995) Low molecular weight heparin versus regular heparin or aspirin in the treatment of unstable angina and silent ischemia. J. Am. Coll. Cardiol. 26:313–318.

101. Antman EM (1996) Hirudin in acute myocardial infarction: thrombolysis and thrombin inhibition in myocardial infarction (TIMI) 9B trial. Circulation 94:911–921.

102. Sherry S (1992) Fibrinolysis, Thrombosis, and Hemostasis: Concepts, Perspectives, and Clinical Applications, Philadelphia, Lea & Febiger, pp. 119–160.

103. Martin GV and Kennedy JW (1994) Choice of Thrombolytic Agent, in Management of Acute Myocardial Infarcation, Julian D, Braunwald ED, eds., Saunders, Philadelphia, 1994.

104. GUSTO. (1993) An international randomized trial comparing four thrombolytic strategies for acute myocardial infarction. The GUSTO Investigators. N. Engl. J. Med. 329(10):673–682.

105. National Heart Attack Alert Program Coordinating Committee, 60 Minutes to Treatment Working Group (1994) Emergency department: rapid identification and treatment of patients with acute myocardial infarction. Ann. Emerg. Med. 23:311–329.

106. International Joint Efficacy Comparison of Thrombolytics (1995) Randomized, double-blind comparison of reteplase double-bolus administration with streptokinase in acute myocardial infarction (INJECT): trial to investigate equivalence. Lancet 346:329–336.

107. Bode C, Smalling RW, Berg G, Burnett C, Lorch G, Kalbfleisch JM, Chernoff R, Christie LG, Feldman RL, Selas AA, and Weaver WD (1986) Randomized comparison of coronary thrombolysis achieved with double-bolus reteplase (recombinant plasminogen activator) and front-loaded, accelerated alteplase (recombinant tissue plasminogen activator) in patients with acute myocardial infarction. Circulation 94:891–898.

108. Fendrick AM, Ridker PM, and Bloom BS (1994) Improved health benefits in increased use of thrombolytic therapy. Arch. Intern. Med. 154:1605–1609.

109. Sane DC, Califf RM, Topol EJ, Stump DC, Mark DB, and Greenberg CS (1989) Bleeding during thrombolytic therapy for acute myocardial infarction: mechanisms and management. Ann. Intern. Med. 111:1010–1022.

110. Fibrinolytic Therapy Trialists' (FTT) Collaborative Group. (1994) Indications for fibrinolytic therapy in suspected acute myocardial infarction: collaborative overview of early mortality and major morbidity results from all randomized trials of more than 1000 patients. Lancet 343:311–322.

111. Anderson JL and Karagounis LA (1994) Does intravenous heparin or time-to-treatment/reperfusion explain differences between GUSTO and ISIS-3 results? Am. J. Cardiol. 74:1057–1060.

112. Cannon CP, McCabe CH, Diver DJ, Herson S, Greene RM, Shah PK, Sequeira RF, Leya F, Kirschenbaum JM, Majorien RD, Palmeri ST, Davis V, Gibson CM, Poole WK, and Braunwald E (1994) Comparison of front-loaded recombinant tissue-type plasminogen activator, anistreplase and combination thrombolytic therapy for acute myocardial infarction: results of the thrombolysis in myocardial infarction (TIMI) 4 trial. J. Am. Coll. Cardiol. 24: 1602–1610.

113. Lincoff AM and Topol EJ (1997) Interventional catheterization techniques. In Heart Disease: A Textbook of Cardiovascular Medicine, 5th ed., Braunwald, E. D., ed., Philadephia, Saunders, pp. 1366–1369.

114. Ryan TJ, Bauman WB, Kennedy JW, Kereiakes DJ, King SB, McCallister BD, Smith SC, and Ullyot DJ (1993) ACC/AHA guidelines for percutaneous transluminal coronary angioplasty: a report of the American College of Cardiology/American Heart Association Task Force on Assessment of Diagnostic and Therapeutic Cardiovascular Procedures (Committee on Percutaneous Transluminal Coronary Angioplasty). J. Am. Coll. Cardiol. 22:2033–2054.

115. Simes JR, Weaaver DW, Ellis SG, and Grines CL (1996) Overview of the randomized trials of primary PTLA and thrombolysis in acute myocardial infarction. Circulation 94(Suppl. 1): KI331.

116. Garrett HE, Dennis EW, and DeBakey ME (1973) Aortocoronary bypass with saphenous vein graft: seven-year follow-up. JAMA 223:792–794.

117. Favaloro RG (1969) Saphenous vein graft in the surgical treatment of coronary artery disease: operative technique. J. Thorac. Cardiovasc. Surg. 58:178–185.

118. Berg R Jr, Selinger SL, Leonard JJ, Grunwald RP, and O'Grady WP (1981) Immediate coronary artery bypass for acute evolving myocardial infarction. J. Thorac. Cardiovasc. Surg. 81:493–497.

119. Kirklin JK, Akins CW, Blackstone EH, et al. (1991) Guidelines and indications for coronary artery bypass graft surgery; a report of the American College of Cardiology/ American Heart Association Task Force on assessment of diagnostic and therapeutic cardiovascular procedures (Subcommittee on Coronary Artery Bypass Graft Surgery). J. Am. Coll. Cardiol. 17: 543–589.

120. Stevens JH, Burdon TA, Peters WS, Siegel LC, Pompili MF, Vierra MA, St. Gour FG, Ribakove GH, Mitchell RS, and Reitz BA (1996) Port-access coronary artery bypass grafting: a proposed surgical method. J. Thorac. Cardiovasc. Surg. 111:567–573.

121. Yusef S, Peto R, Lewis J, Collins R, and Sleight P (1985) Beta blockade during and after myocardial infarction: an overview of the randomized trials. Prog. Cardiovasc. Dis. 27:335–371.

122. The TIMI Study Group (1989) Comparison of invasive and conservative strategies after treatment with intravenous tissue plasminogen activator in acute myocardial infarction: results of the thrombolysis in myocardial infarction (TIMI) phase II trial. N. Engl. J. Med. 320:618–627.

123. First International Study of Infarct Survival Collaborative Group (1986) Randomized trial of intravenous atenolol among 16,027 cases of suspected acute myocardial infarction: ISIS-1. Lancet 2:57–66.

124. The MIAMI Trial Research Group (1985) Metoprolol in acute myocardial infarction: patient population. Am. J. Cardiol. 56: 1G–57G.

125. Pfeffer MA, Braunwald E, Moye LA, Basta L, Brown EJ, Cuddds TE, Davis BR, Geltman EM, Goldman S, Flaker GC, Klein M, Lamas GA, Packer M, Rouleau J, Rouleau JL, Rutherford J, Wetheimer JH, Hawkins CM, and the SAVE Investigators (1992) Effect of captopril on mortality and morbidity in patients with left ventricular dysfunction after myocardial infarction: results of the survival and ventricular enlargement trial (SAVE). N. Engl. J. Med. 327(10):669–677.

126. Latini R, Maggioni AP, Flather M, Sleight P, and Tognoni G (1995) ACE-inhibitor use in patients with myocardial infarction: summary of evidence from clinical trials. Circulation 92:3132–3137.

127. Sigurdsson A and Swedberg K (1994) Left ventricular remodelling, neurohormonal activation and early treatment with enalapril (CONSENSIS II) following

myocardial infarction. Eur. Heart J. 15(Suppl. B):14–19.

128. Aresenia MA (1993) Magnesium and cardiovascular disease. Prog. Cardiovasc. Dis. 35:271–310.

129. Antman EM, Lau J, Kupelnick B, Mosteller F, and Chalmers TC (1992) A comparison of results of meta-analyses of randomized control trials and recommendations of clinical experts: treatments for myocardial infarction. JAMA 268:240–248.

130. Antman EM (1995) Magnesium in acute MI: timing is critical. Circulation 92: 2367–2372.

131. Antman EM (1995) Randomized trials of magnesium in acute myocardial infarction: big numbers do not tell the whole story. Am. J. Cardiol. 75:391–393.

132. Schechter M, Hod H, Chouraqui P, Kaplinsky E, and Rabinowitz B (1995) Magnesium therapy in acute myocardial infarction when patients are not candidates for thrombolytic therapy. Am. J. Cardiol. 75:321–323.

133. Held P, Yusuf S, and Furberg CD (1989) Calcium channel blockers in acute myocardial infarction and unstable angina: an overview. Br. Med. J. 229:1187–1192.

134. Opie LH and Messerli FH (1995) Nifedipine and mortality: grave defects in the dossier. Circulation 92:1068–1073.

135. Held PH and Yusuf S (1993) Effects of beta-blockers and calcium channel blockers in acute myocardial infarction. Eur. Heart J. 14(Suppl. F):18–25.

136. Campbell RWF (1994) Arrhythmias. In: Management of Acute Myocardial Infarction, Julian DG and Braunwald E, eds., London, Saunders, pp 223–240,

137. Cummins RO, ed. (1994) Textbook of Advanced Cardiac Life Support, American Heart Association.

138. Madias JE, Patel DC, and Singh D (1996) Atrial fibrillation in acute myocardial infarction. a prospective study based on data from a consecutive series of patients admitted to the coronary care unit. Clin. Cardiol. 19:180–186.

139. Berger PB, Ruocco NA Jr, Ryan TJ, Frederick MM, Jacobs AK, and Faxon DP (1992) Incidence and prognostic implications of heart block complicating inferior myocardial infarction treated with thrombolytic therapy: results from TIMI-II. J. Am. Coll. Cardiol. 21:533–540.

140. Zehender M, Kasper W, Kauder E, Schonthaler M, Geibel A, Olschewski M, and Just H (1983) Right ventricular infarction as an independent predictor of prognosis after acute inferior myocardial infarction. N. Engl. J. Med. 328:981–988.

141. Marino PL (1991) The ICU Book. Philadelphia, PA, Lea & Febiger, 1991.

142. Powell WJ, Daggett WM, Magro AE, Bianco JA, Buckley M, Sanders CA, Kantrowitz AR, and Austen WG (1970) Effects of intra-aortic balloon counterpulsation on cardiac performance, oxygen consumption, and coronary flow in dogs. Circ. Res. 26:753–764.

143. Cohn LH (1981) Surgical management of acute and chronic cardiac mechanical complications due to myocardial infarction. Am. Heart J. 102:1049–1060.

144. Bengtson JR, Kaplan AJ, Pieper KS, Wildermann NM, Mark DB, Pryor DB, Phillips HR, and Califf RM (1992) Prognosis in cardiogenic shock after myocardial infarction in the interventional era. J. Am. Coll. Cardiol. 20:1482–1489.

145. Lobo RA and Speroff L (1994) International consensus conference on postmenopausal hormone therapy and the cardiovascular system. Fertil. Steril. 61: 592–595.

146. Colditz GA, Hankinson SE, Hunter DJ, and Willett WC (1995) The use of estrogens and progestins and the risk of breast cancer in postmenopausal women. N. Engl. J. Med. 332:1589-1593, 1995.

147. Stanford JL, Weiss NS, Voight LF, Daling JR, Habel LA, and Rossing MA (1995) Combined estrogen and progestin hormone replacement therapy in relation to risk of breast cancer in middle-aged women. JAMA. 274:137–142.

148. Borsky RD, Koplan JP, Peterson HB, and Thacker SB (1994) Relative risks and benefits of long-term estrogen replacement therapy: a decision analysis. Obstet. Gynecol. 83:161–166.

149. National Cholesterol Education Program (1994) Second report of the expert panel on detection, evaluation, and treatment of high

blood cholesterol in adults (Adult Treatment Panel II). Circulation 89:1333–1445.

150. Gaziano JM, Buring JE, Breslow JL, Goldhaber S, Rosner B, Van DenBurgh M, WIllett W, and Hennekens CH (1993) Moderate alcohol intake, increased levels of high-density lipoprotein and its subfractions, and decreased risk of myocardial infarction. N. Engl. J. Med. 329:1829–1834.

151. Burling TA, Singleton EG, Bigelow GE, Baile WF, and Gottlieb SH (1984) Smoking following myocardial infarction: a critical review of the literature. Health Psychol. 3:83–96.

152. Ruberman W, Weinblatt E, Goldberg JD, and Chaudhary BS (1984) Psychosocial influences on mortality after myocardial infarction. N. Engl. J. Med. 311:552–559.

4

Markers of Myocardial Injury in the Evaluation of the Emergency Department Patient with Chest Pain

Gary B. Green and Sol F. Green

INTRODUCTION

In recent years, the approach used in the evaluation of the emergency department (ED)* patient with suspected myocardial ischemia has undergone dramatic changes. Data-gathering, treatment, and disposition patterns that had been accepted for decades are now being intensely scrutinized and often abandoned in favor of assessment protocols based on new diagnostic technologies (1). Foremost among these new technologies are the many new methods for the laboratory measurement of markers of myocardial injury.

The recent advances in laboratory medicine related to markers of myocardial injury and the current "revolution" in the overall approach to the ED patient with suspected cardiac ischemia are directly linked. As each technical advancement in marker assays occurs, previously existing limitations on the scope, accuracy, and availability of data are removed. This improvement in information, in turn, allows the emergency physician to enact new protocols that surpass previous limitations on the accuracy and timeliness of decisions concerning patient care. At the same time, ever-increasing pressures on EDs

to continue to improve the rapidity and quality of the care delivered further drives the laboratory technology industry to generate faster and more accurate assays. Owing to this dynamic, the clinical chemist and the clinician are increasingly interdependent. Therefore, in order to provide the best care, the emergency physician must maintain an understanding of the capabilities and limitations of the laboratory, including a working knowledge of the currently available laboratory techniques. Conversely, in addition to knowing the physiologic processes occurring within the patient during myocardial ischemia, the clinical chemist will benefit from an understanding of the unique environment in which the initial evaluation and treatment of the ED patient occurs, as well as knowledge of the constraints on and the priorities of the emergency physician.

THE ED ENVIRONMENT

Unlike most other clinical settings, patients usually present to the ED soon after onset of their symptoms and without previous medical evaluation. In many of these patients, their symptoms represent slow or moderately progressive disease states that

---

*See p. 87 for list of abbreviations used in this chapter.

From: Cardiac Markers   Edited by: Alan H.B. Wu
© Humana Press Inc., Totowa, NJ

do not require immediate intervention. However, initially similar presentations in other patients will represent manifestations of rapidly progressive, catastrophic pathology requiring immediate recognition and action. Because the emergency physician is constantly faced with patients with this wide range of pathologies and variable rates of disease progression, which are often difficult or impossible to differentiate initially, every patient must be approached with the assumption that he/she is presenting with an immediate life threat. Although physicians in other clinical settings are able to rely on a differential diagnosis based on the probability of the presentation representing a given disease, emergency physicians must always first consider and rule-out those pathologies that carry the greatest potential for early morbidity and mortality, even if they are statistically improbable.

The necessity of this type of approach is most apparent during the evaluation of the patient presenting with chest pain. Chest pain is one of the most common complaints faced by the emergency physician, causing five million visits a year and representing approx 5% of all ED visits *(2,3)*. Despite this, caring for these patients remains one of the emergency physician's greatest challenges. Among the 1.5 million patients admitted each year to coronary care units (CCUs) for suspected acute ischemic heart disease, the false-positive rate is exceedingly high (35–70%) *(4–6)*. Conversely, it is estimated that from 2–10% of patients with acute myocardial infarction (AMI) who present to EDs with chest pain are inappropriately discharged or admitted to nonmonitored beds *(7–9)*. These "missed AMI" patients may have a higher mortality than those admitted to the CCU *(10–12)*. Additionally, missed AMI is the leading cause of malpractice lawsuits and settlements in the ED setting *(13)*.

Many of the difficulties encountered are attributable to factors inherent to the complaint. There are a multitude of diverse pathologies that may initiate an ED visit for chest pain (Table 1). Confounding the physician's evaluation is the fact that most internal thoracic structures are innervated by visceral rather than somatic nerve fibers. This results in the fact that pain caused by many different intrathoracic pathologies is poorly localized and can often be described only in vague terms. Complicating matters further is the fact that wide variations in the perception and communication of pain exist because of physiologic, cultural, and individual differences. The result is a situation in which patients with unrelated pathologies, which require completely different assessment and treatment strategies, frequently present with similar or even identical signs and symptoms. For example, the initial presentation of myocardial ischemia and esophageal pain owing to acid reflux are often indistinguishable. Conversely, patients with identical pathology may present with dramatically different symptoms. Although many patients experiencing a myocardial infarction will present with the "classic" complaint of substernal chest pain, some AMI patients will complain only of epigastric, jaw, or arm pain, or will be completely pain-free.

Because of these factors, when faced with an ED patient with chest pain, the initial stages of the evaluation must be spent assessing the possibility of any immediately life-threatening pathology, including but not limited to AMI. Other pathologies that must be considered that may require immediate lifesaving action include pulmonary embolism, aortic dissection, and tension pneumothorax. Additionally, several other disease processes commonly manifest as chest pain, which, although not immediate life threats, may place the patient at risk of

Table 1
Common Causes of Chest Pain
___

Cardiac
  Ischemic syndromes
    Stable angina
    Unstable angina
    Variant angina
    AMI
  Valvular disease
    Mitral valve prolapse
    Aortic stenosis
    Subaortic stenosis
  Cardiomyopathy
  Pericarditis
Pulmonary
  Bronchitis
  Bronchospasm
  Empyema
  Pleural effusion
  Pleuritis
  Pneumonia
  Pneumothorax
  Pulmonary edema
  Aortic dissection
  Pulmonary embolism
  Pulmonary hypertension
Vascular
  Aortic dissection
  Pulmonary embolism
  Pulmonary hypertension
Gastrointestinal
  Esophageal spasm
  Gastroesophageal reflux disease (GERD)
  Mallory-Weiss tear
  Esophagitis/gastritis
  Gastric/duodenal ulcer
  Biliary colic
Musculoskeletal
  Costochondritis
  Muscle strain/spasm
  Cervical radiculopathy
Neurologic
  Herpes Zoster
___

subsequent serious morbidity or mortality if not recognized and treated in a timely manner. Examples of these diseases include

pneumonia, peptic ulcer disease, and neoplasm. Because of the possibility of immediate life threats, initial diagnostic and treatment maneuvers must often be based only on a clinical suspicion rather than a confirmed diagnosis. By necessity, more detailed data-gathering and the determination of definitive diagnoses, treatment, and disposition plans may not be the first consideration. Accordingly, during the initial evaluation of these patients, data that allow assessment of prognosis will often prove more valuable than that which aids only in diagnosis.

It must be noted that there are several factors not directly related to the individual patient that also influence the nature of the ED evaluation. Unlike other areas of the hospital, the entry of patients into the ED cannot be controlled. New patients continue to arrive at all times and must be evaluated with minimal delay. Therefore, in order to deliver quality care to all patients, patient flow through the department must be constantly maintained. To do this, the emergency physician must manage multiple patients simultaneously, and must always keep in mind the number and acuity of patients who are waiting to be seen. The result is that significant time constraints are placed both on the overall length of stay in the ED and on the time the physician is able to spend in data-gathering for a given patient. Additional factors indirectly but significantly influence the nature of the ED evaluation as well. Awareness of rising health care costs creates ever-increasing pressure to limit the number of diagnostic tests and to decrease admissions, especially to the highest levels of care (i.e., the CCU). Simultaneously, the desire to avoid adverse outcomes and the related fear of malpractice litigation have the opposite effect.

The overall result of these concerns, constraints and influences, is a constant drive to improve the speed and accuracy of treatment and disposition decisions. Therefore, the value of a diagnostic test must always be weighed against the time added to the patient's ED stay while awaiting test results. Any testing that is included as part of the ED evaluation must be immediately relevant to clinical decision making, and must improve the ability of physicians to match the patient optimally with the most appropriate therapy and/or the required level of subsequent care.

THE TRADITIONAL APPROACH TO THE CHEST PAIN PATIENT

The classic paradigm used for decades in evaluation of a patient's complaint is based on the Oslerian belief that the most useful data will always derive from an exhaustive history and physical examination. Following this, an inclusive differential diagnosis is generated, succeeded by collection of additional data, if needed, through directed supplementary testing. After all data are collected, a definitive diagnosis is made based on the clinician's interpretation of his/her findings, followed by the determination of a treatment plan. Applied to the ED patient with chest pain, the standard evaluation has traditionally consisted of eliciting a detailed account of the presenting symptoms as well as determining the presence or absence of "risk factors" for coronary artery disease, such as smoking, hypertension, and so forth. A thorough physical exam is then followed by an electrocardiogram (ECG) and chest radiograph.

Unfortunately, these traditional modalities are unable to lead consistently to an accurate diagnosis (AMI, unstable angina, stable angina pectoris, noncardiac diagnosis) or to predict reliably the risk of subsequent untoward events. Although the classical text's declaration that the history is "the single most important tool" in the initial evaluation of chest pain patients may be true, it is equally true that patients often present with atypical or even misleading symptoms (2,7). The physical exam and the chest X-ray are sometimes useful to confirm the presence of specific noncardiac causes of chest pain and to identify certain complications of myocardial ischemia. However, in the majority of patients, neither modality will help the clinician to identify those patients whose symptoms represent myocardial ischemia or to differentiate myocardial infarction from other acute ischemic syndromes. Further, although the ECG is clearly helpful when positive, it is initially nondiagnostic in up to 50% of AMI patients presenting to the ED (12).

Analysis of cardiac enzymes has been the gold standard for the in-hospital diagnosis of AMI since the 1960s. Despite this fact, it has not been a traditional part of the ED evaluation of chest pain patients. Publications as recently as a decade ago dismissed the use of cardiac isoenzyme determination in the management of ED patients as being "impractical" (14), "unhelpful" (15), and even potentially dangerous (16). These statements were based on the fact that previously available assay systems were technically complex and slow, often requiring several hours. Test results were therefore not available for consideration within the initial hours of the patient's visit, when the emergency physician is required to make major treatment and disposition decisions. Furthermore, before the advent of immunochemical and other modern laboratory techniques, the diagnostic accuracy of available assays was not sufficient to allow decision making to be based on them. Additional concerns were voiced by those who feared that misinterpretation of results by inexperienced clinicians would lead to patients being inappropriately discharged on the basis of a single negative enzyme measurement.

During the 1980s, a gradual recognition of these factors, as well as the high costs of the "rule-out AMI" CCU admission and increasing concern about ED patients being

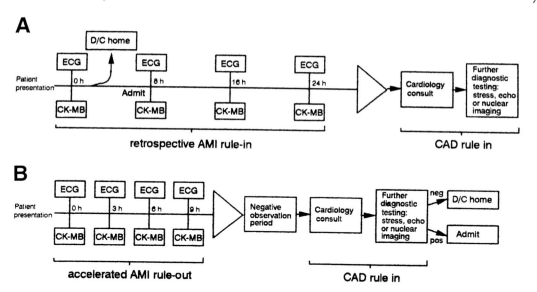

Fig. 1. (A) Conventional ED rule in protocol. **(B)** Cincinnati Chest Pain Emergency Unit protocol.

sent home with "missed AMI" led to scrutiny of the traditional approach. This resulted in a search for better diagnostic tools, including a re-evaluation of cardiac enzyme use. Simultaneously advances in laboratory technology rapidly removed many of the barriers to real-time utilization of myocardial marker assays in the ED and led to the availability of increasing numbers of unique myocardial markers *(17)*. The result has been a rapid evolution in both the laboratory techniques and the ED applications of marker assays. In recent years, the role of ED measurement of markers of myocardial injury has become firmly established and continues to become increasingly important. The most recent step in this process is the incorporation of the available markers into new cardiac assessment protocols, which allow earlier and more accurate decision making at lower costs. Today, it is typical for cardiac marker testing to be conducted at admission and at a frequency of every 8–12 h/d for the first few days (Fig. 1A) *(18)*. A decision to admit or discharge is made on a combination of enzyme results, clinical history, and ECG. Although serial measure-

ments are ideal for interpretation of results, the pressures to move patients in and out of the ED (either discharge or admit) often necessitates making a management decision prior to the establishment of a definitive diagnosis (Fig. 1A).

COMPUTER PROTOCOLS

In an effort to achieve more appropriate triaging of chest pain patients who present to the ED, several investigators have developed decision aids and computer-based triaging protocols *(11,19,20)*. These protocols were designed to reduce the number of inappropriate admissions to the coronary care unit. Perhaps the most well-known algorithm was developed by Goldman et al. *(11)*. Figure 2 illustrates an abridged version of this algorithm. When prospectively applied to 4770 patients presenting at six different hospitals, the algorithm produced a reduction of admissions to the CCU by 11.5% for non-AMI patients, as compared to decisions made by attending physicians. For chest pain patients with AMI, there was no difference in the sensitivity of detecting AMI, and there were no adverse effects to those who

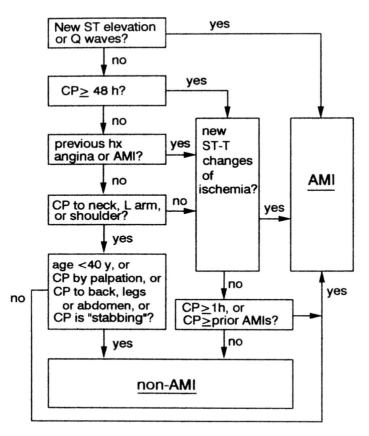

Fig. 2. An abridged version of the Goldman algorithm for triaging ED patients with chest pain *(11)*.

required intensive care. Although medical informatics is an emerging discipline, computer algorithms and intelligent ("expert") systems cannot replace clinical judgment in individual cases, particularly those with complications.

THE CHEST PAIN ED

It is now widely recognized that physician judgment alone is inadequate to differentiate acute myocardial ischemia from nonischemic causes of chest pain. This has led to a growing trend to utilize written evaluation and treatment protocols to guide the care of these patients. These protocols, also referred to as guidelines or critical pathways, are being rapidly developed and applied at departmental, institutional, and even national levels in order to standardize the assessment and treatment of chest pain patients *(21,22)*. Utilization of a protocolized approach offers several advantages. The protocols are generally developed by clinicians with acknowledged expertise in the field, and are based on knowledge of the most recent literature and therefore ideally represent the "state of the art." Protocols can be developed using a multidisciplinary approach with input from cardiologists, laboratory medicine, and imaging specialists in addition to ED physicians, assuring that all available resources will be coordinated and utilized to the patient's greatest benefit. Most importantly, compliance with the protocols and the effect of their utilization on patient outcomes can be monitored, easily allowing constant re-evaluation and improvement. Because of wide variation in individual clinician's management style, resource utilization, and decision patterns, this type of systematic outcome analysis is difficult or impossible under the traditional approach.

Although ED chest pain protocols take many different forms, they can be broadly classified into two groups: those governing initial evaluation and those based on some period of ED observation. The first protocols developed were designed to reduce the time delay for eligible acute AMI patients to receive thrombolytics in the ED *(22)*. The recognition that earlier thrombolytic drugs led to improved outcomes has led to continued attempts to reduce the "door to treatment time" within the ED. Protocols were therefore developed that single out chest pain patients as a group requiring immediate and intensive evaluation. Although the initial motivation and the primary goal of these protocols have been to identify those chest pain patients who require thrombolytic therapy, it quickly became apparent that an early systematic approach can benefit those patients who do not receive lytic therapy as well. These algorithms often call for the triaging of chest pain patients into a distinct geographic area within the ED where they are treated by dedicated personnel. The perception of earlier and improved disposition decisions has led to increasing acceptance of this approach as evidenced by the recent proliferation of distinct ED chest pain units. In 1992, there were 116 such units in the US. Today there are approx 700 ED chest pain centers, and it is estimated that this number will increase *(23)*.

The second type of algorithm is more comprehensive in scope. They encompass the care of the patient beyond the initial hours after presentation and aim to provide a more definitive evaluation of chest pain patients during an extended ED visit. During a period of observation, patients are ruled out for AMI using serial myocardial marker measurements. After AMI is excluded, further diagnostic studies are performed to assess whether the patient's symptoms were owing to acute ischemia or other pathologies. By using this approach, patients are able to undergo a complete cardiac evaluation within 12–24 h as an outpatient in place of the 2–5 d hospitalization previously typical for a rule-out AMI admission *(24)*.

MYOCARDIAL MARKERS IN THE INITIAL ED EVALUATION

The inclusion of myocardial marker measurements in algorithms for the early evaluation of ED chest pain patients is a relatively recent occurrence. After the first descriptions of CK-MB use in the early 1970s, many investigators focused on legitimate, but somewhat exaggerated concerns about the dangers of misinterpretation of single negative cardiac enzyme measurements in the ED. This resulted in a common view until the mid-1980s that stat enzyme tests early in the patient's ED course were contraindicated and established the widespread belief that only serial enzyme measurements (a full enzyme "curve" over 24–48 h) gave clinically useful results *(14–16)*.

In 1987, two independent studies demonstrated that CK-MB measurement in the ED could identify some chest pain patients with myocardial infarction that would have been otherwise missed *(9,10)*. At about the same time, several publications appeared describing rapid, immunochemical laboratory techniques that would allow CK-MB testing to be done on a stat basis so that results could be available within the time frame required for ED decision making (real time) *(17)*. These reports led many clinical investigators to reconsider the role of myocardial marker measurement in the ED, thus leading to the recent proliferation of investigations in this area. The resulting literature supports the inclusion of myocardial marker measure-

Table 2
Summary of Investigations of Myocardial Markers in ED Evaluation

Purpose	Marker	Hours from presentation	n	Reference
Initial ED evaluation	CK-MB	0, 3	183	25
Early MI diagnosis	CK-MB	0, 1, 2, 3	313	26
	CK-MB	0, 1, 2, 3	616	27
	Myoglobin	0, 3	59	28
	Myoglobin	0, 1, 2	198	29
Identification of "missed" MI	CK-MB	Single sample	773	9
	CK-MB	Single sample	271	7
	CK-MB	0, 3	1042	30
Early risk stratification	CK-MB	0, 2	449	31
	CK-MB	0, 2	5120	32
	Troponin T	Single sample	113	33
	Troponin T	Single sample	131	34
Comprehensive ED evaluation	CK-MB	Variable	2684	35
	CK-MB	0, 8, 16, 24	512	36
	CK-MB	0, 3, 6, 9	1010	37

ments in protocols governing the initial ED evaluation of chest pain patients for three distinct purposes (Table 2): first, the ability of myocardial markers to confirm or rule in suspected AMI within the first hours after presentation in patients with nondiagnostic ECGs *(25–30)*, second, the ability of markers to identify some patients with otherwise unrecognized AMI from among the many patients with atypical presentations and non-diagnostic ECGs *(7,9)*, and third, to risk stratify patients early in their ED course, i.e., to identify those patients at particularly high risk for subsequent adverse events *(31–34)*.

Ruling in AMI

In the past decade, the use of thrombolytic agents has dramatically improved the prognosis of AMI. Acute angioplasty, antithrombin and antiplatelet drugs, and other new treatments promise to reduce AMI mortality further in the near future. However, the effectiveness of these treatments is dependent on their early initiation. It is therefore imperative that patients with AMI are identified as soon as possible after presentation to the ED. In those patients whose initial ECG is diagnostic for AMI, no further testing is required and appropriate therapy can be initiated. However, as stated previously, approximately half of AMI patients will have an initially nondiagnostic ECG. The release kinetics of currently available markers generally require 6 h or more after coronary occlusion to exclude infarction, and therefore AMI cannot be definitively ruled out within the first few hours of the ED visit. However, some AMI patients with nondiagnostic initial ECGs will have positive marker tests on ED arrival, and many more will develop positive tests soon after presentation. Therefore, early, rapid serial sampling of myocardial markers can identify many AMI patients with nondiagnostic ECGs (rule-in AMI) and thus allow earlier utilization of time-dependent treatments.

Studies of single CK-MB measurement on ED presentation have demonstrated a sensitivity for AMI of <60%, and single measurements are therefore not considered useful for this purpose *(14–16)*. However, several investigators have demonstrated much higher sensitivity using rapid serial sampling. In a 1987 pilot study, CK-MB was measured on presentation, and 3 h later using three immunochemical assays and a sensitivity for AMI of 92–96% was produced *(20)*. In a larger study, CK-MB measured on presentation and every hour for 3 h in 313 chest pain patients resulted in a sensitivity for AMI that increased with each subsequent measurement, reaching a peak of 92% at 3 h *(26)*. In the largest investigation of CK-MB use to date, the Emergency Medicine Cardiac Research Group studied hourly CK-MB measurement for the first 3 h after presentation in 616 patients from eight hospitals. This protocol yielded a sensitivity for AMI of 79.7% among patients with nondiagnostic ECGs. The combined use of serial CK-MBs and the initial ECG was able to identify 88.4% of AMI patients within 3 h after presentation *(27)*.

Because of its earlier release into serum after coronary occlusion compared to CK-MB, the heme-containing protein, myoglobin, has a potential advantage over CK-MB for early diagnosis of AMI and has also been studied for this purpose. In a study of 59 chest pain patients, myoglobin and CK-MB were measured on presentation and at 3 h after admission *(28)*. A sensitivity of 62% for myoglobin was produced at presentation, compared to 14% for CK-MB. At 3 h, the sensitivity for AMI increased to 90% for CK-MB and to 100% for myoglobin *(28)*. In a subsequent similar study, CK-MB and myoglobin were measured on presentation and hourly for 2 h in 198 patients *(29)*. In this study, assays were considered positive if they reached a specified threshold value or if they doubled in value during subsequent measurements. The sensitivities at 2 h were 82.1% for CK-MB and 100% for myoglobin.

Identifying Missed AMI Patients

As previously stated, single-sample myocardial marker measurements have a low sensitivity for AMI and therefore cannot be used to exclude this diagnosis in the ED.

However, several investigations have assessed the use of early, single-sample CK-MB measurement in the ED in order to identify patients with AMI that was clinically unsuspected. These studies have aimed to address the continued problem of patients presenting to the ED with AMI being inadvertently sent home. Their results support the inclusion of marker measurement into patient care algorithms for low-risk patients at the end of their ED evaluation in order to identify patients with unsuspected AMI prior to discharge.

In one early study, stored serum samples were tested for CK and CK-MB from 482 chest pain patients discharged from the ED *(9)*. Of five discharged patients with a missed AMI, three were found to have had a positive CK-MB in the ED. In a later investigation, the potential utility of single-sample CK-MB measurement was evaluated for identification of unsuspected AMI among patients presenting to the ED with chest pain as well as with other symptoms consistent with possible ischemia *(7)*. Among the 271 patients studied, five discharged patients had positive CK-MB values, with four of these having clear evidence of an acute AMI on follow-up. Additionally, two patients admitted to nonmonitored beds with noncardiac diagnoses were identified by a positive ED CK-MB value and were later determined to have had a clinically unsuspected AMI. All seven of these patients had nondiagnostic initial ECGs, and three of them had presented with symptoms other than chest pain. The results suggest that ED patients to be sent home or admitted to nonmonitored beds after presenting with chest pain as well as with other presentations of possible ischemia could benefit from prerelease "screening" for AMI using CK-MB *(7)*.

The Emergency Medicine Cardiac Research Group prospectively assessed the effect of performing two CK-MB measurements drawn 3 h apart on ED physician decision making *(31)*. This has been the only study to date that reported the actual clinical use of CK-MB testing for this purpose. In this investigation, of 265 enrolled patients who had been slated for discharge by the ED physician, three patients with unsuspected AMI were identified and admitted solely on the basis of a positive CK-MB *(30)*.

Early Risk Stratification

The number and efficacy of treatment modalities available to the physician caring for the patient with an acute ischemic event continue to grow rapidly. As use of these newer therapies, such as early angiographic interventions and antithrombotic drugs, becomes common, it is expected that the overall morbidity and mortality associated with this condition will decline. However, it must also be recognized that as physicians become more aggressive in their utilization of the various modalities, patients are put at greater risk of therapy-related complications. Additionally, the high cost of these interventions as well as the costs of the associated higher level of in-patient care required for their successful utilization necessitate a selective approach to their use. It is therefore imperative that methods be developed to aid the physician in identifying those patients who are most likely to benefit from a more aggressive treatment approach and intensive in-patient care. A tool that could select those patients at high risk for subsequent morbidity and mortality early in their presentation would allow this group to benefit from more invasive therapies while sparing low-risk patients their associated increased costs and potential complications. Several recent investigations suggest that markers of myocardial injury can successfully be used for this purpose.

CK-MB testing was performed on presentation and 2 h later in a two-center study of 449 chest pain patients without diagnostic ECG changes *(31)*. Ischemic events

occurring within 1 wk of presentation were recorded. Patients with a positive CK-MB value were significantly more likely to have a subsequent ischemic complication, regardless of diagnosis. The risk ratio for ischemic events in those with a positive CK-MB test compared to those testing negative was 5.2. These findings have been subsequently confirmed by a large multicenter study, The National Cooperative CK-MB Project Group *(32)*. In this investigation, 5120 patients were enrolled from 53 EDs utilizing similar methodology. In all patients, regardless of final diagnosis, the reported relative risk of complications was 16.1 in those with a positive CK-MB vs those patients with a negative test.

Initial reports suggest that early testing of troponin T (TnT) may also be of value for this purpose. In a pilot study, single samples were tested for cTnT for prediction of adverse events within a 2-wk period among 113 patients presenting to the ED with chest pain or other symptoms of potential ischemia *(33)*. The relative risk of a positive troponin test for adverse events was 1.76 compared to a negative test. In a study of 131 unstable angina patients, cTnT was associated with major adverse events during the subsequent 3 wk *(34)*. Among this higher-risk group, the relative risk ratio for an adverse event of a positive cTnT vs a negative test result was 14 to 1. Several trials are now being planned that assess the utility of ED chest pain treatment protocols using early ED testing of cTnT and troponin I (cTnI) for identification of high-risk patients who will then be targeted for various aggressive treatment strategies.

MYOCARDIAL MARKERS IN THE CHEST PAIN EVALUATION UNIT

From the development of the modern CCU in the 1960s and well into the 1980s, the accepted standard of care dictated that all patients with suspected myocardial infarction be admitted to the CCU for 24–48 h of monitoring, serial ECGs, and completion of a cardiac enzyme curve. The initial challenge to this dictum was motivated by the need to control the skyrocketing medical costs associated with intensive care unit stays during the 1980s. Recognizing the need to identify lower cost strategies for care of ED patients presenting with chest pain, the Multicenter Chest Pain Study Group was formed in 1984. In 1991, this group published the results of a seven-center study of 2684 patients admitted for chest pain and reported that among those patients deemed to be at low risk for AMI, the diagnosis of infarction could have been safely excluded within a 12-h observation period *(35)*. Shortly thereafter, the use of a two-bed, monitored, nonintensive care unit adjacent to the ED for admission of low-risk chest pain patients was reported *(36)*. A strategy of admitting low-risk patients to such a unit was recommended and resulted in an average length of stay of 1.2 d, significantly shorter than standard in-patient care. Routine predischarge stress testing in order reduce the risk of premature discharge of patients who were ruled out for AMI, but who may have unstable coronary syndromes was recommended for consideration.

The new approach has been further refined by investigators at the University of Cincinnati *(37)*. This group has published a study on a series of 1010 patients who were admitted to an ED based chest pain evaluation and treatment unit over 32 mo. In this protocol (Fig. 1B), patients with known coronary artery disease (CAD), hemodynamic instability, ECG changes diagnostic of ischemia, or a clinical syndrome thought to represent unstable angina were directly admitted to the in-patient service. Other patients with symptoms suggestive of possible acute coronary ischemia were observed for 9 h with continuous 12 lead ST-segment ECG monitoring and serial CK-MB measurements at 0, 3, 6, and 9 h after presentation. During the observation period, any signs of instability, ischemic symptoms, ST changes, or a positive enzyme measurement necessitated immediate admission. Patients who had a negative 9-h workup then underwent echocardiography and, if normal, graded exercise stress testing in the ED prior to discharge (Fig. 1). Utilizing this approach, 82.1% of patients were able to be released home from the ED unit. The group concluded that their approach was an effective and safe method for evaluation of low- to moderate-risk patients. The same group has also reported that this method results in significantly lower costs when compared to a group of similar patients being evaluated using the traditional approach (38).

In the five years since the first reports of accelerated AMI exclusion algorithms, many institutions have embraced this basic strategy. Most have chosen to relocate the focus of evaluation of low-risk patients to the ED. However, some continue to use an in-patient unit for this purpose. Additionally, within the ED, some centers have constructed distinct observation areas specifically for this purpose, but others utilize a cardiac protocol without physically separating chest pain patients from the general ED population. Further, although the basic concept of an accelerated AMI rule-out during an extended ED stay followed by diagnostic testing is retained by all of these units, the protocols used are not standardized with respect to selection and timing of either myocardial marker measurements or other diagnostic tests. In an effort to clarify the role of ED chest pain units, the American College of Emergency Physicians has issued an information paper listing the recommended components of these units *(39)* (Table 3). Evaluations of both the clinical and cost-effectiveness of various cardiac evaluation unit protocols continue to be a very active

Table 3
Recommended Components of a Chest Pain Evaluation Unit*a*

Emergency Chest Pain Area—Designated area in the ED for immediate evaluation and treatment initiation of patients with AMI

Rule Out MI Program—Protocol to exclude MI and evaluate risk in chest pain patients

Unit Design—Appropriate space and equipment including monitoring ability and availability of "real time" myocardial marker testing

Unit Staffing—Adequate staffing of physicians, nurses and technicians with specific experience and training in emergency cardiac care.

Management System—Unit management based upon a system of continuous monitoring of relevant clinical and financial indicators

Outreach Program—Program of patient education and public outreach aimed at reduction in treatment delays and risk factor modification

*a*Modified from ref. *39.*

area of investigation and are likely to demonstrate in the near future which algorithms are most efficient.

THE FUTURE OF EMERGENCY CARDIAC CARE

Currently, when establishing cardiac care protocols, many institutions choose to focus initially on either high-risk or low-risk patients, depending on which group is more prevalent in the population they serve. However, as the body of evidence supporting a systematic approach for patients in all risk groups continues to grow, it is likely that increasing numbers of EDs will adopt a more comprehensive approach, which integrates aspects of the selective protocols already described. These care plans will cover all of the various subgroups of chest pain patients, and will guide their management from arrival at the triage desk through the initial physician's assessment and into the definitive evaluation and treatment phase. A flowchart summarizing how myocardial marker

use would be integrated into this type of care plan is shown in Fig. 3.

This type of systematic approach can provide the framework necessary to maximize the benefits offered by myocardial marker testing. However, several important questions remain concerning the specifics of ED marker use. Although the release kinetics, cardiac specificity, and other properties of each of the available markers offers a unique profile, it is not yet clear what the optimum role of each marker will be within such a protocol. Further, although many investigators have evaluated the clinical utility of a single marker, there are still few data available to aid in determining the usefulness of measuring two or more of these markers simultaneously during a patient's ED visit. Simultaneous measurements of various markers may allow more accurate prediction of patient outcomes and may therefore be justified. This concept is currently being marketed to EDs and diagnostic laboratories in the form of a myocardial ischemia or chest pain panel. Unfortunately, it remains unknown whether there is a cumulative benefit or only a cumulative cost when a second, third, or fourth marker is added to such a panel. Alternatively, the unique properties of each marker may allow selective use of multiple markers, allowing the maximum diagnostic benefit of each marker within a specific subgroup of patients while eliminating the necessity of multiple tests yielding redundant information.

Another problem that must be further explored is to determine the optimal format for incorporation of the additional data derived from myocardial injury marker assays into the physician's decision-making process. Most investigations currently report on the predictive values of a single myocardial marker in isolation. However, when faced with the need to make rapid treatment and disposition decisions, the ED physician must consider data from multiple sources.

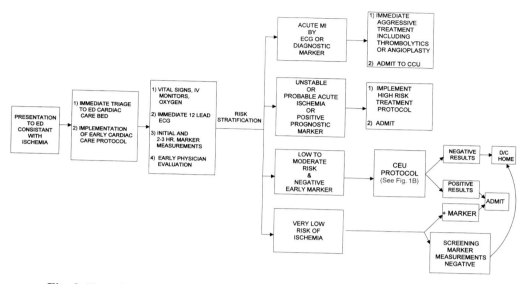

Fig. 3. Use of myocardial markers in the Cincinnati Emergency Unit protocol.

Additional studies are needed in order to aid the clinician in integrating marker results with clinical and ECG data as well as data from other new technologies (such as imaging studies) to yield information that will have a positive impact on decision making. In response to this need, integration of myocardial marker results into currently existing computer-generated decision aides for ED chest pain patients is currently another active area of investigation.

ABBREVIATIONS

AMI, acute myocardial infarction; CCU, coronary care unit; CK, creatine kinase; cTnI, cTnT, cardiac troponins I and T; ECG, electrocardiogram; ED, emergency department; CAD, coronary artery disease.

REFERENCES

1. The Cardiology Roundtable (1994) Perfecting MI ruleout. Best practices for emergency evaluation of chest pain. The Advisory Board Company, Washington, D.C.
2. American Heart Association (1987) Heart Facts. American Heart Center, Dallas, TX.
3. McCaig LF (1994) National hospital ambulatory medical care survey: 1992: emergency department summary. Adv. Data 245:12.
4. Singer DE, Carr PL, Mulley AG, and Thibault GE (1983) Rationing intensive care—physician responses to a resource shortage. N. Engl. J. Med. 309:11,155–11,160.
5. Selker HP, Griffith JL, Dorey FJ, and D'Agostino RB (1987) How do physicians adapt when the coronary care unit is full? JAMA 257:1181–1185.
6. Schor S, Behar S, Modan B, Barell V, Drory J, and Kariv I (1976) Disposition of presumed coronary patients from an emergency room: a follow-up study. JAMA 236:941–943.
7. Green GB, Hansen KN, Chan DW, and Guerei AD, Fleetwood DH, Sivertson KT, and Kelen GD (1991) The potential utility of a rapid CK-MB assay in evaluating emergency department patients with possible myocardial infarction. Ann. Emerg. Med. 20:954–960.
8. Tierney WM, Fitzgerald J, McHenry R, Roth BJ, Psaty B, Stump DL, and Anderson FK (1986) Physicians' estimates of the probability of myocardial infarction in emergency room patients with chest pain. Med. Decis. Making 6:12–17.

9. Hedges J, Rouan GW, Toltzis R, Goldstein-Wayne B, and Stein EA (1987) Use of cardiac enzymes identifies patients with acute myocardial infarction otherwise unrecognized in the emergency department. Ann. Emerg. Med. 16:248–252.

10. Lee TH, Rouan G, Weisberg M, Brand DA, Acampora D, Stasinlewicz C, Walshonk J, Terranova G, Gottlieb L, Goldstein-Wayne B, Copen D, Daley K, Brandt A, Mellors J, Jakubowski R, Cook EF, and Goldman L (1987) Patients with acute MI sent home from the emergency room. Am. J. Cardiol. 60:219–224.

11. Goldman L, Cook EF, Brand DA, Lee TH, Rouan GW, Weisberg MC, Acampora D, Stasinlewicz C, Walshon J, Terranova G, Gottlieb L, Kobernick M, Goldstein-Wayne B, Copen D, Daley K, Brandt AA, Jones D, Mellors J, and Jakubowski R (1988) A computer protocol to predict myocardial infarction in emergency department patients with chest pain. N. Engl. J. Med. 318: 797–803.

12. Zarling EJ, Sexton H, and Milnor P (1983) Failure to diagnose acute myocardial infarction: the clinicopathologic experience at a large community hospital. JAMA 250: 1171–1181.

13. Rusnack RA, Stair TO, Hansen D, and Fastow JS (1989) Litigation against the emergency physician: Common features in cases of missed myocardial infarction. Ann. Emerg. Med. 18:1029–1034.

14. Diagnosis of the doubtful coronary [editorial]. 1982. Lancet 1:661–662.

15. Lee TH, Cook EF, and Weisberg M (1985) Acute chest pain in the emergency room: identification and examination of low-risk patients. Arch. Intern. Med. 145:65–69.

16. Eisenberg JM, Horowitz LN, Busch R, Arvan D, Rawnsley H (1979) Diagnosis of acute myocardial infarction in the emergency room: A prospective assessment of clinical decision marking and the usefulness of immediate cardiac enzyme determination. J. Commun. Health 4:190–198.

17. Green GB, Chan DW, Chandra NC, Pietrzak MP, and Sayers DG (1991) Role of the laboratory in the diagnosis of myocardial injury. Crit. Care Rep. 2:318–330.

18. Wu AHB (1997) Use of cardiac markers as assessed by outcomes analysis. Clin. Biochem. 30:339–350.

19. Tierney MW, Roth BJ, and Psaty B (1985) Predictors of myocardial infarction in emergency room patients. Crit. Care Med. 13:526–531.

20. Pozen MW, D'Agostino RB, Mitchell JB (1985) The usefulness of a predictivbe instrument to reduce inappropriate admissions to the coronary care unit. Ann. Intern. Med. 92:238–242.

21. Braunwald E, Mark DB, Jones RH, Cheitlin MD, Fuster V, McCauley KM, et al. (1994) Unstable angina: diagnosis and management. Clinical practice guidelines number 10 (amended) AHCPR publication no. 94-0602. Rockville, MD, Agency for Health Care Policy and Research and the National Heart, Lung, and Blood Institute, Public Health Service, US Department of Health and Human Services, Rockville, MD, May.

22. Smith EE, Braen GR, Cantrill SV, Dalsey WC, Fesmine FM, Green CS, Karas S, Leibovich M, Mackey D, Molzen GW, and Murphy BA (1995) Clinical policy for the initial approach to adults presenting with a chief complaint of chest pain, with no history of trauma. Ann. Emerg. Med. 25:274–299.

23. Shesser R and Smith M (1994) The chest pain emergency department and the outpatient chest pain evaluation center: Revolution or evolution? Ann. Emerg. Med. 23: 334–341.

24. Hoekstra JW, Gibler WB, Levy RC, Sayre M, Naber W, Chandra A, Kacich R, Magorien R, and Walsh R (1994) Emergency-department diagnosis of acute myocardial infarction and ischemia: A cost analysis of two diagnostic protocols. Acad. Emerg. Med. 1:103–110.

25. Gibler WB, Lewis LM, Erb RE, Makens PK, Kaplan BC, Vaughn RH, Biagini, AV, Blanton JD, and Campbell WB (1990) Early detection of acute myocardial infarction in patients presenting with chest pain and non-diagnostic ECGs: Serial CK-MB sampling in the emergency department. Ann. Emerg. Med. 19:1359–1366.

26. Marin MM and Teichman SL (1992) Use of rapid serial sampling of creatine kinase MB

for very early detection of myocardial infarction in patients with acute chest pain. Am. Heart J. 123:354–361.

27. Gibler WB, Young GP, Hedges JR, Lewis LM, Smith MS, Carleton SC, Aghababian RV, Jorden RO, Allison ES, Otten EJ, Makens PK, and Hamilton C (1992) The Emergency Medicine Cardiac Research Group: Acute myocardial infarction in chest pain patients with nondiagnostic ECGs: Serial CK-MB sampling in the emergency department. Ann. Emerg. Med. 21:504–512.

28. Gibler WB, Gibler CD, Weinshenker E, Abbottsmith C, Hedges JR, and Barsan WG (1987) Myoglobin as an early indicator of acute myocardial infarction. Ann. Emerg. Med. 16:851–856.

29. Tucker JF, Collins RA, Anderson RA, Hess M, Farley IM, and Hagemann DA (1994) Value of serial myoglobin levels in the early diagnosis of patients admitted for acute myocardial infarction. Ann. Emerg. Med. 24:704–708.

30. Hedges JR, Gibler WB, Young GP, Hoekstra JW, Slovis C, Aghababian R, and Smith M (1996) Multicenter study of creatine kinase—MB Use: Effect on chest pain clinical decision making. Acad. Emerg. Med. 3:7–15.

31. Hedges JR, Young GP, Henkel GF, Gibler WB, Green TR, and Swanson JR (1994) Early CK-MB elevations predict ischemic events in stable chest pain patients. Acad. Emerg. Med. 1:9–16.

32. Hoekstra JW, Hedges JR, Gibler WB, Robison RM, and Christensen RA (1994) Emergency department CK-MB: A predictor of ischemic complications. Acad. Emerg. Med. 1:17–28.

33. Hamm CW, Ravkilde J, Gerhardt W, Jorgensen P, Peheim E, Ljungdahl L, Goldmann B, Katus HA (1992) The prognostic value of serum troponin T in unstable angina. N. Engl. J. Med. 327:146–150.

34. Wu A, Abbas SA, Green S, Pearsall P, Dhakam S, Azar R, Onoroski M, Senaie A, McKay R, and Waters D (1995) Prognostic value of cardiac troponin T in unstable angina pectoris. Am. J. Cardiol. 76:970–972.

35. Lee TH, Juarez G, Cook F, Weisberg MC, Rouan GW, Brand DA, and Goldman L (1991) Ruling out acute myocardial infarction: A prospective multicenter validation of a 12-hour strategy for patients at low risk. N. Engl. J. Med. 324:1239–1246.

36. Gaspoz JM, Lee TH, Cook F, Weisberg MC, and Goldman L (1991) Outcome of patients who were admitted to a new short-stay unit to rule out myocardial infarction. Am. J. Cardiol. 68:145–149.

37. Gibler WB, Runyon JP, Levy RC, Sayre MR, Kacich R, Hattemer CR, Hamilton C, Grlach JW, and Walsh RA (1995) A rapid diagnostic and treatment center for patients with chest pain in the emergency department. Ann. Emerg. Med. 25:1–8.

38. Hoekstra JW, Gibler WB, Levy RC, Sayre M, Naber W, Chandra A, Kacich R, Magorien R, and Walsh R (1993) Emergency department diagnosis of acute myocardial infarction and ischemia: A cost analysis [Abstract]. Ann. Emerg. Med. 22:941.

39. Graff L, Joseph T, and Andelman R (1995) American College of Emergency Physicians Information Paper: Chest Pain Units in Emergency Departments—A Report from the Short-Term Observation Services Section. Am. J. Cardiol. 76:1036–1039.

5

Ultrastructure of the Striated Muscle Cell

Robert G. McCord and Allen W. Clark

INTRODUCTION

The succeeding chapters deal with the biochemistry and clinical utilization of cardiac markers. This chapter deals with the *source* of these markers as they are released into the blood following injury. To appreciate this, a knowledge of cell anatomy at the ultrastructural level is necessary. Over the past 50 yr, two technologies have evolved that have enabled us to understand cell structure by providing details not possible with the light microscope. These investigative tools are the electron microscope (EM*) and X-ray diffraction. The former has elucidated the substructure of muscle fibers as seen with routine histology (or polarizing optics), whereas the latter has given us knowledge about the molecular structure of the muscular contractile apparatus *(1,2)*.

BASIC STRUCTURE
OF THE MAMMALIAN CELL

The shapes and staining of cells as seen in the light microscope are actually manifestations of cell ultrastructure that can be seen at the level of the EM. This instrument has enabled us not only to see very tiny subcellular structures, but also to see images at low magnifications (comparable to light microscopy) with incredible clarity *(1,3,4)*.

The two most obvious components of a cell are the nucleus and the cytoplasm. The nuclei of different cell types have varying sizes and shapes as well as varying locations within the cell cytoplasm. Likewise, the cytoplasm of the cell is variable in size, shape and staining intensity. Because myocardial markers are found in the cytoplasm, we will only consider the basic ultrastructure of this component of the cell (Fig. 1).

The cytoplasm of the cell is separated from the external environment by a plasmalemma, more commonly referred to as the cell membrane. Internal to the cell membrane is the cytoplasm, which is comprised of a cytoplasmic matrix (cytosol) containing enzymes, and soluble proteins and nutrients. Floating in the cytosol are organelles and inclusions such as mitochondria, rough and smooth-surfaced endoplasmic reticulum (RER and SER), the Golgi apparatus, secretory granules, lysosomes, ribosomes, peroxisomes, microtubules, intermediate filaments, microfilaments, and centrioles *(1,3,4)*.

Mitochondria are the main site of energy production for the cell. The external mem-

---

*See p. 100 for list of abbreviations used in this chapter.

The authors dedicate this Chapter to David B. Slautterback. What is presented in this Chapter represents a mere shadow of his vast knowledge of the subject.

From: Cardiac Markers   Edited by: Alan H. B. Wu
© Humana Press Inc., Totowa, NJ

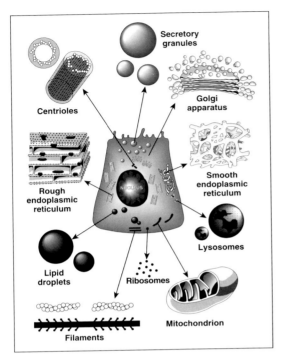

Fig. 1. Components of the mammalian cell, excluding the nucleus. (Reproduced and modified, with permission, from Fawcett: *A Textbook of Histology,* Twelfth Edition, Chapman and Hall, New York, 1994.)

brane has a smooth outline while the internal membrane is folded into shelf-like cristae. In between the cristae is the matrix, containing DNA, RNA, ribosomes, proteins, enzymes of the Krebs cycle, lactate dehydrogenase, and mitochondrial creatine kinase (CK).

Ribosomes are small dense particles comprised of RNA and protein. They are organized into clusters called polyribosomes and participate in the synthesis of cytoplasmic proteins.

The RER is associated chiefly with export protein synthesis. RER is a system of interconnected membranous sacs called cisternae that represent a compartment separated from the cytosol. Ribosomes are attached to the cytoplasmic surfaces of these cisternae. The SER also represents a compartment sep-

arated from the cytosol. SER is usually composed of anastomosing tubules whose cytoplasmic surfaces are devoid of ribosomes. This organelle is associated with synthesis of lipids, the detoxification of drugs, and the sequestration of calcium ions *(1,3,4)*.

The Golgi apparatus plays an important role in secretion because it modifies, packages, and distributes certain products. Lysosomes are membrane-bound structures that contain various hydrolytic enzymes.

Within the cytosol is the cytoskeleton consisting of microtubules and filaments, which contribute to the structural framework of the cell. Microtubules are long tubules believed to provide structural support as well as to contribute to the movement of components within a cell. There are two classes of cytoplasmic filaments: microfilaments such as actin, and intermediate filaments such as keratin, desmin, vimentin, fodrin, and glial fibrillary acidic protein.

The cytosol also contains inclusions such as glycogen and lipid droplets. Both are energy depots: glycogen is the substrate of the enzyme glycogen phosphorylase; lipid droplets contain fatty acids, the major fuel of the heart.

Centrioles are cylindrical structures the walls of which are composed of highly organized microtubules. Centrioles duplicate prior to cell division and migrate to opposite poles of a dividing cell where they participate in the organization of mitotic spindles that are also comprised of microtubules.

STRUCTURE OF STRIATED MUSCLE

Skeletal Myofibers

A striated skeletal muscle fiber is a syncytium (multinuclate giant cell) and is referred to as a fiber because it is long and narrow. On examination of hemotoxylin-eosin- (H&E) stained, longitudinal sections, myofibers are seen to have cross-striations

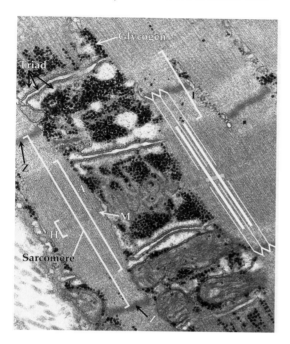

Fig. 2. Electron micrograph of a skeletal muscle fiber showing the I band, A band, H band, M line (creatine kinase and myomesin), sarcoplasmic reticulum (SR), Z lines, and triads (terminal cysterns and T-tubule). (Micrograph by A. W. Clark.)

that are alternating dark and light bands of different refractile index. These are easily seen in H&E stained material and can be accentuated by using phosphotungstic acid hematoxylin (PTAH) stain.

Figures 2 and 3 show the ultrastructure of the skeletal myofiber. The dark staining bands are referred to as the "A" (anisotropic) bands because of their refractive index. The light bands are the "I" (isotropic) bands. The A bands have a midregion known as the "H" (heller or bright) band. The "H" band, in turn, is bisected by the "M" (middle) line or band. The latter band is comprised of ultra-thin filaments that connect the central portions of the myosin thick filaments to one another and keep them in register. These "M" line filaments are largely comprised of CK and myomesin (MM) *(5)*.

The "I" bands are interrupted by a dark line referred to as the "Z" line (from the German zwischenscheibe meaning "in between"). The segment between one "Z" line and another is referred to as the sarcomere.

The sarcomere pattern is due to the presence of two different types of filaments: a thick filament (composed chiefly of myosin molecules) and a thin filament (composed of actin, tropomyosin, and troponin) *(1,6)*. The myosin molecule is long and asymmetric, about 200 nm in length and 2–3 nm in diameter. It is comprised of two heavy chains and four light chains. Myosin molecules self-assemble into thick filaments that are about 1.5 µm in length and 15 nm in diameter.

Each thin filament has an average length of 100 nm and varies from 6 to 7 nm in diameter. One end of each thin filament is anchored to the Z line. The Z line is a woven lattice that contains α-actinin, desmin, vimentin, synemin, and filamin.

Thin filaments have an actin backbone, a double helix of G-actin monomers (Fig. 4). Tropomyosin is a long thin molecule that is comprised of two parallel polypeptide chains wrapped around each other in a coiled helical structure. Tropomyosin wraps around the actin helix over its length. Located at 40 nm intervals along the tropomyosin molecule are groups of the troponin complex consisting of three protein subunits: T, I, and C. The letters of the complex relate to the function of each of its members, i.e., **C** for the calcium-binding component, **I** for the inhibitory component, and **T** for the tropomyosin-binding component.

According to the Huxley sliding filament hypothesis *(7)*, contraction is brought about when the thin filaments slide in between the thick filaments during muscle contraction. The myosin cross bridges move on the surface of the actin in a manner similar to the oars of a boat on the water. This rowing of the myosin cross bridges moves the thin fil-

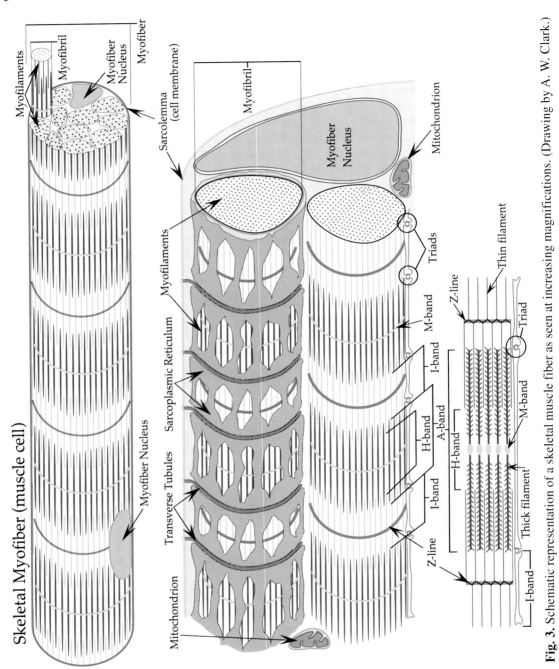

Fig. 3. Schematic representation of a skeletal muscle fiber as seen at increasing magnifications. (Drawing by A. W. Clark.)

aments toward the M-bands, reduces the distance between Z-lines, and shortens the length of sarcomeres.

Because muscle contraction depends on the availability of cytoplasmic calcium ions

and relaxation occurs during the unavailability of cytoplasmic calcium ions, the regulation of sarcoplasmic calcium ion concentrations is of critical importance. The organelle chiefly responsible for this regula-

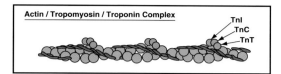

Actin / Tropomyosin / Troponin Complex
TnI
TnC
TnT

Fig. 4. Reproduced and modified, with permission, from Junqueria: *Basic Histology,* Eighth Edition, Appleton & Lange, Stamford, CT, 1995.

tion is a specialization of the smooth endoplasmic reticulum referred to as the *sarcoplasmic reticulum* (SR) *(1,3,4)*. In mammalian skeletal myofibers, sleeves of SR encircle the myofilaments, forming them into long, cylindrical structures called myofibrils. (A useful concept is to think of myofibers as composed of myofibrils which are composed, in turn, of myofilaments: *see* Fig. 3.)

At both junctions of the A band and the I band (the A–I junction) in every sarcomere, there are two expanded SR cisternae. These lateral expansions, or terminal cisternae, of the SR are rich in calsequestrin, a protein that avidly and reversibly binds calcium *(8)*. In between the two terminal cisternae is a transverse tubule also known as a "T" tubule. T tubules are thin, tubular invaginations of the sarcolemma that penetrate throughout the myofiber cytoplasm. A T tubule surrounds each myofibril at every A–I junction (two/sarcomere). When properly sectioned, the two terminal SR cisternae and T tubule form a triple structure referred to as a *triad.* The major role of the terminal cisternae of the SR is the storage, release, and re-accumulation of calcium ions.

As shown in Fig. 3, the SR between the terminal cisternae anastomose extensively over the surface of the myofibril. Since glycogen phosphorylase is associated with the SR *(9,10)* and glycogen particles can easily be discerned in the sarcoplasm adjacent to the SR (Fig. 5), it can be inferred that this organelle also plays a role in the metabolism of this important energy source.

During excitation–contraction coupling, an action potential originating at the neuromuscular junction sweeps over the sarcolemma (plasma membrane) and into the interior of the myofiber via the T- tubules. This induces voltage-gated calcium channels located in the membrane of SR terminal cisternae to open and permit the exit of calcium ions into the sarcoplasm *(12–14)* (Fig. 6). These ions diffuse between the thick and thin filaments. Calcium attaches to binding sites on troponin C with a resultant spatial change in the configuration of the troponin subunits. Tropomyosin is then pulled away from myosin binding sites on the globular actin, freeing the actin to interact with the head of a cross bridge of the myosin molecule *(11,12)* (Fig. 7). The myosin head pulls the actin along with the myosin filament, resulting in contraction.

Conversely, during relaxation, calcium is vigorously transported back into the SR and is removed from troponin C, allowing a reconfigurational change, i.e., tropomyosin is pulled into position to shield the myosin binding sites on the actin filament. Calcium is stored in the interior of the terminal cistern until the next action potential. The energy required for all these contraction processes is derived from adenosine triphosphate (ATP) which, in turn, is derived from the metabolism of glucose, glycogen, or free fatty acids.

In addition to the system of contractile filaments, the sarcoplasm also contain glycogen, myoglobin, ribosomes and mitochondria. As already mentioned, glycogen is usually associated with cisternae of the SR and is visible in electron micrographs as coarse dark granules. Myoglobin, a protein that contains heme and therefore can bind oxygen, subsequently releases oxygen to mitochondria where oxidative phosphorylation and ATP generation occur. An immunoelectron microscopic study has revealed that myoglobin is located in the cytosol of the I-band *(15)*.

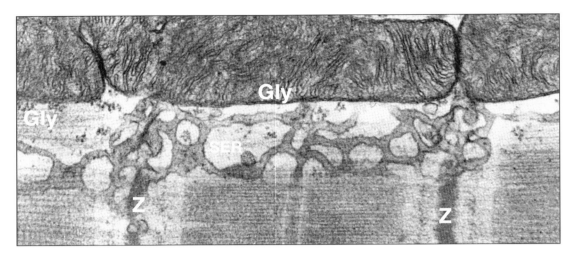

Fig. 5. Electron migrocraph showing smooth endoplasmic reticulum/glycogen relationship. (Reproduced and modified, from Fawcett DW, McNutt NS. *J. Cell Biol,* 1969, **42**:1, by copyright permission from Rockefeller University Press, New York.)

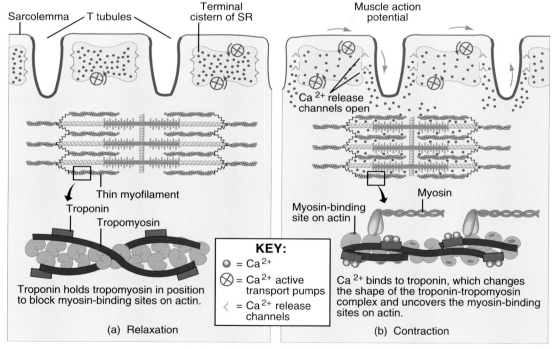

Fig. 6. Schematic representation of the relationship between the T tubules, terminal cisternae, and myofilaments during relaxation (left) and contraction (right) in skeletal muscle. (Reproduced and modified, with permission, from *Introduction to the Human Body,* HarperCollins College Publishers, New York, 1994.)

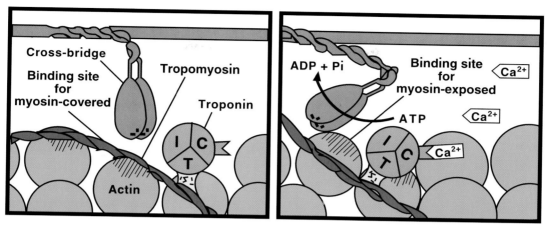

Fig. 7. Schematic representation of calcium binding to troponin C with conformational change of troponin T and resultant exposure of myosin binding site when tropomyosin is moved. (Reproduced and modified, with permission, from Junqueria: Basic Histology, Eighth Edition, Appleton & Lange, Stamford, CT, 1995.)

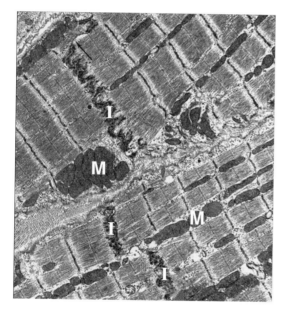

Fig. 8. Electron micrograph demonstrating intercalated disks (I). Note also numerous mitochondria (M). (Reproduced and modified, with permission, from *Junqueria: Basic Histology,* Eighth Edition, Appleton & Lange, Stamford, CT, 1995.)

Skeletal myofibers have many nuclei that are located very close to the sarcolemma. In histologic cross-sections, the nuclei are therefore seen on the periphery of the cell (Fig. 3).

Cardiac Myocytes

At first glance, cardiac muscle appears similar to skeletal muscle. In the past, cardiac muscle tissue was thought to be a syncytium very much like skeletal myofibers. EM has shown that this is not true. In fact, cardiac muscle is composed of individual myocytes separated from one another by cell membranes, although the myocytes are joined together by elaborate, highly modified cell junctions called intercalated disks.

Like skeletal myofibers, the sarcoplasm of cardiac myocytes is subdivided into myofibrils, although these branch and anastomose with each other to a greater extent than the myofibrils of skeletal myofibers. Cardiac myofibrils are composed of thin and thick filaments arranged in sarcomeres, displaying striations comparable to those of skeletal muscle sarcomeres.

As already mentioned, intercalarted disks are the sites where the individual cardiac muscle cells are attached to each other (Fig. 8). In the EM, three types of cell junctions can be seen within the intercalated disks: *fascia adherens, desmosomes,* and *gap junctions (1,3,4)* (Fig. 9).

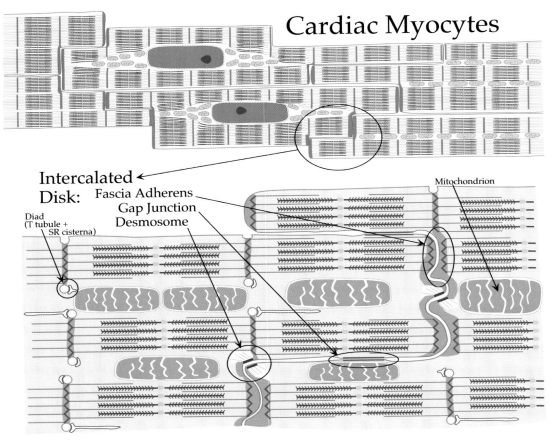

Fig. 9. Schematic representation of intercalated disks between cardiac myocytes. (Drawing by A. W. Clark.)

The fascia adherens is roughly comparable to the zonula adherens, a major component of the junctional complex of epithelial cells. It is comprised of dense, filamentous plaques applied to the cytoplasmic faces of the myocyte plasma membrane. Each plaque is positioned exactly opposite identical dense plaques applied to the cytoplasmic faces of the plasma membrane of the adjacent myocyte. The two plasma membranes (sarcolemmas) are separated, in this region, by a space of approx 20–30 nm and within this space are extracellular glycoproteins that aid in the adhesion of adjacent myocytes. The fascia adherens of the intercalated disk serve as the attachment sites for thin filaments. The other ends of these thin filaments interdigi-

tate with the thick filaments of the inititial myocyte sarcomeres (Fig. 9).

There are two other junctional specializations within an intercalated disk. One of these is the desmosome (macula adherens) another major component of the junctional complex of epithelial cells. Desmosomes also have plaques of dense material applied to the cytoplasmic surfaces of the plasma membrane. These plaques serve as the attachment sites for keratin intermediate filaments. It is inferred that desmosomes assist in maintaining the attachment of myocytes to each other, serving the same function they do in other cell types.

The third component of the intercalated disk is the gap junction that is characterized

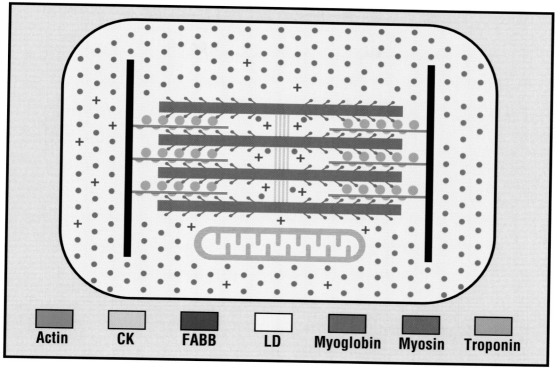

Fig. 10. Schematic summary of the cellular location of markers. (Drawing by R. G. McCord.)

by the very close apposition of adjacent cell membranes. Gap junctions provide ionic continuity between adjacent cells and are thus responsible for the transmission of action potentials from cell to cell.

A major difference between the skeletal myofiber and the cardiac myocyte involves the arrangement of the T tubules and sarcoplasmic reticulum. In cardiac myocytes, T tubules appear at the Z-line of the sarcomere, instead of the A–I junctions. In addition, only one cistern of SR is associated with the T tubule, a configuration called a diad *(17)*.

The SR in cardiac myocytes is not as regularly arranged as the SR of the myofiber and, as a consequence, cardiac myofibrils branch and anastomose with each other to a far greater extent than the myofibrils of skeletal myofibers.

In cardiac muscle, the action potential depends primarily on the entry of calcium

ions from the extracellular space and not from the SR. This is another important difference between cardiac and skeletal muscle.

Because heart muscle is constantly beating and therefore requires a continuous energy source, it is not surprising to see large numbers of mitochondria throughout the myocyte sarcoplasm *(1,3,4)*. Mitochondria account for 40% of the cytoplasmic volume of cardiac myocytes while they account for only 2% of the cytoplasmic volume of many skeletal muscle fibers.

Finally, in contrast to the multinucleate skeletal myofibers, cardiac myocytes usually have a single, centrally placed nucleus, although binucleate myocytes are not that uncommon.

SUMMARY

The intracellular locations of cardiac markers are shown in Fig. 10, CK contributes to the M band. Lactate dehydrogenase (LD) is found in the cytosol and mitochondria. Troponin is found in the sarcoplasm (6%) and as part of the thin filament. Myosin, the major molecular component of the thick filament of the contractile apparatus, is composed of light and heavy chains. Glycogen phosphorylase is located on the inner surfaces of the SR. Fatty acid-binding protein (FABB) and myoglobin are diffusely spread throughout the sarcoplasm. Mitochondrial isoenzymes, such as CK and aspartate aminotransferase, are not currently being investigated as markers for myocardial injury.

ABBREVIATIONS

CK, creatine kinase; EM, electron microscopy; FABB, fatty acid binding protein; H&E, hematoxyline-eosin; LD, lactate dehydrogenase; MM, myomesin; PTAH, phophotungstic acid hematoxylin; RER, rough endoplasmic reticulum; SER, smooth endoplasmic reticulum; SR, sarcoplasmic reticulum

ACKNOWLEDGMENTS

The authors gratefully acknowledge Dr. John Fallon for his suggestions, Dr. Geraldine Gauthier for her reading of the manuscript, and Dr. Alan Wu for the invitation to participate in this book.

REFERENCES

1. Fawcett DW (1994) Bloom and Fawcett: A Textbook of Histology, Chapman & Hall, New York.
2. Squire J (1981) The Structural Basis of Muscular Contraction, Plenum Press, New York.
3. Cormack DH (1993) Essential Histology, J. B. Lippincott Company, Philadelphia, PA.
4. Junqueira LC et al. (1995) Basic Histology, Appleton & Lange, Stamford, CT.
5. Ventura-Clapier R, Veksler V, and Hoerter JA (1994) Myofibrillar creatine kinase and cardiac contraction. Mol. Cell Biochem. 133/134:125–144.
6. Franchi LL, Murdoch A, Brown WE, et al. (1990) Subcellular localisation of newly incorporated myosin in rabbit fast skeletal muscle undergoing stimulation-induced type transformation. J. Musc. Res. Cell. Motil. 11:227–239.
7. Huxley AF and Nierdergerke R (1954) Structural changes in muscle during contraction. Interference microscopy of living muscle fibers. Nature 173:971–973.
8. Jorgensen AO, Shen ACY, Campbell KP, and MacClennan DH (1983) Ultrastructural localization of calsequestrin in rat skeletal muscle by immunoferritin labeling of ultrathin frozen selections. J. Cell Biol. 97:1573–1581.
9. Cuenda A, Nogues M, Gutierrez-Merino C, and de Meis L (1993) Glycogen phosphorolysis can form a metabolic shuttle to support Ca2+ uptake by sarcoplasmic reticulum membranes in skeletal muscle. Biochem. Biophys. Res. Commun. 196:1127–1132.
10. Cuenda A, Henao F, Nogues M, and Gutierrez-Merino C (1994) Quantification and removal of glycogen phosphorylase and other enzymes associated with sarcoplasmic reticulum membrane preparations. Biochim. Biophys. Acta. 1194:35–43.
11. Ganong WF (1995) Review of Medical Physiology, Appleton & Lange, Stamford, CT.
12. Ebashi S, Endo M, and Ohtsuki I (1969) Control of muscle contraction. Q. Rev. Biophys. 2:351–384.
13. Block BA, Imagawa T, Campbell KP, and Franzini-Armstrong C (1988) Structural evidence for direct interaction between the molecular components of the transverse tubule/sarcoplasmic reticulum junction in skeletal muscle. J. Cell Biol. 107:2587–2600.
14. Goodman, SR (1994) Medical Cell Biology, J. B. Lippincott Company, New York.
15. Kawai H, Nishino H, Nishida Y, et al. (1987) Localization of myoglobin in human muscle cells by immunoelectron microscopy. Muscle & Nerve 10:144–149.
16. Widnell CC and Pfenninger KH (1990) Essential Cell Biology, Williams & Wilkins, Baltimore, MD.
17. Willerson JT (1995) Cardiovascular Medicine, Churchill Livingstone, New York.

Part II
Cytoplasmic Markers

6

Myoglobin and Carbonic Anhydrase III

Hemant C. Vaidya and H. Kalervo Vaananen

INTRODUCTION

Currently, the diagnosis of acute myocardial infarction (AMI)* in the first 6–8 h after the infarction is based on the clinical presentation of the patient with typical chest pain and electrocardiogram (ECG). However, chest pain is a nonspecific presentation. Only about 32.5% of patients admitted with chest pain are eventually diagnosed as having AMI. Among the patients with chest pain, typical ECG abnormalities, such as Q-wave changes and ST-T-wave elevation, are observed in 73% of AMI patients (sensitivity 73%) (1–3). Thus, a clinical need has been created to have an adjunctive biochemical marker that can aid in more efficient early diagnosis of AMI. In response to this need, several biochemical markers, such as myoglobin, CK-MM isoforms, CK-MB isoforms, and myosin light chain, are being evaluated for their early diagnostic utility (4,5). Attempts are also being made to enhance the diagnostic efficiency of myoglobin by combining its results with ECG (6–8), CK-MB (9), or carbonic anhydrase III (CAIII) (10–12). Myoglobin is a 17.8-kDa oxygen binding heme protein present in both cardiac and skeletal muscle. It constitutes about 2% of the total muscle protein

and is located in the cytoplasm. Although structurally similar to hemoglobin subunits, its physiological role is not well understood. Cell injury during AMI releases myoglobin into the blood circulation. The relationship between myoglobinemia and myocardial infarction was first reported in 1975 (13).

ANALYTICAL TECHNIQUES

Measurement of Myoglobin in Serum

Myoglobin can be measured in serum specimens by radioimmunoassay (RIA) (14,15), latex agglutination (16–18), or two-site immunoassay (19,20). The first RIA for myoglobin was developed in 1975 with the use of polyclonal antibodies that recognized myoglobin (14). The analytical sensitivity of the assay was 0.5 ng/mL. Since then, several commercial RIAs have been developed.

In an RIA, a sample is mixed with radioactive myoglobin and antimyoglobin antibodies. The antimyoglobin antibodies are then precipitated with the use of a second antibody, and the amount of precipitated radioactivity is measured. The precipitated radioactivity is inversely proportional to the myoglobin concentration in the specimen. The RIAs have intra- and interrun imprecision (coefficient of variation [CV]) of 5 and

---

*See p. 111 for list of abbreviations used in this chapter.

From: Cardiac Markers Edited by: Alan H. B. Wu
© Humana Press Inc., Totowa, NJ

10%, respectively. The long turnaround time to obtain the result, the need for a skilled operator, lack of automation, and the use of radioactive material restrict the use of RIAs in a stat mode that is required for myoglobin.

In the latex agglutination assays, the antimyoglobin antibodies are immobilized on latex particles. When the particles are mixed with a serum sample, they aggregate proportionally to the myoglobin concentration in the specimen. Most of the earlier versions of this particle-based assay gave a semiquantitative result. More recently, turbidimetric (e.g., the Turbitime, Behring Diagnostics, Westwood, MA) (18) and nephelometric (e.g., Nephelometer, Behring) (16) assays have been made available that are quantitative, have rapid turnaround time of <20 min, and show good analytical performance. These rapid assays could potentially be used in an emergency department for the early diagnosis of AMI. However, turbidity of the specimens could interfere in the assays.

Myoglobin can also be measured by monoclonal antibody- (MAb) based two-site immunoassays that can be performed on serum or plasma samples (19,20). In these assays, two MAbs recognizing different epitopes on the myoglobin molecule are used. One of the antibodies is immobilized on a solid support, whereas the other is conjugated to an enzyme or fluorescein. The test specimen is incubated with the antibodies, and the amount of conjugate bound to the particles is measured using appropriate detection systems. The analytical performance claims by the manufacturers of some of the immunoassays are listed in Table 1.

Measurement of Myoglobin and CAIII in Serum

A dual-label, time-resolved fluorometric immunoassay for simultaneous detection of myoglobin and CAIII from the same specimen has been recently reported (21). In this assay, serum sample, europium- (Eu) labeled

CAIII, samarium- (Sm) labeled myoglobin, rabbit antimyoglobin, and anti-CAIII polyclonal antibodies are added to microtiter wells coated with antirabbit IgG antibodies. After a 2-h incubation period, the unbound label is washed, and Eu and Sm bound to the well are measured by time-resolved fluorometry. The selective fluorescence of each analyte bound to the well is inversely proportional to the analyte concentration in the sample. The mean within- and between-run precision (CV) was 4.6 and 6.2% for CAIII and 5.9 and 7.3% for myoglobin, respectively. Although, unique in nature, the current format of this simultaneous assay takes 2 h. It needs to be modified to yield results in a shorter time to meet the stat need for these assays.

CLINICAL UTILITY OF MYOGLOBIN

Normal Levels of Myoglobin

The upper limit of normal for serum myoglobin has been reported to be between 31 and 80 ng/mL (13,16,19). The variation in the values may be owing to the lack of standardization of the analyte or differences between the assay configurations. The normal level of myoglobin is about 25% higher in men than in women (22). Myoglobin values are also known to increase with age in both sexes (19).

Myoglobin Levels in Patients with AMI

In patients with myocardial infarction, the myoglobin level could rise approx 10 times above the upper limit of normal. Myoglobin exhibits a temporal release into the blood circulation. As shown in Fig. 1, the myoglobin level in patients with AMI becomes abnormal within 2 h, peaks in 6–9 h, and returns to normal 24–36 h after the infarction. CK-MB, on the other hand, becomes abnormal in about 6 h, peaks in 12–24 h, and returns to baseline concentrations 48 h after AMI. The early rise in the serum levels of

Table 1
Some Features of Myoglobin Immunoassays[a]

	Stratus	OPUS	RIA	Access®	Technicon Immuno 1
Manufacturer	Behring-Dade, Miami, FL	Behring-Dade, Westwood, MA	Biomerica, Newport Beach, CA	Beckman-Sanofi, Chaska, MN	Bayer Diagnostics, Terrytown, NY
Format	Immunofluorometric assay	Immunofluorometric assay	Radioimmunoassay	Chemiluminescent	Enzyme immunoassay
Antibodies	MAb pair	MAb/polyclonal antibody pair	Polyclonal-antibody	MAb pair	MAB/polyclonal antibody
Assay range, ng/mL	0–1000	0–500	0–250	0–4000	0–3000
Sample type	Serum	Serum	Serum	Serum or EDTA plasma	Serum or plasma
Sample size, µL	200	25	50	10	3
Analytical sensitivity, ng/mL	1.2	1.0	20.0	8.9	1.3
Interassay precision	3.6–6.8%	4.3–5.9%	6.1–8.6 %	2.1–3.7%	2.8–4.2%
Intra-assay precision	1.3–6.3%	3.2–6.9%	2.5–4.7%	4.5–6.4%	5.1–6.1%
Recovery range	92.1–102.3%	93.2–104.8%	79–112%	95.6–104.5	NA
Time to first result	10 min	20 min	~2 h	15 min	24 min
Reference range ng/mL	110	Males: 10–33 Females: 8–31	6–85	70	Males: <84 Females: <50

[a]Information from product insert sheets. NA = not available.

myoglobin compared to CK-MB is attributed to its small molecular size. In patients with myocardial cell injury, intracellular myoglobin is released into the surrounding vascular space. The small molecular size allows myoglobin to translocate rapidly into the systemic blood circulation without going through lymphatic vessels. CK-MB, on the other hand, with a mol wt of about 80 kDa, is translocated into the circulation strictly through the lymphatic system.

Since serum levels of myoglobin become abnormal in patients with AMI beginning about 2 h after the infarction and thrombolytic therapy is most effective within the first 6 h in these patients, several investigators have evaluated the possibility of using myoglobin measurement for the early diagnosis of AMI. In one study, myoglobin levels were determined in 289 patients suspected of having AMI during their stay in the cardiac care unit *(23)*. On the basis of WHO criteria, 162 of 289 patients were found to be non-AMI, whereas 127 patients were confirmed to have AMI. When myoglobin was measured within 8 h after admission ($n = 164$), the clinical sensitivity and specificity for detecting AMI were 97.1 and 97.9%, respectively. However, when myoglobin was measured anytime after admission, the clinical sensitivity and specificity for detecting AMI dropped to 77.2 ($n = 289$) and 96.3%, respectively. The loss of sensitivity was owing to 29 patients in whom myoglobin was measured within 2 h or after 15 h of the infarction. The authors also reported six

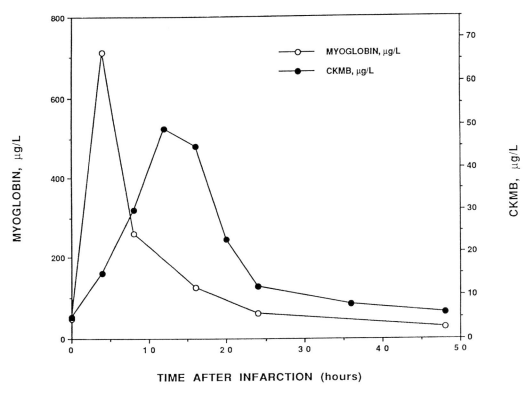

Fig. 1. Typical temporal pattern of serum myoglobin and CK-MB in patients with AMI.

false-positive results because of renal failure ($n = 3$), shock ($n = 2$), and angina ($n = 1$).

Similar clinical performance of myoglobin has also been reported using a rapid immunonephelometric assay for myoglobin *(24)*. These studies suggests that myoglobin may be a good screening assay in an emergency department for the early diagnosis of AMI. However, elevated myoglobin values should be cautiously interpreted if the patient under evaluation for AMI has renal dysfunction or skeletal muscle injury. Because of these limitations of the myoglobin test, a negative myoglobin result in a patient admitted within 2–12 h after the onset of chest pain may help in ruling out AMI, but a positive myoglobin value in a patient suspected of AMI may need confirmation by a more definitive cardiac marker.

Myoglobin and CK-MB

Diagnosis and management of AMI within 48 h of infarction can be greatly improved by the concomitant measurement of myoglobin and CK-MB. This is because the temporal patterns of these two markers complement each other in this time period (Figs. 1 and 2). To improve the clinical performance of the myoglobin assay, CK-MB can also be measured on single or sequential samples collected on admission and 4 h later from patients with and without AMI *(9)*. Patients with cardiogenic shock, cardiac arrest, or electrical defibrillation were excluded from the study. In this study, the diagnostic sensitivity, specificity, positive predictive value (PPV), and negative predictive value (NPV) of myoglobin and CK-MB on the two samples (collected at 0

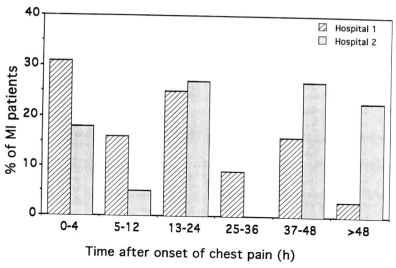

Fig. 2. Time between onset of chest pain and first serum sample for CK-MB and LD1 analysis at two major (>500 bed) hospitals. The percentage of AMI patients is plotted against the time when the first sample was drawn in the emergency department.

and 4 h) was computed along with the diagnostic performance of increase in myoglobin and/or CK-MB values in 4 h. The results of this study suggest that 100% NPV (to rule out AMI) can be obtained by measuring the change of myoglobin or CK-MB values during the first 4h after admission of patients for AMI evaluation. In addition, the authors found that abnormal myoglobin values for samples collected on admission or at 4 h after admission had 100% PPV (to rule in AMI). Similar results were obtained when the clinical utility of myoglobin and CK-MB was measured over a 12-h period in an emergency department population *(25)*.

Myoglobin and Electrocardiography

Electrocardiography is routinely performed on patients suspected of having AMI. If the history of the patient suggests that the onset of typical chest pain was within 6 h before admission and the ECG is abnormal, the clinicians may treat the patient with thrombolytic agents. However, as stated ear-

lier, chest pain is a nonspecific presentation, and some 27% of the patients with AMI do not show typical ECG changes. Therefore, a significant number of AMI patients may not receive thrombolytic therapy because of the inability of early disease diagnosis. Since myoglobin has been shown to be an early biochemical marker, attempts have been made to use ECG along with myoglobin to improve the efficiency of early AMI diagnosis *(6–8)*. In one study, 70 patients admitted to the emergency department with chest pain were evaluated by stepwise use of ECG and serum myoglobin values *(8)*. The efficiency of AMI diagnosis was found to be 62% with the use of ECG alone and was increased to 82% with the multivariate use of ECG and myoglobin. These results strongly suggest that myoglobin is a good adjunct to ECG for the early diagnosis of AMI. Similar studies on a larger scale are required to convince the clinicians to use myoglobin along with ECG for the early diagnosis of AMI. Inclusion of mid to late markers, like CK-MB, cardiac troponin I (cTnI), and lactate dehydrogenase 1 (LD1) measurement, in such studies may help to identify the patients admitted after 6 h of the onset of chest pain *(24)*.

Myoglobin and CAIII

CAIII is a 28-kDa cytoplasmic protein present in skeletal muscle, but not in cardiac muscle *(10)*. Myoglobin, on the other hand, is present in both skeletal and cardiac muscle. Release of myoglobin from skeletal muscle decreases its specificity in the diagnosis of AMI. Several recent studies have shown the appearance and disappearance of CAIII closely follow the release of myoglobin from skeletal muscle (Fig. 3) *(11,26,27)*. These studies demonstrate that the ratio of myoglobin to CAIII in serum remains constant after skeletal muscle injury, yet displays a temporal pattern following myocardial injury. In a pilot study, the myoglobin to CAIII ratio in the serum of AMI patients was found to be clearly elevated when compared to patients with neuromuscular disease or healthy controls before and after physical exercise *(11)*. In a follow-up study, serum myoglobin to CAIII ratio was measured at the time of admission in 267 patients admitted to a hospital with a history of symptoms suggesting AMI *(12)*. The specificity, sensitivity, PPV and NPV of the ratio for diagnosis of AMI were 96, 84, 76, and 97%, respectively. The diagnostic performance of the myoglobin to CAIII ratio was better than that of CK, CK-MB, or myoglobin alone. In another recent study with 251 consecutive patients presenting to the emergency department within 12 h of chest pain, myoglobin/CAIII ratio was significantly more sensitive and equally specific as CK-MB for the early diagnosis of patients with AMI *(28)*.

Elevation of Myoglobin Levels in Non-AMI Conditions

The serum level of myoglobin is elevated in various conditions other than AMI as

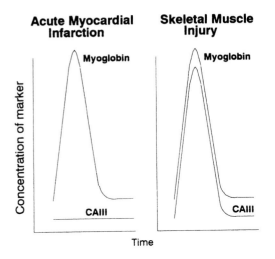

Fig. 3. Comparison of myoglobin and CAIII in AMI and acute skeletal muscle injury. Although myoglobin is increased in both, CAIII is more specific to skeletal muscles and is normal in patients with AMI.

listed in Table 2. As stated earlier, myoglobin is present in both skeletal and cardiac muscle. Thus, the patients with AMI and heart surgery release myoglobin from heart muscle, whereas people who perform exhaustive exercise, have skeletal muscle injury, or are genetic carriers of progressive muscular dystrophy release myoglobin from skeletal muscle *(29,30)*. Since serum myoglobin is eliminated from the circulation through kidneys, renal failure could also elevate the levels of serum myoglobin *(24)*. Extensive release of myoglobin from skeletal muscles will result in rhabdomyolysis-induced renal failure *(30,31)*. Failure to clear myoglobin by the kidneys further aggrevates and perpetuates this condition. Measurement of urine myoglobin concentrations and calculation of the ratio of urine to serum, or if urine volume is known, the myoglobin clearance rate, are useful in identifying rhabdomyolysis patients who are at high risk for developing renal failure *(32,33)*. Serum myoglobin concentrations coupled with a low clearance rate put the

Table 2
Serum Myoglobin Concentration in Various Conditions

Conditions in which serum myoglobin levels are increased:
AMI
Open heart surgery
Exhaustive exercise
Skeletal muscle damage
Patients and genetic carriers of progressive muscular dystrophy
Shock
Severe renal failure
Following intramascular injections (variable)
Conditions in which serum myoglobin levels remain normal:
Healthy adults
Chest pain without AMI
Congestive heart failure with AMI
Cardiac catheterization
Moderate exercise

patient at greatest risk. These patients should be immediately treated with alkalinization and mannitol *(34)*.

Myoglobinemia cause by skeletal muscle damage and renal disease limits the use of myoglobin as a diagnostic test for AMI. However, clinical presentation and renal function tests of patient being evaluated for AMI can help rule out some of the non-AMI conditions that can cause elevation of myoglobin concentration in blood.

Myoglobin Levels after Reperfusion

It is now well established that the patients with AMI who present to the emergency room within 6 h of the onset can be managed effectively by thrombolytic therapy. However, the success of the therapy is not complete. Approximately 20% of the infract-related arteries fail to open following the treatment. To assess the success or failure of thrombolysis, patients are often evaluated by coronary arteriogram. This procedure is

highly sensitive, but is invasive, requires cardiac catheterization, and is expensive to perform. It is not available at many hospitals. Alternately, several noninvasive and less expensive parameters to determine the recanalization of the artery have been suggested. These include relief of chest discomfort, occurrence of reperfusion arrhythmia, normalization of ST-segment elevation, and rapid rise of biochemical markers, such as myoglobin, CK-MB, and cTnI *(30,35,36)*. Among these parameters, biochemical markers are the most sensitive. Since myoglobin is a smaller mol-wt protein than CK-MB and cTnI, its temporal release pattern is earlier than others. Serial measurement of serum myoglobin in patients undergoing thrombolytic therapy has shown that the myoglobin level peaks approx 2 h after reperfusion of the occluded artery. Prediction of the success or failure of reperfusion can be determined by the myoglobin concentration–time curves using two indices. The time required for myoglobin concentration to rise from 25–100% of the peak value has been reported to be 71 ± 7.9 min in reperfused population and 341 ± 35.3 min for the nonreperfused population *(37)*. Alternately, when the rate of rise of myoglobin in 2 h is calculated, 85% of the reperfused patients had a >4.6-fold increase in myoglobin values over their initial myoglobin values, and in 100% of the nonreperfused patients, this increase in myoglobin values was <4.6-fold *(37)*. A typical temporal pattern of myoglobin in reperfused and nonreperfused patients is shown in Fig. 4. Thus, measurement of myoglobin following thrombolytic therapy is a good noninvasive alternative to evaluate successful recanalization of the occluded artery, especially when coronary arteriogram is not available or appropriate for a given patient. It should be mentioned that the coronary artery patency is very dynamic, and can spontaneously reocclude or reperfuse at any moment. Thus, the clinical impression of

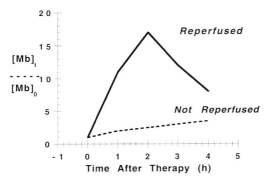

Fig. 4. Typical temporal pattern of serum myoglobin following thrombolytic therapy in reperfused and nonreperfused patients. $[Mb]_t$, myoglobin concentration at time "t" and $[Mb]_0$, myoglobin concentration just before thrombolytic therapy.

reperfusion must also be considered when evaluating patients.

Myoglobin in Reinfarction

The rapid clearance of myoglobin from blood following AMI enables this marker to be useful in the detection of reinfarction and myocardial extensions. Table 3 illustrates two such cases. In case #1, the diagnosis of AMI is initially established with the 8-h specimen, since all markers are above their respective cutoff concentrations. By 50 h, the myoglobin result has returned to normal, whereas each of the other markers remains increased. Beginning at 58 h and especially at 82 h, the myoglobin result has increased above the cutoff concentration, indicating the presence of new myocardial injury owing to a reinfarction. Results for CK-MB and cTnI may still reflect the presence of injury from the original infarction.

Case #2 is an AMI patient who suffered complications. Essentially all cardiac markers are elevated at each time-point from 4–96 h after AMI. The presence of complications cannot be discerned by examining the results for CK-MB or cTnI, since they appear typical for AMI. However, results for myoglobin

Table 3
Use of Myoglobin for Detection of Reinfarction and Extension[a]

Time, h	cTnI	Myoglobin	CK-MB
Case #1			
2	0.95	15	4.0
8	5.5	52	29
41	7.9	58	31
50	5.6	16	8.6
58	4.8	40	5.1
70	2.8	31	2.2
82	2.6	128	4.5
Case #2			
4	1.8	102	2.8
7	97	>625	161
12	>150	>625	177
20	>150	309	66
28	96	>625	161
48	23	291	7.8
96	85	>625	22

[a]All results in ng/mL and were obtained on the Opus Plus (Behring). Cutoff time given after onset of AMI concentrations: cTnI 2.5, CK-MB 5.0, and myoglobin 33 ng/mL.

clearly show that in the absence of new skeletal muscle or renal disease, cardiac injury is ongoing. These cases illustrate the role myoglobin has in clinical management.

CONCLUSIONS

Myoglobin is a controversial biochemical marker for the diagnosis of AMI. Myoglobin, if measured within 2–12 h after infarction, offers high clinical sensitivity and specificity. However, false-positive results can be seen owing to skeletal muscle injury or renal failure. False-positive results owing to skeletal muscle damage can be identified by careful clinical history, and may be eliminated by determining the myoglobin to CAIII ratio. False-positive results owing to renal failure can be identified by the kidney function tests, like serum creatinine, blood urea nitrogen, and urine myoglobin testing. False-negative results owing to late admissions (12–24 h after infarction) can be identified by concomitant measurement of CK-MB and LD1. The efficiency of early diagnosis of AMI can be improved when clinical history and ECG are taken into account along with the myoglobin values. Efficiency could also be improved by measuring sequential samples within 4 h after admission. A serum myoglobin level can be a useful indicator of successful reperfusion following thrombolytic therapy. The utility of myoglobin should be greatly enhanced with the availability of rapid commercial assays for the early diagnosis and management of patients with AMI.

ABBREVIATIONS

AMI, Acute myocardial infarction; CAIII, carbonic anhydrase III; CK, creatine kinase; CV, coefficient of variation; ECG, electrocardiogram; Eu, eurpoium; kDa, kilodaltons; LD, lactate dehydrogenase; NPV, negative predictive value; PPV, positive predictive value; RIA, radioimmunoassay; Sm, samarium; WHO, World Health Organization.

REFERENCES

1. Anderson HV and Willerson JT (1993) Thrombolysis in acute myocardial infarction. N. Engl. J. Med. 329:703–709.
2. Jagger JD, Murray RG, Davies MK, Littler WA, and Flint EJ (1987) Eligibility for thrombolytic therapy in acute myocardial infarction. Lancet i:34–35.
3. Lott JA (1984) Serum enzyme determinations in the diagnosis of acute myocardial infarction: an update. Hum. Pathol. 15: 706–716.
4. Puleo P and Roberts R (1989) Early biochemical markers of myocardial necrosis. Cardiovasc. Clin. 20:143–154.
5. Kaplan LA and Stein EA (1985) In search for biochemical marker of MI. Diagn. Med. 8:25–33.
6. Sederholm M and Sylven C (1983) Relation between ST and QRS vector changes and myoglobin release in acute myocardial infarction. Cardiovasc. Res. 17:589–594.
7. Grottum P, Sederholm M, and Kjekshus JK (1987) Quantitative and temporal relation between the release of myoglobin and creatine kinase and the evolution of vectorcardiographic changes during acute myocardial infarction in man. Cardiovasc. Res. 21: 652–659.
8. Ohman EM, Casey C, Bengston JR, Prior D, Tormey W, and Horgan JH (1990) Early detection of acute myocardial infarction: additional information from serum concentration of myoglobin in patients without ST elevation. Br. Heart. J. 63:335–338.
9. van Blerk M, Maes V, Huyghens L, Derde MP, Meert R, and Gorus FK (1992) Analytical and clinical evaluation of creatine kinase MB mass assay by IMx: comparison with MB isoenzyme activity and serum myoglobin for early diagnosis of myocardial infarction. Clin. Chem. 38:2380–2386.
10. Kato K and Mokuno K (1984) Distribution of immunoreactive carbonic anhydrase III in human tissue, determined by a sensitive enzyme immunoassay method. Clin. Chim. Acta. 141:169–177.
11. Vaananen HK, Syrjala H, Rahkila P, Vuori J, Melamies LM, Myllyla V, Takala TE (1990) Serum carbonic anhydrase III and myoglobin concentrations in acute myocardial infarction. Clin. Chem. 36:635–638.
12. Vuori J, Syrjala H, and Vaananen HK (1996) Myoglobin carbonic anhydrase III ratio: Highly specific and sensitive early indicator for myocardial damage in acute myocardial infarction. Clin. Chem. 42:107–109.
13. Kagen L, Scheidt S, Roberts L, Porter A, and Pau H (1975) Myoglobinemia following myocardial infarction. Am. J. Med. 58: 177–182.
14. Stone MJ, Willerson JT, Gomez-Sanchez CE, and Waterman MR (1975) Radioimmunoassay of myoglobin in human serum. Results in patients with acute myocardial infarction. J. Clin. Invest. 56:1334–1339.
15. Kubasik NP, Guiney W, Warren K, D'Souza JP, Sine HE, and Brody BB (1978) Radioimmunoassay of serum myoglobin: evaluation of a commercial kit and assessment of its usefulness for detecting acute myocardial infarction. Clin. Chem. 24:2047–2049.
16. Massoubre C, Chivot L, Mainard F, Bridjii B, and Madec Y (1991) Immunonephelo-

metric assay for myoglobin. Clin. Chim. Acta. 201:223–230.

17. Chapelle JP and Heusghem C (1985) Semi-quantitative estimation of serum myoglobin by a rapid agglutination method: an emergency screening test for acute myocardial infarction. Clin. Chim. Acta. 145: 143–150.

18. Delanghe J, Chapelle JP, el Allaf M, and De Buyzere M (1991) Quantitative turbidimetric assay for determining myoglobin evaluated. Ann. Clin. Biochem. 28:474–479.

19. Chapelle JP, Lemache K, el Allaf M, el Allaf D, and Pierard L (1994) Fast determination of myoglobin in serum using a new radial partition immunoassay. Clin. Biochem. 27:423–428.

20. Silva DP, Landt Y, Porter SE, and Ladenson JE (1991) Development and application of monoclonal antibodies to human cardiac myoglobin in a rapid fluorescence immunoassay. Clin. Chem. 37:1356–1364.

21. Vuori J, Rasi S, Takala T, and Vaananen K (1991) Dual-label time resolved fluoroimmunoassay for simultaneous detection of myoglobin and carbonic anhydrase III in serum. Clin. Chem. 37:2087–2092.

22. Delanghe JR, Chapelle JP, and Vanderschueren SC (1990) Quantitative nephelometric assay for determining myoglobin evaluated. Clin. Chem. 36:1675–1678.

23. Reese L and Uksik P (1981) Radioimmunoassay of serum myoglobin in screening for acute myocardial infarction. Can. Med. Assoc. J. 124:1585–1588.

24. Collins R and Tucker J (1991) Myoglobin and CK-MB for the diagnosis of acute myocardial infarction in emergency room patients. Clin. Chem. 37:978.

25. Brogan GX, Friedman S, McCuskey C, Cooling DS, Berratti L, Thorde HC, and Bock JL (1994) Evaluation of a new rapid quantitative immunoassay for serum myoglobin versus CK-MB for ruling out myocardial infarction in the emergency department. Ann. Emerg. Med. 24:665–671.

26. Takala TES, Rahkila P, Hakala E, Vuori J, Puranen J, and Vaananen K (1989) Serum carbonic anhydrase III, an enzyme of type I muscle fibers and the intensity of physical exercise. Pflugers Arch. 413:447–450.

27. Syrjala H, Vuori J, Huttunen K, and Vaananen HK (1990) Carbonic anhydrase III as a marker for diagnosis of rhabdomyolysis. Clin. Chem. 36:696.

28. Borgan GX, Vuori J, Friedman S, McCuskey CF, Thorde HC, and Vananen HK, Coolin DS, Bock JL (1996) Improved specificity of myooglobin plus carbonic anhydrase assay versus that of creatine kinase MB for early diagnosis of acute myocardial infarction. Ann. Emerg. Med. 27:22–28.

29. Stone MJ and Willerson JT (1983) Myoglobinemia in myocardial infarction. Int. J. Cardiol. 4:49–52.

30. Varki AP, Roby DS, Watts H, and Zatuchni J (1978) Serum myoglobin in acute myocardial infarction: A clinical study and review of the literature. Am. Heart J. 96:680–688.

31. Hamilton RW, Hopkins MB, and Shihabi ZK (1989) Myoglobinuria, hemoglobinuria, and acute renal failure. Clin. Chem. 35: 1713–1720.

32. Wu AHB, Laios I, Green S, Gornet TG, Wong SS, Parmaley L, Tonnesen A, Plaisier B, and Orlando R (1994) Immunoassays for serum and urine myoglobin: myoglobin clearance assessed as a risk factor for acute renal failure. Clin. Chem. 40:796–802.

33. Laios I, Caruk R, and Wu AHB (1995) Myoglobin clearance as an early indicator for rhabdomyolysis-induced acute renal failure. Ann. Clin. Lab. Sci. 25:179–184.

34. Eneas JF, Schoefeld PY, and Humphreys MH (1979) The effect of infusion of mannitol-sodium bicarbonate on the clinical course of myoglobinuria. Arch. Intern. Med. 139:801–805.

35. Ellis AK, Little T, Mansud ARZ, and Klocke FJ (1985) Pattern of myoglobin release after reperfusion of injured myocardium. Circulation 72:639–647.

36. Apple FS, Henry TD, Berger CR, and Landt YA (1996) Early monitoring of serum cardiac troponin I for assessment of coronary reperfusion following thrombolytic therapy. Am. J. Clin. Pathol. 105:6–10.

37. Ellis AK, Little T, Mansud ARZ, Livermann HA, Morris DC, and Klocke FJ (1988) Early non-invasive detection of successful reperfusion in patients with acute myocardial infarction. Circulation 78:1352–1357.

7

Creatine Kinase, Isoenzymes, and Variants

Alan H. B. Wu

TOTAL CREATINE KINASE

Biochemistry

Creatine kinase (CK)* (EC 2.7.3.2, adenosine triphosphate:creatine N-phosphotransferase) exists as a dimer, and is an important enzyme regulator of high-energy phosphate production and utilization within contractile tissues. Recent studies suggest that CK also has a more general role in shuttling high-energy phosphate bonds via creatine phosphate (CP) from the site of ATP production in the mitochondria to the site of utilization within the cytoplasm *(1)*. The "shuttle hypothesis" is supported by observations that CK is found in some tissues, such as the distal tubules of the nephron, that have high energy needs. Although the distal tubules have no contractile function, they nevertheless require ATP for maintenance of ionic gradients through the ATP-dependent sodium-potassium membrane pump *(2)*.

CK catalyzes the phosphorylation of creatine (produced in the kidneys, liver, and pancreas) by adenosine triphosphate (ATP) to form CP and adenosine diphosphate (ADP):

$$\text{Creatine} + \text{ATP} \xrightarrow{\text{CK}} \text{CP} + \text{ADP} \quad (1)$$

In the mitochondria, ATP generated by oxidative phosphorylation is converted to CP by this forward reaction by mitochondrial isoenzymes (Fig. 1). CP is transported to the cytoplasm and stored. During muscle contraction, the cytoplasmic isoenzymes catalyze the reverse CK reaction and the *in situ* regeneration of ATP needed to support muscle metabolism. The use of CP as an energy storage form has advantages over ATP directly. Use of CP makes ADP produced from the above reaction immediately available for reoxidative phosphorylation within the mitochondria, thereby eliminating the delay for ADP to diffuse back into the mitochondrial matrix *(3)*.

Because of its size (>80 kDa), CK is not filtered through the glomerulus, and therefore, it is not cleared through the kidneys. Unlike amylase and lipase, total CK is not increased in patients with acute renal failure. Some investigators have suggested that CK and other enzymes, such as aspartate aminotransferase and lactate dehydrogenase, are cleared through the reticuloendothelial (RE) system, such as in the liver *(4)*. This hypothesis is supported by studies using zymosan, a polysaccharide that is an inhibitor of particle uptake by the RE system. Zymosan has

---

*See pp. 122–123 for list of abbreviations used in this chapter.

From: Cardiac Markers   Edited by: Alan H. B. Wu
© Humana Press Inc., Totowa, NJ

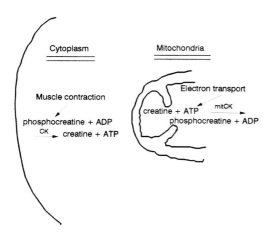

Fig. 1. Biologic functions of mitochondrial and cytolic isoenzymes of CK. (Used with permission from Wu AHB (1991) Enzymes in cardiovascular and skeletal muscle diseases. In: Clinical Chemistry, Wu AHB, Chan KM, Hursting MJ, Lott JA, Spillman T, and Wheaton D. eds. Bethesda, MD, Health and Education Resources.)

been shown to reduce the in vivo clearance rate of CK *(5)*. Other clearance mechanisms, however, may also be involved, since the removal of the liver does not appear to alter the clearance rate of CK *(6)*. For example, the clearance of lactate dehydrogenase isoenzymes appears to be related to macrophage activity *(7)*.

Laboratory Analysis

The analysis for total CK in serum requires coupling of the reverse reaction to hexokinase and glucose-6-phosphate dehydrogenase (G-6-PD) to produce NADPH. The rate of product formation is monitored spectrophotometrically. There have been many methods described for the analysis of CK. The method described by Oliver and revised by Rosalki, however, has been universally accepted and is used in clinical laboratories worldwide:

$$\text{Creatine phosphate + ADP} \xrightarrow{\text{CK}} \text{creatine + ATP} \quad (2)$$

$$\text{ATP + glucose} \xrightarrow{\text{hexokinase}} \text{glucose-6-phosphate + ADP} \quad (3)$$

$$\text{Glucose-6-phosphate + NADP}^+ \xrightarrow{\text{G-6-PD}} \text{6-phosphogluconate + NADPH + H}^+ \quad (4)$$

The activities of the coupling enzymes are present in excess concentrations, so that the CK reaction is rate-limiting. The production of NADPH per unit of time is computed by measuring its absorptivity in a spectrophotometer at 340 nm. The forward reaction has an optimum pH between 6.5 and 6.7. (The reverse reaction has an optimum of 9.0 and can proceed some six times faster.) CK requires magnesium ions and use of an activator for maximum recovery of enzyme activity. Thiols, such as *N*-acetyl-L-cysteine (NAC), β-mercaptoethanol, dithiothreitol, dithioerythriotol, and glutathione, have been used so that reactive thiol groups on CK remain oxidized. EDTA is added to prevent auto-oxidation of activators, and to chelate calcium and ferric ions, which can inhibit the CK reaction. Adenosine monophosphate (AMP) and diadenosine-5-pentaphosphate (DAPP) are added to inhibit adenylate kinase (AK). This enzyme is found in erythrocytes and the liver, and can produce falsely increased apparent CK activity when present in appreciable concentrations:

$$2\text{ADP} \xrightarrow{\text{AK}} \text{ATP + AMP} \quad (5)$$

Numerous national committees have made recommendations for a standardized CK assay. The assays recommended by these organizations are very similar to one another with only minor changes in reagent concentrations and conditions. Those recommended by the International Federation of Clinical Chemistry (IFCC) assay are listed in Table 1 *(8)*. As shown in Fig. 2, the IFCC and most of the others describe a two-step assay.

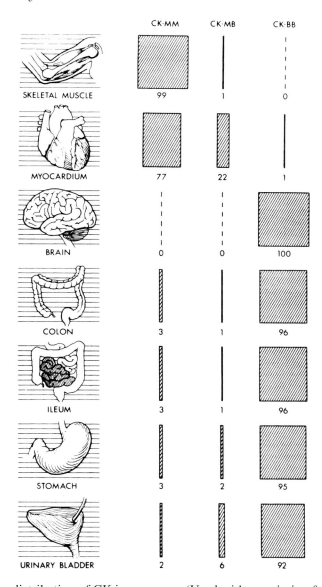

Fig. 4. Tissue distribution of CK isoenzymes. (Used with permission from ref. *20.*)

smooth muscles, including the stomach, colon, bladder, uterus, and prostate, and is the major CK isoenzyme found in the fetus. CK-BB is also released in some cases of breast, colon, and prostate cancers *(22)*, although the clinical utility of CK-BB, a tumor marker, has been questioned *(23)*.

The heart has the third highest concentration of total CK at about 500 U/g wet wt. It is also the organ with the highest concentration of CK-MB activity, estimated to be between 15 and 40%, with the remaining activity being largely owing to CK-MM. Following acute myocardial infarction (AMI), there is an increase in total CK activity in serum, and an absolute and relative increase in the CK-MB isoenzyme. For the past several decades, analysis of CK-MB has been the hallmark for the biochemical diagnosis of AMI.

Normal Range for CK Isoenzymes

The reference interval for CK-MB is dependent on the methods used. For activity-based assays (electrophoresis, column chromatography, or immunoinhibition), the upper limit of normal (ULN) ranges between 10 and 20 U/L or 4 and 6% of total activity. For immunoassays (mass measurements), the ULN is between 5 and 10 ng/mL or 2 and 4% of total. Individuals who train for long distance races (e.g., marathon running) have very high resting concentrations of CK-MB. This may be owing to an adaptation by the athlete to produce a higher relative content of CK-MB within the skeletal muscles themselves (24). The normal CK-BB activity in serum, as measured by electrophoresis, is below the detection limit (i.e., <5 U/L). There are currently no commercial immunoassays specific for CK-BB. However, it is likely that normal concentrations of CK-BB are under 1 ng/mL.

The reference range for total CK is higher in children than adults (25). Values are about twice as high in neonates and gradually decline as the child grows older. The pediatric CK isoenzyme distribution also changes from CK-BB found predominately *in utero*, to CK-MB, and then to the CK-MM form, which predominates in adults. Unlike measurement of total CK, which is useful for monitoring children with muscular dystrophies, assay of isoenzymes has questionable clinical significance.

CK-MB in Myocardial Infarction

An AMI is characterized by the release of cardiac enzymes and proteins from ischemic areas to the blood. The activity of total CK begins to increase within 4–6 h after the onset of chest pain, and remains abnormal for 48–72 h. For patients without electrocardiographic (ECG) evidence of AMI (non-Q-wave subendocardial), total CK activity ranges from the ULN to about a threefold increase. Because the reference limit is very broad, an AMI occuring in small, sedentary individual may have a peak total CK activity that is within the ULN. This is possible if the baseline CK is very low prior to the onset of injury.

For AMI patients with positive ECG results (transmural), total CK activities can be as high as 10–20 times the upper reference limit. Peak enzyme activities for AMI patients with permanent coronary artery occlusions usually occur between 18 and 24 h. For those AMI patients who have spontaneous or thrombolytic therapy-induced recanalization, an accelerated release of CK and other cardiac proteins is observed ("wash-out phenomenon"). This results in peak concentrations that occur a few hours sooner and at higher activities than patients with permanent occlusions. Total CK has high clinical sensitivity for diagnosis of AMI (>90%), but results are not specific for myocardial injury. As described in Table 2, various nonmyocardial conditions will increase total CK.

The CK-MB isoenzyme has been considered the "gold standard" for diagnosis of AMI. CK-MB can be measured either by enzyme activity (column chromatography, electrophoresis, or immunoinhibition) or mass concentrations (immunoassays). These assay methods are described in Chapters 8 and 9. The release of CK-MB from damaged myocytes parallels release of total CK from these tissues. As such, the clinical sensitivity for CK-MB in AMI patients is similar. For clinical specificity, CK-MB is decidedly better than total CK. High activity or concentration of CK-MB is indicative of myocardial injury, especially when the amount of this isoenzyme relative to total CK ("relative index") is also increased. The clinical sensitivity of this marker may be higher than for total CK, even though both are simultaneously released from injured tissues. This is because measurement of

Table 3
Myocardial Sources of Abnormal CK-MB in Serum

Cardiovascular diseases	Surgical procedures	Skeletal muscle
AMI	Open heart surgery	Normal children
Unstable angina pectoris	Coronary artery bypass graft	Acute skeletal muscle injury
Congestive heart failure	Valve replacement	Chronic skeletal muscle injury
Arrhythmia and tachycardia	Coronary angioplasty	Myositis
Pulmonary emboli	w/complications	Cocaine use
	Directional atherectomy	

CK-MB in serum is more indicative of myocardial injury than total CK and a lower cutoff concentration can be used.

Abnormal CK-MB Concentrations Not Associated with AMI

The assay for CK-MB is one of the few enzyme tests that historically has been directly linked to a single disease rather than being indicative of several related and unrelated disorders of a particular organ. The exclusive association of CK-MB with AMI, however, has no pathophysiological basis. CK-MB is increased in any diagnostic or surgical condition that is associated with myocardial injury. Abnormal concentrations can also be the result of release from skeletal muscles. Table 3 lists conditions other than AMI that can produce increases in CK-MB (9). In addition to these, there have been two cases of ectopic production of CK-MB by malignancy (26,27).

Clinical Significance of CK-BB in Brain Injury

CK-BB is found in high concentrations in the central nervous system and smooth muscles. Therefore, an increase in this isoenzyme is expected in the cerebral spinal fluid (CSF) and serum of patients with injuries to these tissues (see Table 4). In one study, 14 of 15 patients with brain contusions had increases in CSF CK-BB (28). Increased CSF CK-BB has been linked to the Liege

coma scale with high activity linked to a poor prognosis (29). The increase in CK-BB in blood of patients with injury to the brain and central nervous system may be caused by a breakdown in the blood–brain barrier and leakage of enzymes from the CSF. Under normal circumstances, this barrier should exclude leakage of this protein into the blood. In 26 patients with brain injury, half had detectable concentrations of CK-BB by electrophoresis (30). The significance of CK-BB in serum is unknown, however, since one study using a sensitive and specific immunochemical assay for CK-BB showed no correlation with CK-BB activity with the size of brain lesions (31). As such, CK-BB is not routinely used in clinical practice.

CK ISOENZYME VARIANTS

The origins of the classical isoenzymes of CK-MM, MB, and BB in serum can be traced to release from selected organs that contain these isoenzymes. CK-MM and MB isoforms are natural serum degradation products of single tissue isoenzymes. The biochemistry and clinical significance of isoforms will be described in Chapter 10. Atypical or isoenzyme variants do not have a tissue origin and are not normally observed in healthy individuals. Two major high-mol-wt forms have been identified and have been termed as "macro-CK" types 1 and 2 (32). These isoenzymes are not routinely measured, since they do not appear to have

Table 4
Causes of Abnormal CK-BB in Serum

Central nervous system disorders	Neoplasms
Seizures	Breast
Brain infarction	Prostate
Head injury	Colon
Delirium tremens	
Hypoxic shock	

clinical utility. However, their presence will interfere with some methods of analysis for CK-MB, including immunoinhibition and electrophoresis. Further details of these interferences are discussed under the corresponding chapters.

Macro-CK Type 1

The presence of a CK variant was first identified in the late 1970s as a band migrating between CK-MM and CK-MB by electrophoresis (33). Subsequent studies with specific antibodies have shown that this isoenzyme consists of CK-BB linked with the Fab portion of immunoglobulin IgG. Table 5 shows the characteristics of this variant. A diagrammatic representation of the type 1 variant is shown in Fig. 3. Gradient gel electrophoresis studies showed that macro-CK has a mol wt of about 340 kDa. Since monomeric IgA has a mol wt of 160 kDa, the stoichiometry of macro-CK is probably 2:1 (BB:IgG). Unlike CK-MB and BB, which are very labile, macro-CK type 1 is very resistant to heat denaturation. This may help explain why the type 1 variant tends to persist in blood at increased activities for many months or years. The prevalence of macro-CK type has been estimated to be under 4% of hospitalized patients (34). It is observed most frequently in elderly women. Macro-CK type 1 is not associated with any particular disease and has been observed in normal individuals (35). A rarer form of

macro-CK is the linkage of CK-BB with IgA (36). The finding of this form is more significant for laboratories performing CK isoenzyme measurements by electrophoresis, since this variant comigrates with CK-MB. Linkage of CK-MM with IgA and CK-MB to IgG has also been described, with electrophoretic migration near CK-MM.

Macro-CK Type 2

The characteristics of the type 2 variant are also shown in Table 5. Like type 1, this isoenzyme is rarely seen, has a high molecular weight, and is heat-stable. This atypical isoenzyme, however, is not linked to immunoglobulins and is not affected by anti-CK-M or B antibodies, and is thought to be a oligomeric complex of mitochondrial CK. The occurrence of macro-CK type 2 with clinical diseases has been studied by a number of investigators. In adults, this variant isoenzyme is seen almost exclusively in patients with hepatic cirrhosis and metastatic disease, and its presence is associated with a poor prognosis (34,37). In many malignant patients, CK-BB has also been found with macro-CK type 2 (34). However, this enzyme does not appear to have any clinical significance, since it has poor sensitivity for disease and lacks prognostic value in nonmalignant liver diseases (38). Macro-CK can also be observed in neonates (34,39). Unlike adults with malignancies, the enzyme correlates with the presence of myocardial injury, and neonates with macro-CK type 2 have a good prognosis.

ABBREVIATIONS

ADP, adeonsine diphosphate; AK, adenylate kinase; AMI, acute myocardial infarction; AMP, adeonsine monophosphate; ATP, adenosine triphosphate; CBM, Commission on Biochemical Nomenclature; CK, creatine kinase; CP, creatine phosphate; CSF, cerebrospinal fluid; DAPP, diadenosine-

Table 5
Characteristics of Macro-CK Types 1 and 2

Parameter	Type 1	Type 2
Isoenzyme form	CK-BB, MM	Mitochondrial
Molecular weight	340,000	Variable, from 250→750,000
Stability at 45°C	Stable	Stable
Electrophoretic migration	Usually between MM and MB	Cathodic to CK-MM
Immunoglobulin bound	IgG, IgA (rarer)	None
Presence in serum	Persistent	Transient
Prevalence	<4%	<4%
Clinical significance	None	Adults: metastatic disease
		Neonates: myocardial injury

5-pentophosphate; DMD, Duchenne muscular dystrophy; ECG, electrocardiogram; G-6-PD, glucose-6-phosphate dehydrogenase; IFCC, International Federation of Clinical Chemistry; kDa, kilodaltons; NAD(P), nicotine adenine dinucleotide (phosphate); PCR, polymerase chain reaction; RE, reticuloendothelial; ULN, upper limit of normal.

REFERENCES

1. Bessman SP and Carpenter CL (1985) The creatine-creatine phosphate energy shuttle. Ann. Rev. Histochem. 54:831–862.
2. Hamburg JJ, Friedman DL, and Perryman MB (1991) Metabolic and diagnostic significance of creatine kinase isoenzymes. Trends Cardiovasc. Med. 1:195–200.
3. Friedman DL and Perryman MB (1991) Compartmentation of multiple forms of creatine kinase in the distal nephron of the rat kidney. J. Biol. Chem. 266: 22,404–22,410.
4. George S, Ishikawa Y, Perryman MB, and Roberts R (1984) Purification and characterization of naturally occurring and *in vitro* induced multiple forms of MM creatine kinase. J. Biol. Chem. 259:2667–2674.
5. Fleisher GA and Wakim KG (1963) The fate of enzymes in body fluids: an experimental study. 1. Disappearance rates of glutamic-pyruvic transaminase under various conditions. J. Lab. Clin. Med. 61:76–85.
6. Roberts R and Sobel BE (1977) Effect of selected drugs and myocardial infarction on the disappearance of creatine kinase from the circulation of conscious dogs. Cardiovasc. Res. 11:103–112.
7. Hayashi T and Notkins AL (1994) Clearance of LDH-5 from the circulation of inbred mice correlates with binding to macrophages. Int. J. Exp. Pathol. 75:165–168.
8. Horder M, Elser RC, Gerhardt W, Mathieu M, and Sampson EJ (1991) Approved recommendation on IFCC methods for the measurement of catalytic concentration of enzymes. Part 7. IFCC method for creatine kinase. Eur. J. Clin. Chem. Clin. Biochem. 29:435–456.
9. Chan KM, Ladenson JH, Pierce GF, and Jaffe AS (1986) Increased creatine kinase MB in the absence of acute myocardial infarction. Clin. Chem. 32:2044–2051.
10. Hollander JE (1995) The management of cocaine-associated myocardial ischemia N. Engl. J. Med. 333:1267–1272.
11. Siegel AJ, Silverman LM, and Holman L (1981) Elevated creatine kinase MB isoenzyme levels in marathon runners. Normal myocardial scintigrams suggest noncardiac source. JAMA 246:2049–2051.
12. Symanski JD, McMurray RG, Silverman LM, Smith BW, and Siegel AJ (1983) Serum creatine kinase and CK-MB isoenzyme responses to acute and prolonged swimming in trained athletes. Clin. Chim. Acta. 129:181–187.
13. Yasmineh WG, Ibrahim GA, Abbasnezhad M, and Awad EA (1978) Isoenzyme distroi-

bution of creatine kinase and lactate dehydrogenase in serum and skeletal muscle in Duchenne muscular dystrophy, collagen disease, and other muscular disorders. Clin. Chem. 24:1985–1989.

14. Silverman LM, Mendell JR, Sahenk Z, and Fontana MB (1976) Significance of creatine phosphokinase isoenzymes in Duchenne dystrophy. Neurology 26:561–564.

15. Gruemer HT and Prior T (1987) Carrier detection in Duchenne muscular dystrophy: a review of current issues and approaches. Clin. Chim. Acta. 162:1–18.

16. Prior TW, Papp AC, Synder PJ, Sedra MS, Western LM, Bartolo C, Moxley RT, and Mendell JR (1994) Heteroduplex analysis of the dystrophin gene: application to point mutation and carrier detection Am. J. Med. Genet. 50:68–73.

17. Ma TS, Ifegwu J, Siciliano MJ, Roberts R, and Perryman MB (1991) Serial Alu sequence transposition interrupting a human B creatine kinase pseudogene. Genomics 10; 390–399.

18. Perryman MB, Strauss AW, Buettner TL, and Roberts R. (1983) Molecular heterogeneity of creatine kinase isoenzymes. Biochim. Biophys. Acta. 747:284–290.

19. Klein SC, Haas RC, Perryman MB, Billadello JJ, and Strauss AW (1991) Regulatory element analysis and structural characterization of the human sarcomeric mitochondrial creatine kinase gene. J. Biol. Chem. 266:18,058–18,065.

20. Lott JA and Nemesanszky E (1996) Creatine kinase. In: Clinical enzymology: a case-oriented approach, Lott JA and Wolf PL, eds., New York, Field and Rich/Yearbook, p. 166.

21. Hamburg RJ, Friedman DL, Olson EN, Ma TS, Cortez MD, Goodman C, Puleo PR, and Perryman MB (1990) Muscle creatine kinase isoenzyme expression in adult human brain. J. Biol. Chem. 265:6403–6409.

22. Silverman LM, Dermer GB, Van Steirteghem AC, and Tokes ZA (1979) Creatine kinase BB: a new tumor-associated marker. Clin. Chem. 25:1432–1435.

23. Wong SS, Wu AHB, and Fritsche HA (1987) Re-evaluation of creatine kinase BB as a tumor marker. Clin. Chem. 33:809–811.

24. Apple FS, Rogers MA, Casal DC, Lewis L, Ivy JL, and Lampe JW (1987) Skeletal muscle CK-MB alterations in women marathon runners. Eur. J. Appl. Physiol. 56: 49–52.

25. Lang H and Wurzburg U (1992) Creatine kinase, an enzyme of many forms. Clin. Chem. 28:1439–1447.

26. Annesley TM and McKenna BJ (1983) Ectopic creatine kinase MB production in metastatic cancer. Am. J. Clin. Pathol. 79: 255–259.

27. Wu AHB, Feng YJ, and Fiedler PN (1997) Ectopic production of creatine kinase MB: updated evaluation by mass assays. Clin. Chem. 43:2006,2007.

28. Norby HK and Urdal P (1982) The diagnostic value of measuring creatine kinase BB activity in cerebrospinal fluid following acute head injury. Acta Neurochirurgica 65:93–101.

29. Han P, Born JD, Chapelle JP, and Milbouw G (1983) Creatie kinase isoenzyes in severe head injury. J. Neurosurg. 58:689–692.

30. Kaste M, Hernesniemi J, Somer H, Hillborn M, and Konttinen A (1981) Creatine kinase isoenzymes in acute brain injury. J. Neurosurg. 55:511–515.

31. Schwartz JG, Bazan C, Gage CL, Prihoda TJ, and Gillham SL (1989) Serum creatine kinase isoenzyme BB is a poor index to the size of various brain lesions. Clin. Chem. 35:651–654.

32. Stein W, Bohner J, Steinhart R, and Eggstein M (1992) Macro creatine kinase: determination and differentiation of two types by their activation energy. Clin. Chem. 28: 19–24.

33. Urdal P and Landaas S (1979) Macro creatine kinase BB in serum, and some data on its prevalence. Clin. Chem. 25:461–466.

34. Wu AHB, Herson VC, and Bowers GN Jr (1983) Macro creatine kinase type 1 and 2: Clinical significance in neonates and children as compared with adults. Clin. Chem. 29:201–204.

35. Whelan PV and Malkus H (1983) A macro creatine kinase isoenzyme in serum of apparently healthy individuals. Clin. Chem. 29:1411–1414.

36. Wong SS, Earl R, and Wu AHB (1987) Simultaneous presence of IgA- and IgG-CK-BB in a patient without myocardial infarction. Clin. Chim. Acta. 166:99–100.

37. Stein W, Bohner J, Renn W, and Maulbetsch R (1985) Macro creatine kinase type 2:

results of a prospective study in hospitalized patients. Clin. Chem. 31:1959–1964.

38. Castaldo G, Salvatore F, and Sacchetti L (1990) Serum type-2 macro creatine kinase isoenzyme is not a useful marker of severe liver diseases or neoplasia. Clin. Biochem. 23:523–527.

39. Rizzotti P, Cocco C, Burlina A, Marcer V, Plebani M, and Burlina A (1995) Macro creatine kinase type 2: a marker of myocardial damage in infants? Clin. Biochem. 18: 239–241.

Alan H. B. Wu

INTRODUCTION

The earliest methods for creatine kinase-(CK)*MB isoenzyme analysis were column chromatography and electrophoresis. These two techniques remain as the only tests routinely available for measurement of all three CK and five lactate dehydrogenase (LD) isoenzymes. Most laboratories have abandoned the manual column chromatography assay, as originally described in 1974 (1). However, because the Dupont *aca* immunoinhibition/column chromatography assay is still used by some laboratories, both the manual and automated methods are described in this chapter. On the other hand, CK isoenzyme analysis by agarose gel electrophoresis is still in use today. Although many laboratories have switched to mass assays for CK-MB, there has been a resurgence of electrophoresis users with the development of automated equipment. Both the manual and automated methods are described.

Immunoinhibition assays were first developed in the 1975 (2) and continue to be in widespread use today. The CK immunoinhibition assay makes use of polyclonal antibodies that are added to a serum sample to bind and inhibit CK-M subunits specifically.

The residual enzyme activity following antibody inhibition is measured using conventional reagents for total CK. The major advantage of immunoinhibition assays is that they can be adapted to automated high-throughput clinical chemistry analyzers. Therefore, results can be obtained conveniently and rapidly. The costs for immunoinhibition are also the lowest of all assays for CK-MB, because reagents are inexpensive and there is no incremental amount of labor associated with the CK-MB immunoinhibition assay linked to automated analyzers. The disadvantage of these assays is that they are not specific for the CK-MB isoenzyme. As a result, it is customary for many laboratories to follow up positive results with a more definitive CK-MB confirmation assay, such as electrophoresis or immunoassay (3). Therefore, although the turnaround time for the screening assay is rapid, the follow-up confirmation assay is usually delayed.

COLUMN CHROMATOGRAPHY

Figure 1 illustrates the manual column chromatography assay for CK isoenzymes. A 0.5 × 6 cm column containing an anion-exchange resin (DEAE-Sephadex A-50, Pharmacia, Piscataway, NJ) is constructed

---

*See p. 141 for list of abbreviations used in this chapter.

From: Cardiac Markers Edited by: Alan H. B. Wu
© Humana Press Inc., Totowa, NJ

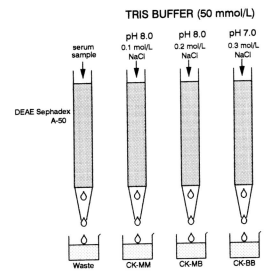

TRIS BUFFER (50 mmol/L)

Fig. 1. Manual column chromatography for CK-MB isoenzymes.

from a 12.5-cm Pasteur pipet *(4)*. The column is equilibrated with 50 mmol/L Tris buffer, pH 8.0, containing 100 mmol/L NaCl. The analysis begins with the addition of a 1.0-mL serum sample. For optimal performance, the sample is diluted such that total CK activity is between 600 and 2000 U/L. This is followed by 1.0-mL aliquots of the equilibration buffer. After each stepwise addition, fractions eluting from the column are collected and combined for further analysis for CK. The CK-MM isoenzyme is not sufficiently charged under these equilibrium conditions to be retained by the resin and, therefore, passes through the column. The next step is to add 1.0-mL aliquots of 50 mmol/L Tris buffer, pH 8.0, containing 200 mmol/L NaCl. Under these conditions, the higher salt concentration is able to displace the CK-MB isoenzyme from the column. As before, individual fractions are collected and combined. In the last chromatographic step, 1.0-mL aliquots of 50 mmol/L Tris buffer, pH 7.0, containing 300 mmol/L NaCl are added to the column. The pH shift and the further increment in

salt concentration enable elution of CK-BB from the column. If multiple fractions from each eluate are collected as described in the original procedure, they are collated. Each of the collated fractions are then tested for residual CK activity using appropriate reagents. Results must be multipled by the appropriate dilution factor. The fraction corresponds in order of collection: CK-MM, MB, and BB.

The disadvantage of column chromatography is that it is labor-intensive. In addition, the assay is insensitive, because during collection each isoenzyme is diluted by the elution buffer. An increase in sensitivity would be obtained if collected fractions were concentrated prior to analysis for residual CK activity. This would further add to the assay's costs and turnaround times.

ELECTROPHORESIS

Manual Electrophoresis

Electrophoresis assays are widely used in the clinical laboratory for proteins (serum, urine, and cerebrospinal fluid proteins, lipoproteins, and hemoglobin) and isoenzymes (amylase, LD, and CK). The electrophoresis assay for CK isoenzymes was described in 1972 *(5)*. Electrophoresis is normally performed either on agarose gel or cellulose acetate as support. The basic steps needed for the manual electrophoresis assay are shown in Figs. 2–4. Figure 2A illustrates the template method for applying serum samples. A thin acetate film is placed on top of the gel. Individual samples are pipeted through the slot and into the gel. Other methods, particularly those that use of cellulose acetate, have an applicator consisting of a wire that immersed into the serum sample and then transferred to the electrophoresis surface for deposition. An eight-sample applicator is shown in Fig. 2B. Each of these two application methods will produce an electrophoresis gel that contains CK fractions present in "bands." In yet another

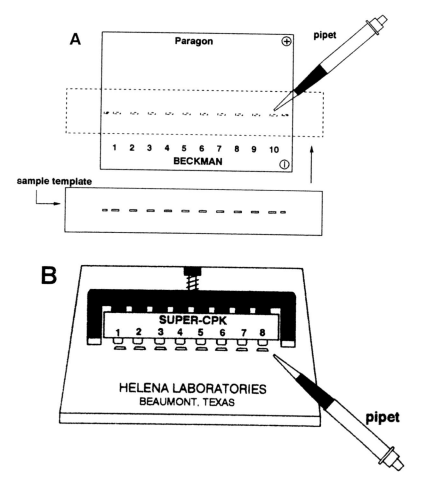

Fig. 2. Sample application methods for manual electrophoresis assay for CK-MB. (**A**) Template method: Serum samples (3–5 µL) are pipeted into the template. The sample incubates for 5 min to allow for diffusion into the gel. The template is blotted and removed. (**B**) Slot applicators: A thin wire is dipped into each sample, which is then transferred to the gel surface for application.

variation of sample application, one manufacturer has agarose gels with preformed wells, whereby samples can be directly applied using an automated pipeter. When stained, the CK bands will present as "dots" ("Isodot," Helena Laboratories, Beaumont, TX).

After all of the sample has been applied, the gels are placed into the electrophoresis chamber. This chamber contains positive (anode) and negative (cathode) electrodes placed in separate compartments, and loaded

with the proper electrophoresis buffer (*see* Fig. 3A). Gels are electrophoresed typically for 20–30 min at 100 V. In order to visualize isoenzyme bands, the gels must be stained for desired enzyme activity. For CK, a blotter is saturated with CK reagents and then placed directly on top of the electrophoresed gel (Fig. 3B). The reagent is identical to that used for measuring total CK using a chemistry analyzer. The overlay and gel incubate at 45°C. The elevated temperature is used to hasten the enzyme-catalyzed reactions. CK

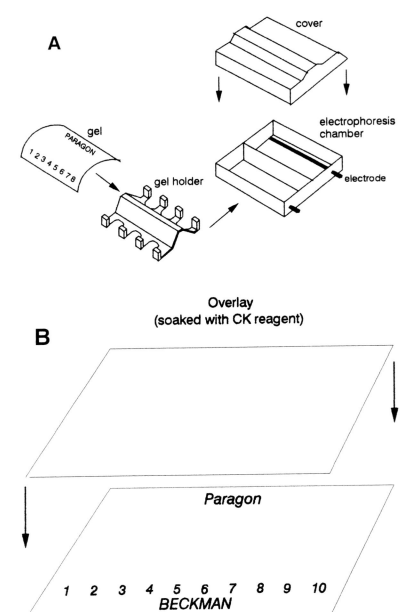

Fig. 3. Electrophoresis process. (**A**) The electrophoresis gel with loaded samples is placed into the chamber and electrophoresed at 100 V for 20 min. (**B**) After electrophoresis, a blotter saturated with CK reagent is placed onto the gel and allowed to incubate for 20 min at 45°C.

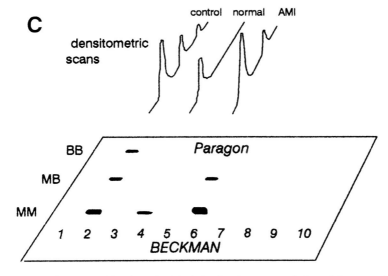

Fig. 3. *(continued)* **(C)** The gel is rinsed with deionized water and placed into a gel dryer (<74°C). The dried gel is then scanned fluorometrically using a densitometer (excitation: 340 nm, emission: 455 nm).

present on the gel reacts with the substrate to produce products that are coupled to other reagents and enzymes:

$$\text{Creatine phosphate} + \text{ADP} \xrightarrow{\text{CK}} \text{creatine} + \text{ATP} \quad (1)$$

$$\text{ATP} + \text{glucose} \xrightarrow{\text{hexokinase}} \text{glucose-6-phosphate} + \text{ADP} \quad (2)$$

$$\text{Glucose-6-phosphate} + \text{NADP+} \xrightarrow{\text{g-6-PD}} \text{6-phosphogluconate} + \text{NADPH} + \text{H+} \quad (3)$$

After 20 min of incubation with the substrate, the overlay is removed, thereby ending the reaction, and the gel is dried in an oven. Individual CK isoenzyme bands can then be visualized by exciting the gel with UV light at 340 nm and observing the resultant fluorescent emission at 455 nm (Fig. 3C). Special UV gel boxes are available for inspecting CK isoenzyme gels. As the fluorescence bands fade over time, gels can be photographed for permanent record keeping. An alternate visualization tech-

nique is to react NADPH produced in the above reaction with a tetrazolium salt to produced a colored product *(6)*. These bands can be seen without use of a UV light source. One such reaction is given below:

$$\text{NADPH} + \text{phenazine methosulfate nitroblue tetrazolium} \xrightarrow{\hspace{2cm}} \text{formazan (purple)} \quad (4)$$

The gels dried to produce a permanent record without the need to photograph them.

Under most electrophoretic conditions, CK-BB migrates furthest from the sample application point toward the anode. CK-MB migrates intermediate between the application point and anode, and CK-MM migrates cathodic to the point of application. The presence of a band migrating into the MB region indicates myocardial damage owing to an infarction. For quantitative measurement, the gels can be scanned by a densitometer. The area under the MB band can be divided into the area for all CK isoenzyme bands, with results expressed as a percentage of total. The normal range for most CK electrophoresis procedures is 0–5%. The absolute activity for the CK-MB band is not determined.

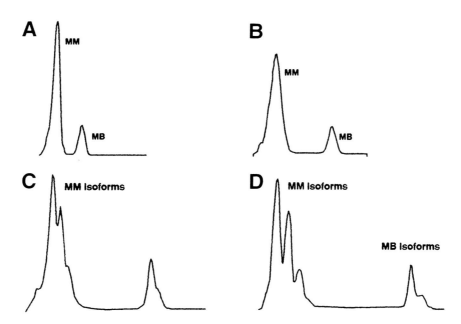

Fig. 4. Resolution of CK isoenzymes and isoforms vs electrophoresis voltage. (**A**) 250 V; (**B**) 500 V; (**C**) 750 V; (**D**) 900 V. (Data obtained from the Helena CardioRep analyzer.)

Automated Electrophoresis

The disadvantage of manual electrophoresis is the 2–3 h needed to perform the assay. In order to reduce the turnaround time, one manufacturer has developed a general automated electrophoresis analyzer (Rep, Helena Labs.) and a specialized analyzer for cardiac isoenzymes (CardioRep) *(7).* These analyzers automate each of the steps necessary for performing CK isoenzymes and isoforms, including sample application, electrophoresis, reagent addition and incubation for band visualization, gel drying, and densitometric scanning. To reduce the time needed to separate CK bands, the gels are electrophoresed at high voltages (900 V). Under these conditions, CK isoenzymes and isoforms (described in Chapters 7 and 10) are resolved. Figure 4 illustrates the effect of electrophoresis resolution as a function of applied electrophoresis voltage. At 250 and 500 V, the MM isoenzyme is adequately separated from MB, but no isoforms are discernible. At 750 V, three isoforms for MM and two for MB

can be seen, although the resolution between bands is not adequate. At 900 V, separate MM and MB isoforms can be observed. Higher voltages enable baseline separation for each isoform band, but such resolution is normally unnecessary, unless the isoforms themselves are to be measured (*see* Chapter 9).

Electrophoresis Performance

The major advantage of electrophoresis is the direct UV visualization of all CK isoenzyme and CK-like isoenzyme bands. Figure 5 summarizes the bands that can be observed by electrophoresis. Each of the major isoenzymes actually consists of isoforms that can only be observed following high voltage or extended time electrophoresis. Under normal (low-voltage) electrophoresis conditions, isoform bands merge into single MM, MB, and BB isoenzyme bands.

The major disadvantage of electrophoresis is analytical sensitivity. Manual electrophoresis assays have a sensitivity of about 5 U/L, which is above the activity of MB

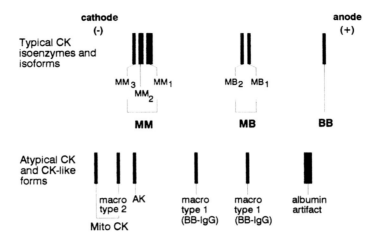

Fig. 5. Diagrammatic representation of CK isoenzymes, isoforms, atypical forms, and artifacts as measured by agarose gel electrophoresis.

found in normal individuals. Therefore, the MB band is absent when serum from normal healthy individuals is tested. For retrospective diagnosis of a typical AMI, the lower sensitivity of electrophoresis does not pose a problem, since AMI patients will have MB activities that will greatly exceed the normal range. However, for early diagnosis or detection of "silent acute myocardial infarctions (AMIs)," higher sensitivity assays are needed, since the MB content is much lower. Electrophoresis is not as sensitive as mass assays for testing under these conditions (8). Moreover, the accuracy of electrophoresis has recently been questioned by the Ontario Laboratory Proficiency Testing Program (9). Despite these criticisms of accuracy, electrophoresis is still considered the standard measure of CK and LD isoenzyme distribution.

Detection of Electrophoretic Artifacts and Atypical Isoenzymes

A fluorescent band can also occasionally be visualized that migrates between MB and BB isoenzymes. This band is owing to the presence of fluorescent metabolites (and possibly drugs) that bind to albumin. Its presence is found most often in patients with chronic renal failure, presumably because of the inability of the kidney to excrete these fluorescent compounds (10). The presence of the albumin artifact can be distinguished from true CK isoenzyme bands on the basis of its different fluorescence emission wavelengths. Adenylate kinase (AK) is a CK-like enzyme that catalyzes the conversion of ADP to ATP, and migrates cathodic to CK-MM:

$$2ADP \xrightarrow{AK} ATP + AMP \qquad (5)$$

ATP produced by this reaction will couple with hexokinase and g-6-PD to produce NADPH. The presence of either the albumin artifact or AK can be recognized by performing electrophoresis and omitting the CK substrate from the formulary of the overlaying reagent. Without creatine phosphate, true CK isoenzymes will not be able to produce NADH, but electrophoretic artifacts will remain detectable.

Macro-CK forms can also be discerned by electrophoresis when they are present. Macro-CK type 1 containing IgG typically migrates between the MM and MB isoenzymes and causes no ambiguities with CK-MB quantitation. On the other hand, the type 1 form containing IgA often comigrates

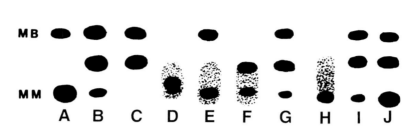

Fig. 6. Use of specific antibodies prior to electrophoresis for detection of suspect bands: macro-IgG (band between MM and MB) and macro-IgA (band at MB) in a case report. Lane A, control sera; B, patient's serum showing CK-MM and two suspect bands; C–I, patient serum mixed with specific antisera; C, anti-CK-M, showing removal of MM; D, anti-CK-B showing removal of both suspect bands; E, anti-IgG showing removal of band between MM and MB; F, anti-IgA showing removal of MB band; G, anti-λ showing no effect; H, anti-K showing removal of both suspect bands. I, anti-IgM showing no effect. (Used with permission from ref. *13.*)

with the MB band, and differentiation may not be possible. Subsequent testing (such as with CK-MB immunoassays; *see* Chapter 9) may be necessary to differentiate it from true CK-MB. Serial samples can be collected over the ensuing few days to document a persistent increase in this "pseudo-MB band" that is typically observed for the presence of this form. Patients with myocardial infarction will have a transient increase in true CK-MB. Bands that migrate cathodic to the application point include mitochondrial CK, macro-CK type 2, and AK. These forms may comigrate with CK-MM and go unrecognized in many electrophoresis systems. The result is an overestimation of the MM activity and a slight decrease in the resulting ratio of MB/total CK. The enzyme activity of dimeric mitochondrial CK is very labile in serum and is not usually observed in human serum. Since mitochondrial CK is found in the brain, mass measurement of mitochondrial CK may have some application in detection of cerebral injury *(11).* Macro-CK type 2 is a polymeric aggregate of mitochondrial CK and also migrates cathodic to CK-MM. The procedure for confirming the presence of macro-CK has been

described by several investigators *(12–15).* These procedures also enable typing of the specific CK isoenzyme and immunoglobulin classes involved. Serum samples containing suspected electrophoretic bands can be mixed (1:1) with various antisera and re-electrophoresed following a 10-min incubation. The electrophoretic migration of suspected CK bands will be altered or their enzymatic activity will be obscured by the binding of antibodies specific to immunoglobulins and/or isoenzymes. Anti-IgG, IgA, and IgM are commercially available in kits for immunofixation electrophoresis (e.g., Paragon, Beckman Instruments, Brea, CA). Antibodies to CK-M are available with the Isomune CK-MB kit (reagent A, Roche Diagnostics, Nutley, NJ), whereas CK-B subunits are available in the Tandem and ICON kits (Hybritech Inc., San Diego, CA). In a case report, Fig. 6 illustrates how specific antibodies were used to denote the presence of IgG- and IgA-macro-CK-BB. Pretreatment with selective precipitation is also effective in confirming macromolecular complexes. Immobilized protein A-sepharose (CL-4B, Pharmacia, Piscataway, NJ) can be used to remove IgG complexes. The two-

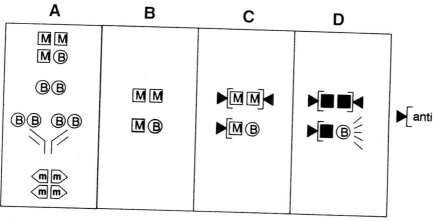

Fig. 7. Diagrammatic representation of the immunoinhibition assay. *See text* for details.

step immunoprecipitation procedure of Iso-mune CK-MB (Roche) can be used to remove isoenzymes containing the M-subunit (CK-MM and CK-MB). These procedures are particularly helpful for atypical isoenzymes that electrophoretically migrate at or near CK-MB (such as IgG macro-CK-BB).

IMMUNOINHIBITION ASSAY

Principle

The general principle for all immunoin-hibition assays is shown in Fig. 7 *(15)*. Panel A shows the classic CK-MM, MB, and BB isoenzymes. Although not shown, each of these isoenzymes consists of several iso-forms (*see* Chapter 10). It is assumed for simplicity that the activities and antigenicity to each isoform of an isoenzyme are identical to one another. Also shown in panel A are macro-CK types 1 and 2 that may be present in a serum sample. However, the immunoin-hibition assay is only an accurate measure of CK-MB activity when CK-BB and the macro forms are absent in serum (panel B). The assay involves the incubation of serum with polyclonal anti-CK-M antibodies (panel C). These antibodies are specifically selected to bind to CK-M subunits in such a way that they inhibit 100% of the CK-MM

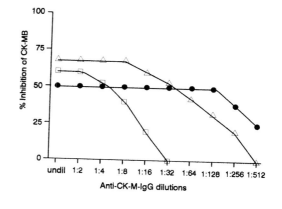

Fig. 8. Inhibition of CK-MB by anti-CK-M antibodies. (Used with permission from ref. *15*.)

activity and precisely 50% of the CK-MB activity. Antibodies raised in goats used for other species, such as rabbit and sheep, do not exhibit the same degree of inhibition (Fig. 8) *(16)*. The use of polyclonal goat anti-bodies also eliminates any potential inter-ferences from the presence of human antimouse antibodies (HAMA) that have been shown to interfere with assays using murine monoclonal antibodies (MAb) *(17)*. The residual CK activity, as measured using total CK reagents, is the result of the B-subunit of MB alone (panel D). To cal-culate the CK-MB activity of the intact

Table 1
Example of an Immunoinhibition Error Caused by Presence of CK-BB,
Macro-CK Type 2, and AK[a]

	Original activity, from sample[b]	Measured residual activity, after immunoinhibition	Calculated activity, residual × 2
CK-MB	50	25	50
CK-BB	25	25	50
Macro-type 2	10	10	20
AK	8	3	6
Total	93	63	126

[a]Error: (actual — calculated/actual) × 100 = (126 − 50)/50 × 100 = 152%.
[b]All results in U/L.

isoenzyme, the residual result must be multiplied by a factor of two.

Accurate calculations of CK-MB by immunoinhibition requires subtraction of background activity owing to the presence of AK. Serum AK activity can exceed 100 U/L at 37°C because of release of AK isoenzymes from red cells, muscle, and liver *(18)*. Therefore, adenosine monophosphate (AMP) and diadenosine-5-pentaphosphate are usually added to CK reagent formulations to inhibit AK. However, residual noninhibited AK activity ranging from 1–3 U/L usually remains. Higher activities are expected in samples that are hemolyzed. For total CK analysis, noninhibited AK activity constitutes a <5% (falsely high) error. In patients with low CK-MB activity, the error caused by AK can be 100% and will limit the sensitivity of the immunoinhibition assay. To correct for presence of this enzyme, the serum sample is incubated with CK reagent that is devoid of CK substrate. Residual activity owing to AK can then be subtracted from the activity of the sample when the substrate, creatine phosphate, is added. The apparent CK-MB activity produced by immunoinhibition is falsely high when either CK-BB or macro-CK types 1 and 2 are present in the serum sample. Table 1 illustrates a hypothetical serum sample containing 50 U/L of CK-MB, 25 U/L of CK-BB, and

10 U/L of macro-CK type 2. Anti-CK-M antibodies are added, and the residual CK activity is measured after a 5-min incubation period. Of the residual activity, the CK-MB isoenzyme contributes 50% of its original activity, since the M-subunit has been inhibited. In contrast, CK-BB and macro-CK type 2 add 100% of their original activity, because neither isoenzyme contains any inhibitable M-subunits. Table 1 also lists 3 U/L of noninhibited AK activity that adds to the residual CK activity. If AK blank is not performed, the total residual activity of this sample after immunoinhibition is 63 U/L. When this is multiplied by 2, the activity of the immunoinhibition tube is 126 U/L, which exceeds the original total CK activity of 93 U/L and produces an error of 152% (Table 1). When the percent MB exceeds typical values seen in AMI (4–25%), as in this example, the presence of an interferrent is inferred. However, falsely high values in the 10–25% range can be produced and are not discernible by immunoinhibition.

Automated Adaptation of CK-MB Immunoinhibition Assay

The CK-MB immunoinhibition assay has been adapted to many automated clinical chemistry analyzers. With the exception of the Roche Isomume-CK (immunoinhibition/immunoprecipitation) and Dupont

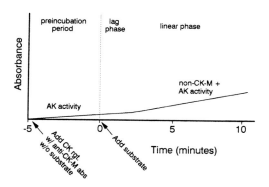

Fig. 9. Reaction vs time curve for the CK-MB immunoinhibition assay.

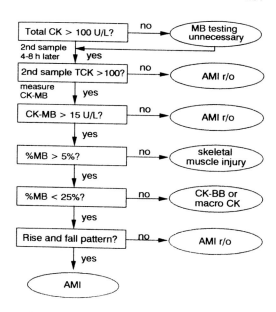

Fig. 10. A typical flow diagram on the utilization of immunoinhibition results for CK-MB. Normal range for CK-MB used in this diagram is 15 U/L and 4% CK-MB/total CK. *See text* for details. (Adapted from the Ektachem 700 package insert, Kodak Co., Rochester, NY.)

aca (column chromatography/immunoinhibition) assays, which are described later in this chapter, all commercial immunoinhibition assays are essentially identical. The optimum automated assay is the two-reagent addition test. Figure 9 illustrates the sequence of these reagent additions. In the first step, the serum sample incubates with anti-CK-M antibodies and the CK reagent minus the substrate (creatine phosphate). A 5-min incubation period is required to establish an equilibrium between the isoenzymes from the serum sample and the added antibodies. This incubation also enables estimation of any noninhibited AK activity present. The substrate is then added to trigger the CK-catalyzed reaction. The non-CK-M subunit activity is determined from the linear portion of the reaction vs time curve (Fig. 9). Enzyme substrate depletion is not a problem in this assay because CK-MM has been inhibited, and high non-M-subunit activity is uncommonly present. Instead, the assay is optimized for higher analytical sensitivity through the use of higher sample volumes than what is normally in use for analysis of total CK. An adjustment in the calculation factor is necessary to account for the increase in sample volume. The upper limit of normal for CK-MB using immunoinhibition is about 10 to 15 U/L at 37°C, and between 4 and 6% relative to total CK.

Interpretation of Immunoinhibition Results

Because of the nonspecificity of immunoinhibition assays for CK-MB, many laboratories use this as a screening test for AMI rule-out. Low activity of CK-MB indicates negative results, which obviate the need for further testing of the sample. Depending on the absolute activity of CK-MB and its ratio relative to total CK, positive results may require additional testing with a more definitive CK-MB assay. Figure 10 illustrates one algorithm regarding how results of CK-MB by immunoinhibition might be interpreted. The analysis begins with measurement of total CK. If the activity is <100 U/L, determination of CK-MB may be unnecessary, because it is likely to be within normal limits. These results are consistent with blood from a non-AMI patient. In the setting of chest pain, it is also possible that the results are consistent with AMI patients with a very small infarct or from whom blood was collected too soon after the onset of symptoms (e.g., within the first 6 h). If either of the latter two situations is suspected based on clinical findings, a second sample should be collected, somewhere between 4 and 8 h after the first sample. If the total CK of the second sample remains low, an AMI has been effectively ruled out. On the other hand, if either or both samples have CK activity exceeding 100 U/L, the high sample(s) should be further tested for CK-MB. A CK-MB result below the upper limit of normal of 15 U/L rules out AMI, particularly when two or more samples are documented to be low. If the CK-MB activity exceeds the upper limit of normal, but the %CK-MB/total CK is <4%, skeletal muscle injury is likely the cause of the high total CK and absolute CK-MB activity. If the %MB exceeds 25%, CK-BB or macro-CK (types 1 and 2) is likely present, because AMI patients rarely have a %MB concentration that exceeds this limit. Although not clinically significant, the presence of these abnormal forms can be confirmed by electrophoresis. The immunoinhibition assay cannot be used to rule out AMI when BB or macro-forms are present. There have been case reports described whereby both AMI and macro-CK are present *(19)*. If the percentage of MB is between 4 and 25%, there is a characteristic rise and fall pattern with serial samples collected over 2–3 d, and a diagnosis of AMI can be made with >90% confidence.

IMMUNOINHIBITION/IMMUNO-PRECIPITATION ASSAY (ROCHE)

To improve on the specificity of immunoinhibition assays for CK-MB, a second immunoprecipitation step can be added. Isomune-CK is a two-tube immunoprecipitation assay developed by Roche Diagnostics *(20)*. As shown in the top three panels of Fig. 11A, 1–3, the first tube is treated in the same way as with the immunoinhibition assay: goat anti-CK-M antibodies are added to a serum sample containing CK isoenzymes. To illustrate how the immunoprecipitation assay corrects for the presence of CK-BB, and macro-CK types 1 and 2, these variants are included in sample calculations (not excluded as in Fig. 11). After a 10-min incubation period, the residual activity of this sample (panel A3) is measured:

$$CK\text{-}BB + macro\text{-}CK\ type\ 1 + macro\text{-}CK \quad\quad (6)$$
$$type\ 2 + \tfrac{1}{2}\ CK\text{-}MB$$

Anti-CK-M antibodies are also added to a second tube containing an aliquot of the serum sample (panel B2). As shown in panel B3, donkey antigoat antibodies linked to an insoluble polymer are then added. This second precipitating antibody will bind to the anti-CK-M antibody that is already linked to CK-MM and MB (panel B3). After a 5-min incubation, the tube is centrifuged. This separates the isoenzymes containing CK-M subunits (CK-MM and MB) from all others (panel B4). The supernatant is removed and assayed for residual activity:

$$CK\text{-}BB + macro\text{-}CK\ type\ 1 + macro\text{-}CK \quad\quad (7)$$
$$type\ 2$$

The calculation of CK-MB is then

$$CK\text{-}MB = (tube\ A - tube\ B) \times 2 \quad\quad (8)$$

One difference in the Roche isomune assay from automated immunoinhibition is that the antibodies are not incorporated within the reagent for measuring residual CK. Therefore, the residual activity of tubes A and B must be corrected for dilution by the volume of antisera added (factors 2 and 1.9, respectively).

Table 2 illustrates how the immunoprecipitation step corrects for the presence of CK-BB and atypical isoenzymes. In tube A, the residual activity after the immunoinhi-

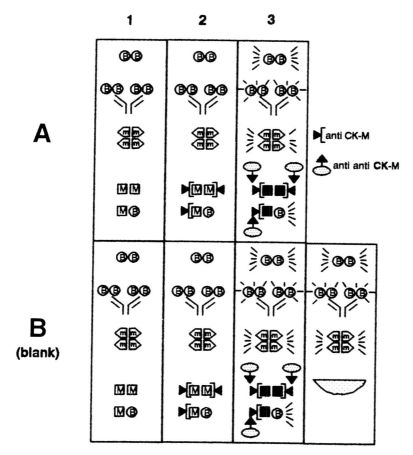

Fig. 11. Diagrammatic representation of the immunoprecipitation assay. *See text* for details.

Table 2
Correction of Immunoinhibition Error by Immunoprecipitation Assays[a]

	Original activity from sample[b]	Tube A, immunoinhibition	Tube B, immunoprecipitation	Calculated activity, A-blank × 2
CK-MB	50	25	0	50
CK-BB	25	25	25	0
Macro-type 2	10	10	10	0
AK	8	3	3	0
Total	93	63	38	50

[a]Error: (actual — calculated/actual) × 100 = (50 − 50)/50 × 100 = 0%.
[b]All in U/L.

bition step (63 U/L after correction by the dilution factor) is the same as the immuno-inhibition step of Table 1. The residual activity of tube B is the sum of CK-BB, macro-CK type 2, and AK (38 U/L after correction). The difference multiplied by 2 produces 50 U/L, which is the correct activity of CK-MB in the original sample.

Table 3
The Effect of Atypical Isoenzymes on Analytical Sensitivity of Immunoprecipitation Assays[a]

	Original activity, from sample[b]	Tube A, immunoinhibition	Tube B, immunoprecipitation	Calculated activity, A-blank × 2
CK-MB	2	1	0	50
CK-BB	25	25	25	0
Macro-type 2	10	10	10	0
AK	8	3	3	0
Total	45	39	38	2
Range[a]	NA	37–41	36–40	–6 to 10

[a]Assuming a 5% precision for residual activity measurement.
[b]All in U/L.

Although the activities of CK-BB and macro-CK variants are accounted for by the immunoprecipitation step, their presence will reduce the sensitivity of CK-MB results. Table 3 illustrates the same case as Table 2, but with a low CK-MB activity in the original sample. Calculation of twice the difference between tubes A and B theoretically produces the correct result of 2 U/L for CK-MB. However, the residual activity of each tube is subject to the imprecision of the residual CK measurement. Using a conservative average precision of 5%, CK-MB activity (calculated from the difference of two relatively large numbers) range from 6–10 U/L (Table 3).

COLUMN CHROMATOGRAPHY/ IMMUNOINHIBITION ASSAY (DuPONT)

One of the first automated CK-MB assay was the *aca* method (Dupont Co., Wilmington, DE) *(21)*. A description of the principles for the column chromatography assay for CK-MB is presented in Chapter 7. Like all *aca* methods, the CK-MB assay is supplied within the reagent pack (Fig. 12). A serum sample is delivered by the analyzer to the pack header. Unique to the CK-MB assay, the pack header contains a chromatographic column containing a mixture of diethy-laminoethyl (DEAE) and carboxylic acid resins. The pH, ionic strength, and resin ratio of the column are set such that the CK-MB isoenzyme separates from CK-MM and CK-BB isoenzyme. The column also retains any red cells and AK that may be present in the serum sample. CK-MB is eluted from the header into the body of the test pack. The *aca* adds reagents to the test pack by breaking the seals to the individual reagent pouches (Fig. 12). To minimize further any contribution by CK-MM that may have been eluted from the column, the first reagent pouch also contains anti-CK-M antibodies. The residual non-CK-M activity is measured using the Rosalki/Oliver reaction scheme, with dithioerythritol as the activator and *N*-2-acetamido-2-aminoethanesulfunoic acid as the buffer. The increase in absorbance owing to the production of NADH is measured spectrophotometrically at 340 nm. Because neither the activator nor the buffer is the same as that recommended by the International Federation of Clinical Chemistry (for total CK), there will be biases between *aca* results and other immunoinhibition assays. The *aca* assay has a turnaround time of 5 min and is useful for stat analysis. Some investigators have been critical of this assay. The assay is directly influenced by protein content and indirectly

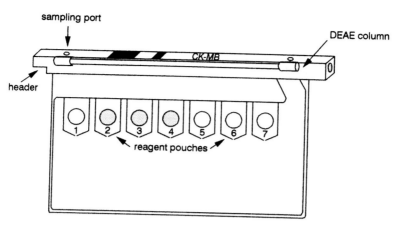

Fig. 12. Reagent pack for the *aca* method for immunoassay for CK-MB. Reagent compartment contents: 1, g-6-PD, hexokinase, anti-CK-M antibody; 2, buffer, ADP, AK inhibitors; 3, creatine phosphate, glucose, dithioerythritol; 4, NAD+; 5–7, empty.

influenced by salt concentrations. Therefore, one investigator has recommended that the *aca* assay is not suited for use with diluted samples *(22)*.

ABBREVIATIONS

aca, Automated clinical analyzer; AK, adenylate kinase; AMI, acute myocardial infarction; AMP/ADP/ATP, adeonsine mono, di- and triphosphate; CK, creatine kinase; DEAE, diethylaminoethyl; g-6-PD, glucose-6-phosphate dehydrogenase; HAMA, human antimouse antibodies; LD, lactate dehydrogenase; NADP+, nicotine adenine dinucleotide (phosphate).

REFERENCES

1. Mercer DW (1974) Separation of tissue and serum creatine kinase isoenzymes by ion-exchange column chromatography. Clin. Chem. 20:36–40.
2. Jockers-Wretou E and Pfleiderer G (1975) Quantitation of creatine kinase isoenzymes in human tissues an sera by an immunological method. Clin. Chim. Acta. 58: 223–232.
3. Wu AHB and Bowers GN Jr (1982) Evaluation and comparison of immunoinhibition and immunoprecipitation methods for dif-

ferentiating MB from BB and macro forms of creatine kinase isoenzymes in patients and healthy individuals. Clin. Chem. 28: 2017–2021.
4. Mercer DW (1975) Simultaneous separation of serum creatine kinase and lactate dehydrogenase isoenzymes by ion exchange column chromatography. Clin. Chem. 21:1102–1106.
5. Roe CR, Limbird LE, Wagner GS, and Nerenberg ST (1972) Combined isoenzyme analysis in the diagnosis of myocardial injury: application of electrophoretic methods for the detection and quantitation of creatine kinase phosphokinase MB isoenzyme. J. Lab. Clin. Med. 80:577–590.
6. Somer H and Konttinen A (1972) A method allowing the quantitation of serum creatine kinase isoenzymes. Clin. Chim. Acta. 36: 531–536.
7. Secchiero S, Altinier S, Zaninotto M, Lachin M, and Plebani M (1995) Evaluation of a new automated system for the determination of CK-MB isoforms. J. Clin. Lab. Anal. 9:359–365.
8. Gadsden RH Sr, Papadea C, and Cate JC IV (1994) Analytical evaluation of methods for serum creatine kinase-MB. Electrophoresis, immunoinhibition and solid phase separation. Ann. Clin. Lab. Sci. 24:110–120.
9. Henderson AR, Stark JA, McQueen MJ, Patten RL, Krishnan S, Wood DE, and Webb S (1994) Is determination of creatine kinase-

2 after electrophoretic separation accurate? Clin. Chem. 40:177–183.

10. Aleyassine H and Tonks DB (1978) Albumin-bound fluorescence: a potential source of error in fluorometric assay of creatine kinase BB isoenzyme. Clin. Chem. 24: 1849–1850.

11. Liu N, Wu AHB, Friedman DL, and Perryman MB (1992) Detection of serum mitochondrial creatine kinase in cerebrovascular accident patients [Abstract]. Clin. Chem. 38:984.

12. Abbott LB and Van Lente F (1992) Procedure for characterization of creatine kinase variant on agarose electrophoretograms. Clin. Chem. 31:445–447.

13. Wong SS, Earl R, and Wu AHB (1987) Simultaneous presence of IgA- and IgG-CK-BB in a patient without myocardial infarction. Clin. Chim. Acta. 166:99–100.

14. Loshon CA, McComb RB, and Bowers GN Jr (1984) Immunoprecipitation and electrophoresis used to demonstrate and evaluate interference by CK-BB and atypical-CKs with CK-MB determinations by immunoinhibition. Clin. Chem. 30:167–168.

15. Wuerzburg U, Hennrich N, and Lang H (1978) Rapid and quantitative determination of creatine kinase-MB activity in serum using immunological inhibition of creatine kinase M subunit activity. In CK-MB immunoinhibition. Gerhardt W, Waldenström J, and Hofvendahl S, eds. Frankfurter, E. Merck, p. 27.

16. Madritsch K (1968) Die myokinase in der diagnostik des herzinfarktes. Schweiz. Med. Wochenscr. 98:646–653.

17. Kricka LJ, Schmerfeld-Pruss D, Senior M, Goodman DBP, and Kaladas P (1990) Interference by human anti-mouse antibody in two-site immunoassays. Clin. Chem. 36: 892–894.

18. Szasz G, Gerhardt W, Gruber W, and Bernt E (1976) Creatine kinase in serum: 2. interference of adenylate kinase with the assay. Clin. Chem. 22:1806–1811.

19. Baum HH, Bohm M, and Neumeier D (1991) Simultaneous occurence of the MB isoenzyme of creatine kinase and macro creatine kinase type 1 in a patient with acute myocardial infarction. Int. J. Cardiol. 31:253–255.

20. Wicks R, Usategui-Gomez M, Miller M, and Warshaw M (1982) Immunological determination of CK-MB isoenzyme in human serum II. An enzymatic approach. Clin. Chem. 28:54–58.

21. Weeks RB and Malhotra HC (1981) Clinical evaluation of an automated column method for CK-MB determinations. Clin. Chem. 27:1024.

22. Stein W and Bohner J (1984) Determination of creatine kinase MB activity with the DuPont *aca:* interferences from the sample matrix. Clin. Chem. 30:238–242.

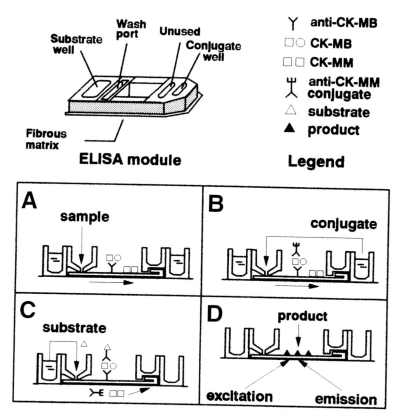

Fig. 2. Fluorogenic ELISA for CK-MB on the Opus Plus. The ELISA module consists of compartments for the conjugate (anti-CK-MM linked to alkaline phosphatase) and substrate (4-methylumbelliferone phosphate). Anti-CK-MB is immobilized onto the fibrous matrix at the base of the module. (**A**) A serum sample containing CK-MM and CK-MB is pipeted by the Opus Plus via the wash port to the fibrous matrix. The incubation period with the sample is 3 min. CK-MB binds to the solid-phase antibody. (**B**) Conjugate is added to the matrix and binds to immobilized CK-MB. (**C**) Substrate is added to react with conjugate immobilized onto CK-MB. The substrate solution also washes unbound proteins, isoenzymes (e.g., CK-MM), and conjugate. (**D**) The fluorescence of 4-methylumbelliferone is measured. (Used with permission from the AACC, ref. *4.*)

CK-MB concentrations is constructed, and unknown sample CK-MB concentrations are calculated using the curve.

The aca® Plus

The DuPont *aca®* plus is a random access, automated processor. The CK-MB mass (MCKMB assay) method for the *aca* plus immunoassay system is an immunoenzymetric assay. The processor pipets and mixes the serum sample, chromium dioxide particles coated with MAb specific for CK-B subunit (solid phase), and conjugate reagent β-galactosidase-labeled MAb for CK-MB isoenzyme in a reaction vessel. After a 15-min incubation period, the processor performs three sequential washings, and then transfers the particle/CK-MB/enzyme conjugate complex into an analytical *aca* test pack. The test pack is then removed from the processor and placed on the *aca* discrete clinical analyzer for quantitation of CK-MB in the sample. β-Galactosidase bound to the antigen/

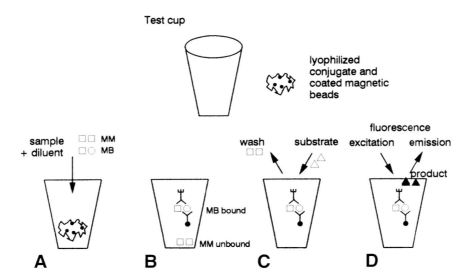

Fig. 3. Fluorogenic ELISA for CK-MB on the Tosoh AIA-1200. The AIA-Pack contains magnetized microbeads coated with anti-CK-BB antibodies. A lyophilized conjugate, anti-CK-MB antibodies conjugated to alkaline phosphatase, is also included in the test cup. The symbols for CK-MM, MB, and antibodies are the same as in Fig. 2. **(A)** A serum sample containing CK-MM and CK-MB and diluent are added to the reaction cup. The conjugate is reconstituted with the diluent. The incubation period with the sample is 40 min. **(B)** CK-MB binds to the solid-phase antibody and the reconstituted conjugate. **(C)** Unreacted sample and unbound enzyme conjugate are washed away. The substrate, 4-methylumbelliferone phosphate, is added. **(D)** The fluorescence of 4-methylumbelliferone is measured. (Used with permission from the AACC, ref. *4*.)

antibody complex catalyzes the hydrolysis of the substrate chlorophenol red-β-*d*-galactopyranoside (CPRG) to chlorophenol red (CPR). The color change read at 577 nm is the result of the production of CPR and is directly proportional to the concentration of CK-MB present in the patient sample.

Abbott IMx

A STAT CK-MB assay has been released by Abbott using the Abbott IMx. The assay is a reformulation of their microparticle enzyme immunoassay (MEIA), cutting down turnaround times from 34 to 15 min. Other changes include the use of an animal-based matrix in their controls and calibration materials from a human-based serum matrix. Sample, diluent, and anti-CK-MB-coated microparticles (latex submicron particles suspended in a sucrose solution) are added

to an incubation well in the reaction cell. Sucrose is used to allow the microparticles to remain in suspension for the duration of the assay. Microparticles coated with anti-CK-MB capture CK-MB molecules forming an antibody/antigen complex. The complex is then transferred to an inert glass fiber matrix in another compartment of the same reaction cell. The microparticles bind irreversibly to the glass fiber matrix. The antigen/antibody complex is retained by the glass fibers, while the reaction mixture flows through the large pores of the matrix into the blotter. The matrix is washed to remove all unbound materials, and anti-CK-MM (goat) alkaline phosphatase conjugate is dispensed onto the matrix, binding with the antibody/antigen complex. The matrix is once again washed to remove any unbound materials. The conjugate catalyzes the hydrolysis of 4-MUP to the fluorescent product 4-MU. The rate at which 4-MU is generated is directly proportional to the concentration of CK-MB in the test sample.

Access

Recently, Sanofi Diagnostics Pasteur has released a CK-MB assay on the Access. The Access is a nonisotopic, automated, random access immunochemistry analyzer. The CK-MB assay is a one-step, two-site sandwich assay. Paramagnetic particles coated with mouse monoclonal anti-CK-BB comprise the solid phase. After the sample containing CK-MB is introduced, mouse monoclonal CK-MB conjugated to alkaline phosphatase is added. The sample is incubated at 37°C for 5 min in order to ensure sandwich formation, followed by three washes. The substrate (dioxetene-P) is added, followed by a second 5-min incubation, and absorbance is read at 530 nm as dioxetene-P is converted to dioxetane. The signal is proportional to the CK-MB concentration in the sample.

Technicon Immuno 1

The Techicon Immuno 1 is also a nonisotopic automated, random access immunochemistry analyzer. In sandwich assays, such as for CK-MB, the Technicon Immuno 1 makes use of anti-CK-MB antibodies conjugated to fluorescein, and anti-CK-B antibody linked to alkaline phosphatase. In the presence of CK-MB from the serum, the two antibodies bind to form a complex that is captured by the magnetic particle linked to antifluorescein. Addition of substrate to the alkaline phosphatase, *p*-nitrophenyl phosphate, provides a means for measurement of the enzyme label by rate absorbance. The Technicon Immuno 1 may be the most precise of immunoassay analyzers with coefficient of variations (CVs) of under 5% for CK-MB at the medical decision limits *(18)*.

CK-MB MASS ASSAY STANDARDIZATION

Although immunoassays have been shown to be accurate and reliable, there have been numerous reports of discrepant results among patients when transferred from one hospital to another. Different hospitals may have very different positive CK-MB cutoff values, causing clinical confusion. Since most of the mass assays make use of the same capture antibody (Conan from Washington University), biases in results are likely owing to differences in the calibration of the instrumentation and the assignment of the standards used in the assay. The standardization of all CK-MB mass assays would have significant clinical benefit when results from one assay are compared to another.

Split patient sample correlation studies reported in the literature show that commercially available CK-MB immunoassays correlate well ($r > 0.98$), but are biased from one another as reflected in the slopes of the analysis (slope range 0.4–1.6) *(19)*. For example, in one study, CK-MB was measured in serum by fluorometric enzyme immunoassay on the Baxter Stratus Analyzer and by immunochemiluminometric assay using the Ciba Corning Magic Lite System *(20)*. Correlations with an immunoradiometric assay (Embria) were: Stratus = 0.999 (Embria) – 3.3; $r = 0.969$, and Magic Lite = 1.225 (Embria) – 3.03; $r = 0.971$. Both methods proved to be highly sensitive and specific in the diagnosis of AMI; however, the need for standardization of CK-MB assays is stressed.

American Association for Clinical Chemistry (AACC) Mass Standardization Subcommittee

In January 1992, the AACC CK-MB Mass Assay Standardization Subcommittee (MB MASS) was formed. The major objec-

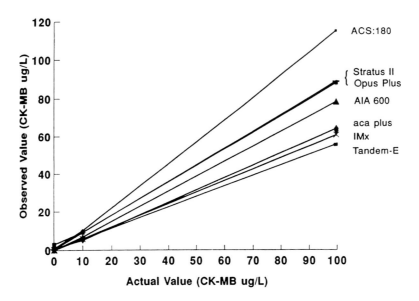

Fig. 4. Calibration curves for CK-MB mass assays using a single set of standards. (Used with permission from the AACC, ref. *4*.)

tive of the subcommittee was to develop a reference material using human CK-MB that can be used to reduce between-laboratory variation in the accuracy of the CK-MB mass assays. Their work involves the identification of a source CK-MB material, establishment of purification and protein determination protocols, and the investigation of various matrices and forms (liquid or lyophilized) in which the standards would be made. With cooperation among manufacturers, it is hoped that this reference material will be used to standardize assay methods so that biases between assays will be reduced or eliminated.

Figure 4 shows results of a study conducted by the subcommittee, where calibration curves were generated using CK-MB standards (0, 10, and 100 ng/mL) run on each of seven immunoassays (DuPont *aca* plus, Behring Diagnostics Opus Plus, Abbott IMx, Hybritech Tandem-E, Ciba-Corning ACS:180, Baxter Stratus II, and Tosoh AIA 600). Table 2 shows the assays have excellent correlation (coefficients are all 0.999).

The immunoassays have similar *y*-intercepts, but slopes vary greatly. The data imply that the principal reason for biases between methods is the lack of a universally accepted CK-MB standard.

Four sources of CK-MB were considered for the development of a CK-MB standard: human heart CK-MB, hybrid CK-MB, recombinant $CK-MB_2$ (tissue isoform), and recombinant $CK-MB_1$ (serum isoform, without the C-terminal lysine on the M subunit) *(21)* and purified with the use of anti-CK-MB MAb-based immunoaffinity chromatography *(22)*. The concentration of the purified CK-MB was determined spectrophotometrically *(23)*.

Four matrices were also evaluated: unprocessed CK-MB-free human serum pool, stripped serum (processed human serum pool that was passed through an ion-exchange column to remove residual CK-MB), synthetic matrix, and manufacturers' recommended diluents. In an attempt to standardize CK-MB mass assay, the subcommittee prepared lyophilized stan-

Table 2
Comparison of Several CK-MB Mass Assays (Regression Analysis Data)

Analyzer	Slope	Y-intercept	r
Ciba Corning ACS:180	1.125	−0.0777	0.9994
Dade Stratus II	0.891	0.3674	0.9999
Hybritech Photon Era	0.563	0.0593	0.9997
Behring Opus Plus	0.894	1.1609	0.9994
Abbott IMx	0.581	0.1493	0.9992
Dupont *aca* plus	0.636	−0.1264	0.9993
Tosoh AIA 600	0.787	−0.4764	0.9999

dards using purified CK-MB spiked into processed human serum. Calibration curves using these standards did not significantly reduce the bias among CK-MB values of the patient samples analyzed on seven immunoassay systems *(24)* (subsequent work has included most of the new assays now available.) The subcommittee found that in some systems, CK-MB recovery was greater in patient samples than in the standards. In other systems, CK-MB recovery was less in patient samples than in the standards. One possible cause of such discrepancy could be alteration of CK-MB during lyophilization. The results indicated that lyophilization caused loss of immunoactivity of CK-MB and recommended the use of frozen material.

Correlation Study

Purified human heart CK-MB standards prepared in processed human serum, unprocessed human serum, and manufacturers' recommended diluent were assayed on each immunoassay analyzer and later used to correct original calibration curves via regression analysis.

In an alternate approach for standardization of CK-MB mass assays, the manufacturers of the assay were provided 20 patient sample pools (not used in the initial correlation study above) and pure human heart CK-MB. Each participating manufacturer prepared 5 CK-MB standards (0, 10, 50, 100,

and 200 ng/mL) in its recommended sample diluent. The standards and the samples were analyzed in duplicate in their respective immunoassay system. Measured CK-MB values of the standards by each immunoassay system were also plotted against the assigned CK-MB values of the standards (0, 10, and 100 ng/mL) to determine each immunoassay's slope bias toward the standards. The initial CK-MB value of patient samples was then divided by the slope bias of each system for the standards to obtain the corrected CK-MB values. The corrected patient results were reanalyzed by linear regression analysis to determine the corrected slope biases (*see* Table 3).

Summary

In summary, the subcommittee found that there is excellent correlation among the CK-MB mass immunoassays, but poor accuracy. Standardization of a primary calibrator alone did not improve accuracy significantly. The major reason for these failures seems to be the sensitivity of certain immunoassays to the matrix differences between the patient samples and the lyophilized and/or processed human serum used in the preparation of the standards. The accuracy of the assays can be significantly improved with the use of CK-MB standards prepared in sample diluent recommended for each assay. Thus, the protocol to standardize CK-MB mass assays centers around the use of a standard pro-

Table 3
Correlation Plots of CK-MB Values from Various Assays vs IMx
Before and After Correction Using MB-MASS Standards

Analyzer	Before correction		After correction	
	Slope	*r*	Slope	*r*
ACS:180	1.37	0.99	0.80	0.99
Stratus II	0.82	0.99	0.99	0.99
aca plus	0.71	0.99	0.89	0.99
AIA 600	0.90	0.99	0.98	0.99
Embria-CK	0.80	0.99	0.92	0.99
Mean (SD)	0.94 (0.26)		0.92 (0.08)	

vided by a national and/or international standard organization (yet to be determined), which each manufacturer would use to calibrate its assay. However, before recommending the protocol for the standardization of CK-MB mass assays, the protocol needs to be confirmed from different heart tissues to understand lot-to-lot variability.

CLINICAL UTILITY OF CK-MB MASS ASSAYS

Historically, patients with AMI have been closely monitored utilizing CK-MB levels, every 8 h over a 48-h period, post onset of chest pain. New-generation immunoassays have offered real-time test results allowing earlier diagnosis.

Early Diagnosis of AMI

The introduction of thrombolytic therapy in the past several years has sparked tremendous interest in early diagnosis of AMI. Several serologic methods have been introduced as well as continuous electrocardiogram (ECG) monitoring and new imaging techniques. Estimates of the initial sensitivity of conventional ECG in the diagnosis of AMI in patients presenting to the emergency department (ED) with chest pain vary up to a maximum of 81% *(25)*. Therefore, at least 20% of AMI patients require further investigation to establish a diagnosis. A conven-

tional cardiac enzyme panel based on serial measurements of total CK, CK-MB, aspartate transaminase, and lactate dehydrogenase (LD) is not useful in the early diagnosis of AMI. Other early serologic methods, such as CK isoforms and myoglobin, are discussed in Chapters 10 and 6, respectively. The performance of single values at optimum diagnostic cutoffs and incremental change (log slope) for total CK was studied using a rapid CK-MB mass assay *(26)*. Total CK slope combined with CK-MB concentration allowed accurate diagnosis at 4 h from admission. CK-MB concentration determination 8 h from admission (12–16 h from onset of chest pain) was the most effective single measurement. Rapid diagnostic categorization and possible selection of patients for thrombolysis in patients with an uncertain admission diagnosis are possible by these techniques. However, slope calculations are not easily available.

The potential of mass assays on patient management was investigated for the administration of thrombolytic therapy *(27)*. When blood is collected on admission to hospital, 10% of patients whom were shown by conventional means to have had AMIs had equivocal ECGs, but positive CK-MB concentration results. In half of these patients (5%), thrombolytic therapy was given on the basis of the clinical features and a positive

CK-MB concentration result alone. The CK-MB mass assay can increase the number of diagnoses of AMI made within the time scale required for the successful administration of thrombolytic therapy and could be used to prompt thrombolytic therapy in AMI. Such a protocol may result in some unstable angina patients receiving thrombolytics. Studies have shown that more than 50% of a series of patients with unstable angina had intracoronary thrombus in major coronary arteries, indicating a theoretical benefit from thrombolytic therapy (28). Unfortunately, larger-scale studies on the use of thrombolytic therapy in patients with unstable angina have shown no therapeutic benefit, and possibly a detriment, with an increase in the incidence of AMI (29,30). Therefore, despite the ability to detect earlier diagnosis of AMI with sensitive markers, such information will not be used to treat AMI patients with thrombolytics, unless there is ECG documentation of the infarct.

Confirmation of Reperfusion

Determination of success of coronary reperfusion following thrombolytic therapy can be used to prompt other treatments, such as rescue percutaneous transluminal coronary angioplasty (PTCA). Indices of coronary artery reperfusion have been identified in patients treated with thrombolytic therapy for AMI by means of characteristics from the serum CK-MB time–activity curve (31). Similarly, early markers, such as CK isoforms and myoglobin, can be used to assess coronary reperfusion and have the advantage of shorter time–activity curves, allowing earlier overall assessment.

Risk Stratification

Five to 20% of unstable angina patients progress to AMI or death within the first year (32–36). Postmortem studies have revealed that these fatal events are frequently preceded by microinfarcts. Pathological evidence shows an atheromatous plaque fissuring with subsequent platelet aggregation, thrombosis formation, and episodic embolization. Sensitive CK-MB mass assays can detect prolonged ischemia in unstable angina patients (37). CK-MB assays has been examined as a tool in patient risk stratification for myocardial infarction (38,39). They concluded that a CK-MB mass assay can detect a subgroup of patients with ischemic heart disease and poor clinical outcome, which are not diagnosed using routine diagnostic procedures.

CK-MB elevations within 3 h of presentation in the ED are associated with subsequent ischemic events in clinically stable chest pain patients without ST-segment elevation (40). They concluded that CK-MB can identify a minority of low-risk patients who develop ischemic events and that additional markers for diagnosing myocardial ischemia in the ED are need.

The clinical usefulness of different immunoenzymetric CK-MB methods have been evaluated on coronary care unit (CCU) patients (41). More than 25% of patients with a suspicion of AMI, but with no standard criteria for AMI were identified with small but significant increase of serum CK-MB (mass concentration) and an increased CK-MB (mass)/total CK ratio. During a 4-yr follow-up, 64% of the patients died within 2 yr, the majority being coronary deaths, as compared to 5% of non-AMI patients with suspicion of AMI, but with normal CK-MB values ($p = 0.001$). The findings of such a high mortality rate among patients with increased CK-MB (mass concentration) have important prognostic value even in patients without standard criteria for AMI. Furthermore, the potential utility of rapid point-of-care assays has been evaluated in ED patients with possible AMI (42). When used for patients in whom a cardiac care unit admission is not considered, the CK-MB mass assay may identify some patients with

unsuspected myocardial infarction and prevent inadvertent discharge or admission to
unmonitored beds. Other cardiac markers,
such as troponin, have also been utilized in
risk stratification *(39,43,44)*, as described in
Chapter 13.

CK-MB Elevations
in Non-AMI Patients

Investigators have shown CK-MB elevations in the pediatric population to be clinically insignificant. These elevations are most
likely owing to the change in CK isoenzyme
distribution from CK-BB to CK-MB and
finally CK-MM, which occurs in development from birth to adulthood.

In patients with coronary artery bypass
graft surgery without any evidence of
myocardial infarction, CK-MB elevations
are significant and mimicked a perioperative myocardial infarction *(45)*. In order to
demonstrate a perioperative myocardial
infarction, it is necessary to determine at
least two cardiac markers (such as CK-MB,
LD, LD_1, and so forth) for a long period and
to correlate these results with the clinical
hemodynamic and ECG findings.

Several investigators have also studied the
release of CK-MB following PTCA, demonstrating that CK-MB is a sensitive indicator
of myocardial injury *(46–49)*. Recently, the
release of CK-MB and cardiac troponin T
have been compared in patients undergoing
PTCA to investigate the clinical, procedural,
and angiographic correlates of abnormal elevations of both of these markers *(50)*. Greater
than 40% of patients undergoing coronary
angioplasty have evidence of minor degrees
of myocardial damage, since evidence of
release of biochemical markers and that elevations of both CK-MB and cardiac troponin
T may be indicative of greater levels of
myocardial injury than elevations of cardiac
troponin T alone.

FUTURE NEEDS
FOR CK-MB ASSAYS

Methods for the analysis of CK-MB have
evolved from manual column chromatographic procedures and electrophoresis to
automated techniques. It is likely that there
will be more laboratories switching from
labor-intensive CK-MB procedures to highly
specific and sensitive immunoassays assays
as these assays become more inexpensive
and available on automated immunoassay
analyzers. However, as with any technology, further improvements are warranted.
Currently, none of the immunoassays
can be implemented onto high-volume clinical chemistry analyzers. Routine analysis
requires sample splitting: total CK measured
from a general analyzer, and CK-MB measured from specific immunoassay analyzer.
Stat analysis necessitates training of second-
and third-shift personnel who might not be
accustomed to immunoassay testing. Implementation of a CK-MB mass measurement
onto a medium-size multipurpose chemistry
analyzer would have an immediate impact
on work flow efficiency.

Bedside analysis for CK-MB may also
become important in the future as more hospitals develop point-of-care approaches.
Bedside testing in hospitals today has largely
been limited to glucose and electrolytes.
Whether or not CK-MB should be included
as a high priority, bedside testing service
is debatable. It may be possible that a
more cardiospecific marker, such as troponin, might be better for point-of-care use.
Recently, Spectral Diagnostics Inc.
(Toronto, Ontario) has announced development of a qualitative test panel for emergency analysis, consisting of CK, CK-MB,
troponin-I, and myosin light chains *(see*
Chapter 15). If this new device becomes
accepted for point-of-care testing, it may significantly alter how laboratories use tradi-

tional laboratory-based testing for cardiac markers.

ABBREVIATIONS

AACC, American Association for Clinical Chemistry; AMI, acute myocardial infarction; CAP, College of American Pathologists; CCU, coronary care unit; CK, creatine kinase; CPR(G), chlorophenol red $(-\beta\text{-}d\text{-galactopyranoside})$; ECG, electrocardiogram; ED, emergency department; ELISA, enzyme-linked immunosorbent assay; immunoinhibition; LD, lactate dehydrogenase; MASS, Mass Assay Standardization Subcommittee; MEIA, microparticle enzyme immunoassay; 4-MU(P), 4-methylumbelliferone (phosphate); PTCA, percutaneous transluminal coronary angioplasty; T_r, room temperature.

REFERENCES

1. Delanghe J, DeMol AM, DeBuyzere ML, DeScheerder IK, and Wieme RJ (1990) Mass concentration and activity concentration of creatine kinase isoenzyme MB compared in serum after acute myocardial infarction. Clin. Chem. 36:149–153.
2. Wu AHB and Schwartz JG (1989) Update on creatine kinase isoenzyme assays. Diagn. Clin. Test. 27(8):16–20.
3. Wu AHB (1985) CK-MB assay methods. A comparison. Laboratory Management 23(1): 44–50.
4. Green S and Wu AHB (1993) Immunoassays and electrophoresis for creatine kinase isoenzymes and isoforms in diagnosis and management of acute myocardial infarction, AACC Endo. Metabol. 11:329–344.
5. Bodor GS, Porter S, Landt Y, and Ladenson JH (1992) Development of monoclonal antibodies for an assay of cardiac troponin-I and preliminary results in suspected cases of myocardial infarction. Clin. Chem. 38: 2203–2214.
6. Wong SS, Earl R, and Wu AHB (1987) Simultaneous presence of IgA- and IgG-CK-BB in a patient without myocardial infarction. Clin. Chim. Acta 166:99–100.
7. Venta R, Geijo SA, Sanchez AC, Bao CG, Bartolome LA, Casares G, Lopez-Otin C, and Alvarez FV (1989) IgA-CK-BB complex with CK-MB electrophoretic mobility can lead to erroneous diagnosis of acute myocardial infarction. Clin. Chem. 35: 2003–2008.
8. Wolfson D, Lindberg E, Su L, Farber SJ, and Dubin SB (1991) Three rapid immunoassays for the detection of creatine kinase MB: an analytical, and interpretive evaluation. Am. Heart J. 122:958–964.
9. Brandt R, Gates RC, Eng KK, Forsythe CM, Korom GK, Nitro AS, Koffler IA, and Ogunro EA (1990) Quantifying the MB isoenzyme of creatine kinase with the Abbott "IMx" immunoassay analyzer. Clin. Chem. 36:375–378.
10. Chapelle J and el Allaf M (1990) Automated quantification of creatine kinase MB isoenzyme in serum by radial partition immunoassay, with use of the Stratus analyzer. Clin. Chem. 36:99–101.
11. Apple F, Preese L, and Fredrickson A (1988) Clinical and analytical evaluation of two immunoassays for direct measurement of creatine kinase MB with monoclonal anti-CK-MB antibodies. Clin. Chem. 34:2364–2367.
12. Green S and Lehrer M (1992) Comparison of three immunoassay analyzers for CK-MB with an electrophoretic method. Presented at CliniChem, Tarrytown, NY.
13. College of American Pathologists, Inc. (1990–1996) EC-C and IE-06 Surveys.
14. Seo H, Miyazaki S, Furuno T, Nonogi H, Haze K, and Hiramori K (1993) Creatine kinase MB protein mass is a better indicator for the assessment of acute myocardial infarction in the lower range of creatine kinase level. Jpn. Heart J. 34:717–727.
15. Wu AHB, Gornet TG, Bretaudiere JP, and Panfili PR (1985) Comparison of enzyme immunoassay and immunoinhibition for creatine kinase MB in diagnosis of acute myocardial infarction. Clin. Chem. 31:470–474.
16. Koch TR, Mehta UJ, and Nipper HC (1996) Clinical and analytical evaluation of kits for measurement of creatine kinase isoenzyme MB. Clin. Chem. 32:186–191.

17. Buttery JE, Stuart S, and Pannall PR (1992) Stability of the CK-MB isoenzyme on routine storage, Clin. Biochem. 25:11–13.

18. Ehresman JJ, Zittel DB, Massman TJ, Levine RP, and Baum J (1996) Quantitative immunoassay of serum and plasma CK-MB on the Technicon Immuno 1. [abstract]. Clin. Chem. 52:S155.

19. Green S, Onoroski M, Moore R, Wu A, Lehrer M, and Vaidya H (1993) Use of proposed CK-MB standardization material for calibration of mass measurements: clinical correlation of patient sera [abstract]. Clin. Chem. 39:1269.

20. McBride JH, Rodgerson DO, Ota MK, Maruya M, and McEveney S (1991) Creatine kinase MB measured by fluorometric enzyme immunoassay and immunochemiluminescence. Ann. Clin. Lab. Sci. 21:284–290.

21. Friedman DL, Wu AHB, Gornet TG, Kesterson R, Chen L, Puleo P, and Perryman MB (1993) Recombinant creatine kinase proteins and proposed standards for creatine kinase isoenzymes and subform assays. Clin. Chem. 35:1598–1601.

22. Landt Y, Vaidya HC, Porter SE, Dietzler DN, and Ladenson JH Immunoaffinity purification of creatine kinase MB from human, dog and rabbit heart with the use of monoclonal antibody specific for CK-MB. Clin. Chem. 35:985–989.

23. Gill SC and von Hippel PH (1989) Calculation of protein extinction coefficients from the amino acid sequence data. Anal. Biochem. 182:319–326.

24. Green S, Onoroski M, Moore R, Wu A, Lehrer M, and Vaidya H Standardization of CK-MB mass immunoassays [Abstract]. Clin. Chem. 40:1032.

25. Rude RE, Poole WK, Muller JE, Turi Z, Rutherford J, Parker C, Roberts R, Raabe DS, Gold HK, Stone PH, Willerson JT, and Braunwald E (1983) Electrocardiographic and clinical criteria for recognition of acute myocardial infarction based on analysis of 3,697 patients, Am. J. Cardiol. 52:936–942.

26. Collinson PO, Rosalki SB, Kuwana T, Garratt HM, Ramhamadamy EM, Baird IM, and Greenwood TW (1992) Early diagnosis of acute myocardial infarction by CK-MB mass measurements. Ann. Clin. Biochem. 29:43–47.

27. Collins DR, Wright DJ, Rinsler MG, Thomas P, Bhattacharya S, and Raftery EB (1993) Early diagnosis of acute myocardial infarction with use of a rapid immunochemical assay of creatine kinase MB isoenzyme, Clin. Chem. 39(8):1725–1728.

28. Gotoh K, Minamino T, Katoh O, Hamano Y, Fukui S, Hori M, Kusuoka H, Mishima M, Inoue M, and Kamata D (1988) The role of intracoronary thrombus in unstable angina: angiographic assessment and thrombolytic therapy during ongoing anginal attacks. Circulation 77:526–534.

29. Freeman MR, Langer A, Wilson RF, Morgan CD, and Armstrong PW (1992) Thrombolysis in unstable angina. Randomized double-blind trial of t-PA and placebo. Circulation 85:150–157.

30. Schreiber TL, Rizik D, White C, Sharma CVR, Cowley M, Macina G, Reddy PS, Kantounis L, Timmis GC, Margulis A, Bunnell P, Barker W, and Sasahara A (1992) Randomized trial of thrombolysis versus heparin in unstable angina. Circulation 86:1407–1414.

31. Grande P, Granborg J, Clemmensen P, Sevilla DC, Wagner NB, and Wagner GS (1991) Indices of reperfusion in patients with acute myocardial infarction using characteristics of the CK-MB time activity curve. Am. Heart J. 122:400–408.

32. Gazes PC, Mobley EM, Faris HM, Duncan RC, and Humphries CB (1973) Preinfarctional (unstable) angina—a prospective study—ten year follow-up. Circulation 48:331–337.

33. Heng MK, Norris RM, Singh BN, and Partridge JB (1976) Prognosis in unstable angina. Br. Heart J. 38:921–925.

34. Mulcahy R, Daly L, Graham L, Al Awadhi AH, De Buitleor M, Tobin G, Johnson H, and Contoy R (1985) Natural history and prognosis in unstable angina. Am. Heart J. 109:753–758.

35. Hugenholz PG (1986) Unstable angina revisited once more. Eur. Heart J. 7:1010–1013.

36. Madsen JK, Thomsen BL, Sorensen JN, Kjeldgaard KM, and Kromann-Andersen B (1987) Risk factors and prognosis after discharge for patients admitted of suspected acute myocardial infarction with and without confirmed diagnosis. Am. J. Cardiol. 59:1064–1070.

37. Botker HE, Ravkilde J, Sogaard P, Jorgensen PJ, Horder M, and Thygesen K (1991) Gradation of unstable angina based on a sensitive immunoassay for serum creatine kinase MB. Br. Heart J. 65:72–76.

38. Ravkilde J, Hansen AB, Horder M, Jorgensen PJ, and Thygesen K (1992) Risk stratification in suspected acute myocardial infarction based on a sensitive immunoassay for serum creatine kinase isoenzyme MB. Cardiology 80:143–151.

39. Ravkilde J, Nissen H, Horder M, and Thygesen K (1995) Independent prognostic value of serum creatine kinase isoenzyme MB mass, cardiac troponin-T and myosin light chain levels in suspected acute myocardial infarction. Analysis of 28 months of follow-up in 196 patients. J. Am. Coll. Cardiol. 25: 574–581.

40. Hedges JR, Young GP, Henkel GF, Gibler WB, Green TR, and Swanson JR (1994) Early CK-MB elevations predict ischemic events in stable chest pain patients. Acad. Emerg. Med. 1:9–16.

41. Pettersson T, Ohlsson O, and Tryding N (1992) Increased CK-MB (mass concentration) in patients without traditional evidence of acute myocardial infarction. A risk indicator of coronary death. Eur. Heart J. 13: 1387–1392.

42. Green GB, Hansen KN, Chan DW, Guerci AD, Fleetwood DH, Silvertso KT, and Kelen GD (1991) The potential utility of a rapid CK-MB assay in evaluating emergency department patients with possible myocardial infarction. Ann. Emerg. Med. 20: 954–960.

43. Hamm CW, Ravkilde J, Gerhardt W, Jorgensen P, Peheim E, Ljungdahl L, Goldmann B, and Katus HA (1992) The prognostic value serum troponin T in unstable angina. N. Engl. J. Med. 327:146–150.

44. Wu AHB, Abbas SA, Green S, Pearsall L, Dhakam S, Azar R, Onoroski M, Senaie A, McKay RG, and Waters D (1995) Prognostic value of cardiac troponin-T in unstable angina pectoris. Am. J. Cardiol 76:970–972.

45. Kutsal A, Saydam GS, Yucel D, and Balk M (1991) Changes in the serum levels of CK-MB, LDH, LDH1, SGOT and myoglobin due to cardiac surgery. J. Cardiovasc. Surg. 32:516–520.

46. Klein LW, Kramer BL, Howard E, and Lesch M (1991) Incidence of clinical significance of transient creatine kinase elevations and the diagnosis on non-Q wave myocardial infarction associated with coronary angioplasty. J. Am. Coll. Cardiol. 17:621–626.

47. Oh JK, Shub C, Ilstrup DM, and Reeder GS (1985) Creatine kinase release after successful percutaneous transluminal coronary angioplasty. Am. Heart. J. 109:122–1230.

48. Ravkilde J, Nissen H, Mickley H, Andersen P, Thayssen P, and Horder M (1994) Cardiac troponin-T and CK-MB mass release after visually successful percutaneous transluminal coronary angioplasty in stable angina pectoris. Am. Heart J. 127:13–20.

49. Talasz H, Genser N, Mair J, Artner-Dworzak E, Friedrich G, Moes N, Muhlberger V, and Puschendort B (1992) Side branch occlusion during percutaneous transluminal coronary angioplasty. Lancet 339:1380–1381.

50. Abbas SA, Glazier JJ, Wu AHB, Green SF, Samedy H, Onoroski M, Pearsall LA, Waters DD, and McKay RG (1996) An analysis of the relative sensitivities of cardiac troponin T and of CK-MB in the detection of myocardial injury during percutaneous transluminal coronary angioplasty. Clin. Cardiol. 19:782–786.

10

CK Isoforms

Sol F. Green

INTRODUCTION

In 1985, the TIMI* study group *(1)* conducted a 5-yr multicenter trial. The study concluded that patients with acute myocardial infarction (AMI) received maximum benefits when they received thrombolytic therapy within 4–6 h after onset of chest pain. Therefore, an early biochemical marker of AMI is crucial in diagnosis of myocardial injury. Currently, CK-MB isoforms are the only cardiac-specific markers satisfying these criteria, although other markers are being developed (*see* Chapter 17). The proceeding discussion is focused on review of pertinent biochemistry, approaches to analytical measurements, and the clinical applications of CK isoforms.

REVIEW OF PERTINENT BIOCHEMISTRY

The separation of tissue and serum isoforms of CK isoenzymes using polyacrylamide gel electrophoresis was first described in 1972 *(2)*. CK isoforms (also known as subisoenzymes, subtypes, or subforms) are variants of CK-MM and CK-MB isoenzymes, which are produced by in vivo changes to the M-subunit. The CK-MM isoenzyme dimer has three possible isoforms (MM_3, MM_2, and MM_1), which are named by their relative migration toward the anode using electrophoresis as shown in Fig. 1. MM_3 is the pure gene form present in skeletal muscle and heart, and is known as the tissue form. Following muscle damage, CK-MM_3 is released into the serum, where carboxypeptidase-N cleaves the carboxy-terminal lysine of one M-subunit *(3)* to produce an intermediate form, CK-MM_2. Subsequently, the second M-subunit will lose its C-terminal lysine, producing the serum form, CK-MM_1 (*see* Fig. 2). The carboxypeptidase-N reactions occur slowly over 24 h, and are irreversible *(4–6)*. In theory, the isoform conversion of MM_3 to MM_2 and MM_1 can be used to back-extrapolate when the onset of AMI occurred. However, because the carboxypeptidase activity in serum can be variable *(7,8)*, precise estimates of AMI onset are not possible in actual practice. Differences in the activation energy for the individual isoforms have also been used to date the age of myocardial injury *(9)* (but are not in routine use). Sera of healthy individuals contain only trace amounts of the tissue isoform, CK-MM_3 (12–18%). The major fraction in serum is the fully converted product, CK-MM_1 (47–60%) *(5)*.

---

*See p. 167 for list of abbreviations used in this chapter.

From: Cardiac Markers   *Edited by:* Alan H. B. Wu
© Humana Press Inc., Totowa, NJ

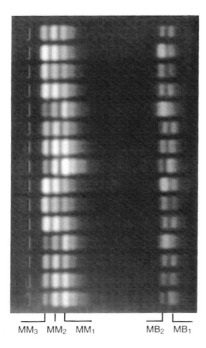

MM₃   MM₂   MM₁   MB₂   MB₁

Fig. 1. Typical electrophoretic agarose gel electrophoresis of CK-MM and MB isoforms (courtesy Helena Laboratories).

Carboxypeptidase-N also acts on the M-subunit of CK-MB. Therefore, there are two CK-MB isoforms: the tissue form, $CK-MB_2$, converted to the serum form $CK-MB_1$ *(10)* *(see* Fig. 1). In normal individuals, the tissue form, $CK-MB_2$ is present in roughly equal concentrations to the converted form, $CK-MB_1$. The biochemistry, kinetics, and clinical utility of CK isoforms have been recently reviewed *(6,11)*.

The tissue form of CK-MB may undergo cleavage of lysine from the B-monomer as well as the M-monomer in vivo, generating at least two more CK-MB isoforms *(12)*. The four possible CK-MB isoforms being generated therefore include: M^+B^+ (tissue form), M^+B^- and M^-B^+ (intermediate forms), and M^-B^- (serum form), where + and − represent the presence and absence of a C-terminal lysine, respectively (*see* Fig. 3). Cleavage of lysine from the carboxyl-terminus of B-monomers occurs first and subsequently from M-monomers in vivo. Development of an assay capable of resolving all of the isoforms of CK-MB that occur in vivo might increase sensitivity for early detection of AMI compared with currently available assays that resolve only two species (MB_2 and MB_1, as seen in Fig. 1). Specific monoclonal antibodies (MAbs) have been used to recognize epitopes on human brain creatine kinase (CK-B) in order to identify its isoforms *(13)*. One antibody, CK-HTB, recognizes the assembled or native CK-B isoform. Two others, CK-END1 and CK-END2, recognize epitopes within 53 amino acids of the C-terminus of CK-B variant, whereas neither antibody binds to native CK-B monomer. Further work needs to be conducted to characterize the in vivo degradation of the CK-B-subunit.

APPROACHES FOR ANALYTICAL MEASUREMENTS OF CK ISOFORMS

Measurement Techniques

Several analytical methods have been developed for measuring CK isoforms, including electrophoresis *(14,15)*, isoelectric focusing *(16)*, chromatofocusing chromatography *(3,17,18)*, and high-pressure liquid chromatography (HPLC) *(19)*. Most methods are deficient in data pertaining to validations, such as for accuracy and precision, although electrophoretic data were the most reproducible, required the shortest analysis time, and appeared to be the most practical method for use in routine clinical analysis. Electrophoresis may also be the most sensitive and least costly technique. The Cardio Rep (Helena Laboratories, Beaumont TX) is a high-voltage automated agarose gel electrophoresis analyzer utilizing a peltier heating and cooling device to control temperature through all processing

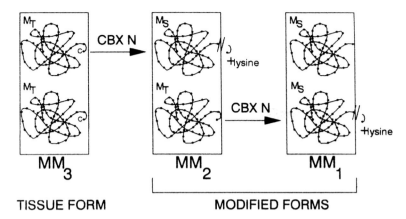

Fig. 2. Diagramatic representation of CK-MM isoform structure, nomenclature, and conversion by carboxypeptidase-N (CBX N). MM3 consists of two unmodified tissue M-subunits. Conversion of one M-subunit to the modified serum form produces MM2 ; conversion of two tissue M-subunits produces MM1. The isoform conversion involves the hydrolysis of the C-terminal amino acid (lysine) from the M chain.

phases. The analyzer runs at 900 V, 60 mA, 24°C, for 6 min. After incubation with CK substrate at 49°C for 5 min, the plate is dried at 54°C for 2 min and fluorescence scanned in a densitometer, producing highly sensitive CK-MB isoform analysis with turnaround times of approx 25 min. The method is linear to 100 U/L CK-MB and sensitive to 1.22 U/L (20).

The Impres-MB-X assay (International Immunoassay Labs, Santa Clara, CA), an immunoextraction assay, is based on an M-subunit antibody that removes CK-MB1 from the specimen. The remaining CK-MB is essentially CK-MB2 and can be measured by traditional methods for CK-MB measurement.

It is important to note that the methods described above are all activity based assays and will not detect MB isoforms if the protein's structure has been altered during release from cardiac tissue and CK becomes inactive. An immunoassay has recently been developed that measures active and inactive forms (21). This assay utilizes a specific monoclonal capture antibody directed against the B-subunit of CK-MB and a specific MAb conjugate directed against the CK-M + lysine-subunit. The analytical sensitivity of the assay was reported to be 0.2 ng/mL. Normal range expressed in %MB2/total MB was from 35–97% when total MB was <3.0 ng/mL.

Factors Affecting Accurate Measurement

There is much debate over CK isoform stability in vitro. CK-MB2 has been shown to have in vitro stability in serum for 6 h postvenipuncture at 4°C and 25°C (22). Losses of MB2 were statistically significant at 37°C. These findings suggest the carboxypeptidase-mediated conversion of CK-MB2 to CK-MB1 is inhibited at temperatures of 25°C or less. However, others have shown that there is significant loss of MB2 activity in the absence of 15 mmol/L EDTA and β-mercaptoethanol (23), prompting the need for preservatives to maintain isoform activity (17,24). Instability issues can be eliminated when testing is performed on a stat basis, since no preservatives are necessary (25–28). In one study (29), CK-MB isoforms were stable at −20°C with no significant

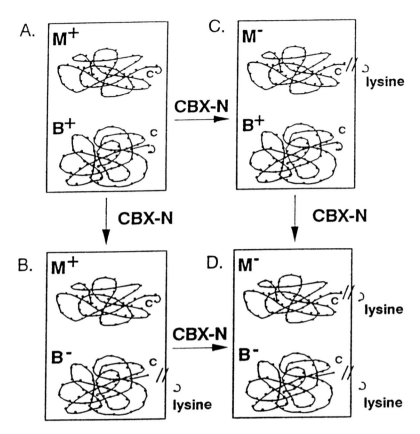

Fig. 3. Conversion schemes of tissue to serum isoforms of MB *(12)*. The conversion of the tissue form of MB (**A**) first proceeds by cleavage of the C-terminal amino acid (lysine) from the B-subunit of MB by carboxypeptidase N (**B**) followed by cleavage of the C-terminal amino acid from the M-subunit (also a lysine, **D**). In contrast, only two MB isoforms are ever observed on agarose gel electrophoresis. These isoforms were thought to arise from cleavage of the tissue form (**A**) to the serum form (**C**) through cleavage of the M-subunit alone.

change in the MB_2/MB_1 ratio after 30 d. Total CK-MB mass or activity degradation was not determined. Other studies have concluded no degradation in activity in EDTA plasma at room temperature for up to 1 h, at 2–6°C for 6 h and at −20°C for 3 d *(30)*.

CLINICAL APPLICATION OF ISOFORM METHODS

CK Isoforms for Early Diagnosis of AMI

The use of an index formulated by summing the concentrations of the M-monomers with intact C-terminal lysines (tissue isoforms), and dividing by the total CK concentration has been suggested *(31)*. This index can help assess early AMI by providing an indication concerning the time of onset of myocardial injury, since coronary artery occlusion produces tissue isoform release, and therefore, an increase in the index and slope on the CK kinetic curve is expected.

Similarly, relative amounts of CK-MM isoforms (MM_3 and MM_1) expressed as the MM_3/MM_1 ratio can be used for early diagnosis of AMI *(26,27,32)*. Ratios of the tissue isoforms to the serum isoforms have greater diagnostic sensitivity than do the individual isoforms *(6,33)*. Evidence of AMI can be detected as early as 1–2 h postinfarction, several hours before CK-MB. MM isoforms can also be used to predict the time of onset of AMI *(34)*. MM_3 is the predominant isoform when tissue necrosis is of relatively recent origin (5–15 h); MM_2 is the dominant subband between 15 and 24 h after AMI, whereas a predominant MM_1 band would indicate that the injury occurred 24 h ago or earlier *(34)*. However, MM isoforms' lack of specificity to cardiac tissue may result in false positives in cases of skeletal muscle trauma or myopathy *(32,35)*. Accordingly, CK-MM isoforms, may be more appropriate for early detection of muscle damage or as one component within a panel of cardiac markers.

Measuring MB_2 activity and the CK-MB tissue form to serum form ratio is a more specific marker of AMI, and can also provide biochemical evidence before the total level of CK-MB exceeds the normal range *(36,37)*. The diagnostic criteria of $MB_2 >$ 1.0 U/L and MB_2/MB_1 ratio of >1.5 have been shown to be specific for AMI within 6 h of infarct in 95% of patients using the Helena Rep System (Helena) *(37)*. More recently, Helena has set its diagnostic criteria for AMI at $MB_2 > 2.6$ U/L and MB_2/MB_1 ratio of >1.7 on the Cardio Rep based on additional clinical trials *(30)*. Figure 4 illustrates several CK densitometer scans, which demonstrate how the MM_3/MM_1 and MB_2/MB_1 ratio change after AMI. The clinical sensitivity of 12.5, 59, and 92% has been reported in patients with AMI when blood was collected 0–2, 2–4, and 4–6 h after onset of chest pain using the MB_2/MB_1 ratio *(37)*. In many conventional assays, CK-MB activity would just be approaching the upper limits of normal during these time intervals *(37)*.

Despite these favorable reports on isoforms for early AMI diagnosis, several other investigators have shown that CK-MB isoforms are not better than or even as good as CK-MB mass assays *(38–40)*. These reports have been critical of the earlier studies where results of isoforms were compared against CK-MB using an insensitive column chromatographic method. In one study *(41)*, the diagnostic utility CK-MM and CK-MB isoform activity assays (as measured by electrophoresis) were compared to a CK-MB mass assay in assessing early AMI. All three tests were ineffective within the first 4 h of onset of chest pain and were most effective at 4–18 hours after onset. Both CK-MM and CK-MB isoform ratios were less effective the CK-MB mass concentrations between 18 and 24 h. In the critical time between 3 and 6 h, the diagnostic performances of all three were comparable. More recently, the clinical utility of a $CK-MB_2$ mass assay, myoglobin, and a total CK-MB mass assay in the diagnosis of AMI have been compared *(22)*. The order of sensitivity at 0–2 h after onset of symptoms was myoglobin > $CK-MB_2$ > CK-MB. Because the release kinetics of $CK-MB_2$ were similar to CK-MB, the use of isoforms is precluded as a sensitive marker of myocardial damage early in the course of AMI.

Although there still remains debate in the clinical utility of CK-MB isoforms as an early marker of AMI, isoforms may play an important role in assessment of reinfarction, reperfusion, decision making in evaluating patients with chest pain, and as a predictive indicator of myocardial injury.

Factors Affecting Accurate Clinical Applications

Other markers, such as total CK, CK-MB, LD, and troponin, are still necessary to access progression of an AMI after initial diagnosis. An isoform assay may produce a false-negative result in a patient if the initial specimen was drawn more than 18–24 h after onset of chest pain *(41)*.

Increases in the ratio MB_2/MB_1 together with an overall increase in CK-MB/total CK

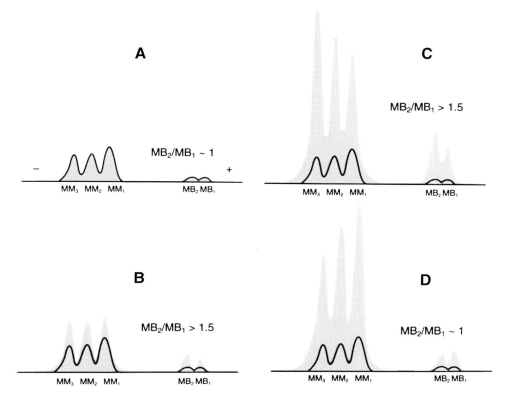

Fig. 4. The CK isoform profile in a typical patient without cardiac injury consists predominately of CK-MM$_1$ (serum form) and smaller amounts of MM$_2$ and MM$_3$. CK-MB$_1$ and CK-MB$_2$ are similar in concentration (<2.6 U/L), and the MB$_2$/MB$_1$ ratio is approx 1 *(36,37)*. **(A)** During the initial hours following AMI, the tissue isoforms (MM$_3$ and MB$_2$) are released from the injured heart tissue. The MM$_3$/MM$_1$ and MB$_2$/MB$_1$ ratio increases rapidly owing to the increase in tissue isoforms entering the serum. Although total CK-MM and total CK-MB will increase during this initial period, their activity may remain in the normal reference range. **(B)** Over the next 24 h, carboxypeptidase-N will cleave the C-terminal lysines of the M-subunits, producing the serum forms (MM$_1$ and MB$_1$). **(C)** The MM$_3$/MM$_1$ and MB$_2$/MB$_1$ ratios will decrease rapidly and return to normal range. **(D)** The MB$_2$/MB$_1$ ratio peaks at 3.1, approx 4–6 h post-AMI and returns to normal levels after 14–18 h, as the tissue form is converted to the serum form.

(relative index) is a highly specific marker for early AMI. Isoforms do not obviate the need to analyze total CK and calculation of a relative index. For instance, in cases of acute trauma or skeletal muscle injury, CK-MB isoforms may be transiently increased owing to release from skeletal muscle (approx 1%), and therefore, total MB, MB$_2$, and the MB$_2$/MB$_1$ ratio may be elevated without cardiac damage. The use of a relative index is essential to rule out AMI in

these patients. Muscle myopathy will cause an increase in total MB, but the % MB will be <4%, and CK-MB isoforms may appear positive *(42)*.

An immunochemical reagent intended for use in fractionating MB$_1$ and MB$_2$ isoforms was examined *(43)*. The reagent C(x) was designed to remove the MB$_1$ isoform present in the patient samples by immunoextraction. Ideally, all of the MB$_1$ activity would be eliminated, leaving only MB$_2$ for quantita-

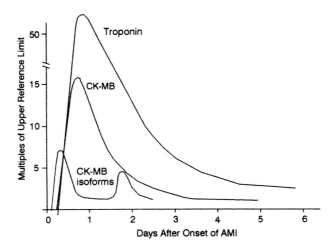

Fig. 5. Use of CK-MB isoforms for detection of reinfarction or extension. CK-MB and cardiac troponin do not return to baseline until >3 d after onset. Isoforms return to normal within 24 h and can be used to detect new onset of injury.

tion. The C(x) reagent eliminated 75% of MB_1 activity while diminishing MB_2 activity by 40%. The reagent could still be useful both for early detection of AMI and accessing reperfusion after thrombolytic therapy. However, it cannot be used to measure the MB_2/MB_1 ratio acurately. Future work should be turned toward the development of more sensitive and faster immunoassays measuring MB_2 in order to aid in early diagnosis of AMI, patient triage, and accessing reperfusion after thrombolytic therapy.

Detection of Reinfarction

CK isoform interpretation can aid in the detection of reinfarction or AMI extension. An MB_2/MB_1 ratio remaining positive 24 h after onset of chest pain is indicative of either reinfarction or AMI extension *(44)*. Other markers, such as total CK, CK-MB, LD, and cardiac troponin T or I, will remain elevated for several days. CK-MB isoforms and myoglobin rapidly return to normal limits (Fig. 5), and this facilitates detection of new injury. Other early markers, such as myoglobin (*see* Chapter 6), are likely to have similar performance, but with less specificity.

Confirmation of Reperfusion

The struggle for new biochemical markers for the determination of success of reperfusion following thrombolytic therapy has been accelerated by modern catheterization techniques, such as rescue (also known as salvage) percutaneous transluminal coronary angioplasty (PTCA). Many cardiologists believe that within the next decade, most major trauma centers will have emergent PTCA techniques available for patients who have failed to achieve reperfusion on treatment with thombolytic therapy. Institutions that may not have a 24-h stat cath laboratory available may opt to treat patients with an additional dose of thrombolytic therapy. In order for these procedures to be successful, biochemical markers of success of reperfusion must be available on a 24-h stat basis with a preferable turnaround time of under 1 h.

Both CK-MM and CK-MB isoforms can be used to detect whether a coronary vessel has reperfused following thrombolysis. The reperfusion of a vessel causes a release of enzymes and proteins previously held back by the blockage. This release, known as the "washout phenomenon," can characterize the success of thrombolytic therapy depending on the rate of enzyme release into circulation *(45–48)*. After thrombolytic therapy, CK-MM or CK-MB isoforms can be used to detect reperfusion by monitoring peak enzyme levels. An isoform pattern that reaches peak levels within a few hours after therapy would indicate successful reperfusion *(49–51)*. Conversely, isoforms reaching peak levels 12 h after therapy would indicate an occluded vessel. The data suggest that criteria based on rates of change in % MB_2 are more sensitive than those based on % MM_3. However, criteria based on % MM_3 are more likely to identify patients in need of interventions to maintain coronary patency. Conventional enzymes, such as total CK-MB or total CK, and proteins, such as troponin T, troponin I, and myosin light chains, can also be used to access reperfusion. However they reach peak levels at slower rates. Myoglobin has release kinetics similar to CK isoforms and may be an alternative early marker of successful reperfusion.

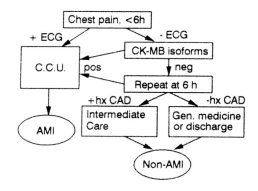

Fig. 6. Proposed triaging system using CK-MB isoforms. (Used with permission from ref. *35*.)

Use of Isoforms for Decision Making in Evaluating Patients with Chest Pain

Presently, AMI is diagnosed by the triad of evidence consisting of chest pain, electrocardiogram (ECG), and CK-MB data (WHO criterial; *see* Chapter 1). However, in many patients, these results are nondiagnostic within the initial 6-h period after infarction. This situation may lead to non-AMI patients being admitted to the coronary care unit (CCU), and remain until CK-MB or some other marker is used to rule out AMI. The consequence of this is not only the tremendous cost of a CCU bed, but it also means a bed may not be available for another patient who is having an AMI. Furthermore, true AMI patients may be misdiagnosed and discharged *(52)*. Several algorithms have been proposed using CK-MB isoforms in addition to conventional rule-in/rule-out criteria in order to improve triage effectiveness *(30,53)*. One proposal involves using CK-MB isoforms with ECG and chest pain in order to reduced non-AMI CCU admissions (*see* Fig. 6) *(35)*. Using this protocol, a large prospective study on 1110 patients was conducted to determine the impact of isoforms on triaging of chest pain patients from the emergency department (ED) *(54)*. The availability of isoforms within 1.2 h after patient arrival in the ED produced a sensitivity of 95.7% and specificity of 93.9% at 6 h after onset of chest pain. It was estimated that use of isoforms for triaging patients would reduce unnecessary CCU admissions by up to 70%.

Implementation of isoforms will require a new "diagnostic mind set" to be adopted *(55)*. Future protocols, such as those described here, will need to be validated. Ideally several different triage protocols may be in place in a given hospital. Depending on environmental factors, such as patient time of arrival after onset of chest pain, clinical symptoms, ECG findings, and the availability of an on-call catheterization team, different protocols may be put to use.

It is important to note that even when early cardiac markers are elevated (CK-isoforms or myoglobin), in patients presented to the ED with non-Q-wave AMI, there is no

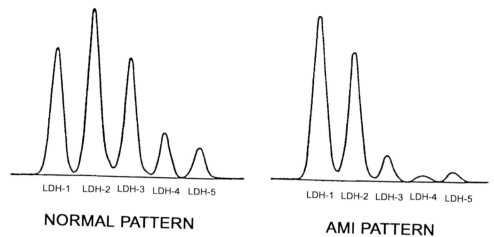

NORMAL PATTERN

AMI PATTERN

Fig. 2. Electrophoretic pattern of serum LD isoenzymes before and after AMI.

Table 1
Final Reaction Mixture Concentrations and Conditions for the IFCC Method for LD[a]

Parameter	Value
Temperature	30.0°C
Wavelength	339 nm
pH	9.40
L(+)-Lactate	50 mmol/L
Buffer	N-methyl-D-glucamine, 325 mmol/L
Serum fraction	0.050 mL
Preincubation phase	180 s
NAD+	10 mmol/L
Lag phase	30 s
Measurement phase	>240 s

[a]Total final volume=1.05 mL. Molar absorption coefficient (30°C, 339 nm) = 630 m²/mol. Most commercial clinical chemistry analyzers set the wavelength to 340 nm.

339 nm, bandwidth ≤ 2 nm, in a recording spectrophotometer equipped with a constant temperature control.

Sample should be collected by venipuncture with minimal manipulation and stasis. Serum is the preferred specimen since plasma may be contaminated with platelets.

A reagent blank reaction using water as sample should be run as a background control. The overall rate of the reaction, A_{all}/min, is the difference between the two reactions:

$$A_{all}/min = A_s/min - A_b/min \qquad (3)$$

where A_s/min is the change of absorbance/min for the reaction with serum sample, and A_b/min is that for the water sample. The concentration of the enzyme activity may be calculated by the following equation:

$$LD = 3333 \times A_{all}/min \text{ U/L} \qquad (4)$$

Assay Performance

The within-run precision of the method for three LD levels ranging from 140–470 U/L is about 0.97%. A reference range of 135–225 U/L was obtained at 37°C *(24)*.

Determination of Isoenzymes

The LD isoenzymes can be analyzed by several different methods. Detection of all isoenzymes can only be achieved by electrophoresis *(26)*. For the heart specific isoenzyme, LD1, immunological, heat inactivation, chemical inhibition, and other chaotropic procedures have been developed.

Table 2
Comparison of Different Commercially Available Electrophoresis Systems

Method	Support medium	Electrophoretic conditions	Detection method
Helena (Beaumont, TX)			
LD-VIS	Cellulose acetate	Tris-barbital, 300 V, 10 min	Colorimetric
LD-FLUR	Cellulose acetate	Tris-barbital, 300 V, 10 min	Fluorometric
Gel-PC	Agarose	Barbital/AMPD, 100 V, 20 min	Colorimetric
Iso-Dot Vis	Agarose	Barbital, 100 V, 20 min	Colorimetric
Iso-Dot Flur	Agarose	Barbital, 100 V, 20 min	Fluorometric
Corning (Corning, NY)			
LD Vis	Agarose	Barbital, 200 V, 35 min	Colorimetric
LD Flur	Agarose	Barbital, 200 V, 35 min	Fluorometric
Gelman (Ann Arbor, MI)			
LD Isozyme	Cellulose acetate	Tris-Barbital, 210 V, 25 min	Colorimetric
Beckman (Brea, CA)			
Paragon	Agarose	Barbital/AMPD, 100 V, 20 min	Colorimetric

Electrophoresis

Electrophoresis followed by densitometry is the method of choice for separation of LD isoenzymes and the detection of the LD1/LD2 flip in AMI *(27)*. In outline, the serum sample is applied onto the gel surface. After the isoenzymes have been separated by electrophoresis, a reaction mixture is layered over the separation medium. The mixture (typically 500 mmol/L L-Lactate, and 13 mmol/L NAD+, dissolved in a suitable pH 8.0 buffer) may be applied as a liquid or in the gel. The overlay and medium are incubated at 37°C. The NADH generated over the LD zones is detected either by its fluorescence, when excited by long-wave UV light (365 nm), or by its reduction of a tetrazolium salt (nitroblue tetrazolium; 3-[4,5-dimethylthiazolyl-2]-2,5-diphenyl-2H-tetrazolium bromide; or 3-[4-iodophenyl]-2-[4-nitrophenyl]-5-phenyl-2H-tetrazolium chloride) to form a colored formazan. Different supporting media, such as agarose, cellulose acetate, polyacrylamide, and starch, have been used *(28)*. Routine analysis kits have become available commercially. They differ in the support medium, electrophoresis conditions, and method of detection. A comparison of these methods is listed in Table 2. These methods have been compared to the reference method *(29)*, and have been shown to give comparable results with underestimation of LD1, LD3, and LD3, and overestimation of LD4 and LD5 *(27)*. Recently, Helena Laboratories (Beaumont, TX) has introduced an automated electrophoresis system, Helena REP, which performs sample application, electrophoresis, development, and densitometry under the control of an integral computer. The whole process of producing isoenzyme results is achievable in less than 25 min.

Heat Stability

LD isoenzymes can be differentiated by means other than electrophoresis. Each fraction differs in thermal stability such that LD4 and LD5 are unstable at temperatures above 45°C, whereas LD1 is stable up to 65°C. LD4 and LD5 are also unstable in the cold (−20°C) *(30)*. Serum rich in LD5 will show some loss of activity on refrigeration. Evidence of heart or liver fraction predominance can be obtained by measuring the total LD activity before and after exposure to 65°C for 30 min. The difference in activity represents the heat-labile (LD4 and LD5) fractions, which is about 10–25% in normal sera, increasing to 33–80% in patients with liver disease. The 65°C stable fraction is about 20–40% in normal, rising to 45–65% in patients with AMI.

α-Hydroxybutyrate Dehydrogenase (HBDH) Activity

LD isoenzymes have different substrate specificities. When α-oxobutyrate is used as substrate in place of pyruvate, the reduction of substrate proceeds at an appreciable rate only when LD1 and LD2 are present, other isoenzymes have much less activity. HBDH activity in serum represents that of the LD1 and LD2. Thus, HBDH measurement may be used as an indicator for myocardial lesions *(12)*.

Ion-Exchange Chromatography

A chromatographic separation procedure using a DEAE-Sephadex ion-exchange minicolumn allowed the discrete estimation of LD1 and LD2 activities *(31)*. In the first step, LD3-5 isoenzymes were eluted, followed by LD2 and LD1. The LD1/LD2 ratio has been shown to have a diagnostic sensitivity for acute myocardial infarction (AMI) of 96% and a specificity of 97% when a decision threshold of 0.76 was used *(31)*. LD isoenzymes have also been separated using Cu-iminodiacetate-PEG. The separation is probably owing to chelation of accessible histidine residues on the protein surface. LD1 displayed weak binding to chelated copper, whereas LD5 bound strongly to this ligand. Resolution of the isoenzymes is possible *(32)*.

Immunoprecipitation

Each LD isoenzyme differs in its immunological reactivity. In 1979, an immunoinhibition assay was developed in which a goat antibody to human LD-M subunit was used to precipitate all the isoenzymes containing the subunit (i.e., LD2–LD5) by means

of a second antigoat antibody *(33)*. Since this second antibody was conjugated to polyvinylidine fluoride particles, the immune complexes were readily centrifuged out of solution, leaving only LD1 in the supernatant. The LD1 activity was assayed by reaction rate methods. The results correlated well with those obtained with the electrophoretic assay ($r = 0.983$). Reported diagnostic sensitivity for myocardial infarction of this technique was 94%. Roche Diagnostics (Nutley, NJ) has used this principle to device a commercially available Isomune LD assay kit. There is disagreement regarding the predictive value of the LD1/total LD ratio in patient with suspected AMI *(34,35)*. A predictive value of 96% and false-positive results in <1% of 65 patients were reported. Others, however, found six false-positive and six false-negative results in 47 patients *(35)*.

Inhibition Method

Substrate inhibition of LD1 by pyruvate at pH 7.1 has been used to estimate the concentration of the isoenzyme *(15)*. Total LD activity is first measured by a standard assay procedure followed by a second assay in the presence of high pyruvate concentrations to inhibit the H-subunit. The decrease in activity represents that of the LD1 isoenzyme. Studies with patients suspected of AMI showed good correlation with Roche Isomune immunological assay as a function of LD1/total LD ratio.

Various chemical inhibitors have been used to inactivate the M- or H-subunit selectively. Oxalate and urea have been employed with varying degrees of success *(16)*. Oxalate 0.2 mol/L in the reaction mixture inhibited 55–68% LD activity. The inhibitory effect was greatest with sera containing an excess of the LD1 isoenzyme. On the other hand, 2 mol/L urea inhibited sera with M-subunit containing LD isoenzymes as in liver disease *(36)*.

A method for assaying LD1 was devised by preincubation with α-chymotrypsin and guanidine *(17)*. Presumably the proteolytic enzyme hydrolyzed phenylalanine bonds in LD3, LD4, and LD5. Guanidine further inactivates LD2, leaving LD1 to be assayed. The results correlated well with the Isomune procedure.

Sodium perchlorate has been used as a chaotropic chemical to inhibit selectively all of the LD isoenzymes containing the M-subunit. LD1 activity can be measured after incubation with this inhibitor *(18)*. This method was adapted in the Abbott A-Gent LD1 isoenzyme assay. Studies reveal that there is an excellent correlation to electrophoresis *(37)*. In addition to perchlorate, 1,6-hexanediol (HD) specifically inhibits the M-subunits *(19)*. The perchlorate method was the most precise, but both correlated well with immunoprecipitation and electrophoretic methods *(38)*. Inhibition with 1,6-HD seemed to have a slightly higher activity and showed greater variability than the electrophoretic method *(39)*. In addition to 1,6-HD, guanidinium thiocyanate (GSCN) has been found to inhibit the M-subunit. GSCN rapidly inactivates all the isoenzymes within 1 min, except LD1, which is further protected by the presence of lactate. It is speculated that GSCN selectively denatures the M-subunit, leaving LD1 undamaged *(20)*.

Assays based on chaotropic inhibitors have become automated. The sodium perchlorate-based A-Gent LD1 assay has been adapted onto the Cobas-Fara (Roche) centrifugal analyzer *(40)*. Recently, commercial kits are available for direct implementation on fully automated chemistry analyzers. Trace America Inc. (Miami, FL) has a kit based on 1,6-HD and Boehringer Mannheim Diagnostics (Indianapolis, IN) provides a LD1 assay based on inhibition by GSCN *(19,41)*. These two commercial assays were compared after implementation on DuPont Dimension AR (Wilmington, DE) and Hitachi 717 (BMC) *(96)*. Intrainstrument assays showed excellent correlation. However, DuPont Dimension consistently gave about 30% lower values than Hitachi 717 independent of which reagent was used. Similarly, DuPont has developed an inhibitory method for the ACA discrete clinical analyzer. This method employs lithium dodecyl sulfate to inactivate selectively isoenzymes containing the M-subunit *(42)*. The remaining LD1 activity is measured by the lactate to pyruvate procedure.

Current Method of Choice

Historically, clinical laboratories measure LD isoenzymes by electrophoretic techniques. For the diagnosis of AMI, the ratio of LD1/LD2 is the preferred parameter. As an easier immunological method of Roche Isomune became available, laboratories began to use selectively the LD1 isoenzyme. This assay was shown to be diagnostically equivalent to the electrophoretic methods. In fact, recent studies have shown that LD1 level alone, even when measured by electrophoresis, is a more efficient parameter for the diagnosis of AMI *(43)*. With this confidence, the measurement of LD1 has become popular. The most recent technology of chemical inhibition has fully automated this analysis, which has been increasingly employed for AMI diagnosis. However, the automation of electrophoresis by Helena REP has assured its application to LD isoenzyme measurements. The decision regarding which assay to use will be determined by economical factors.

CLINICAL UTILITY

Since LD concentration in the cells are about 500-fold higher than that in the serum, any increase in LD activity in the blood suggests tissue injury, and the predominant isoenzyme fraction may identify the organ source *(44)*. The half-life of serum LD has been estimated to be 52–69 h *(14)*. Thus, the enzyme activity remains elevated for several days after tissue injury. Elevations of LD activity in serum may be found accompanying myocardial disease and other miscellaneous organ involvements. It has also been evaluated in urine, cerebrospinal fluid, and effusions.

Diagnostic Utilization for AMI

Acute injury to the myocardium can lead to loss of cell membrane integrity, followed by leakage of the intracellular contents into the intercellular space and, ultimately, into the peripheral blood. Serum activities of creatine kinase (CK) and CK-MB appear before LD (*see* Chapter 1). LD1 often parallels the total LD activity, rises 8–12 h after the onset of chest pain, and peaks at 24–72 h *(30,45,46)*. Since the half-life of LD1 activity in blood ranges from 57–170 h (average 99 h) *(47)*, it does not return to preinfarction levels for 7–12 days *(30,45–48)*. Thus, LD1 is a useful late marker of AMI *(30,45)*. The sequence of events for the release of LD in relation to other serum enzymes after AMI is discussed in Chapter 1. During the course of serum enzyme elevation, LD1 increases faster than LD2 and begins to exceed LD2 about 2–3 h later *(49)* (Fig. 2). Approximately 80% of patients show the highly specific "flipped" pattern within 48 h of chest pain *(30,50)*. In addition to the LD1/LD2 ratio, the measurement of absolute LD and LD1, and the LD1/total LD ratio have been used for the diagnosis of AMI *(51)*. Appropriate timing of blood sampling for enzyme measurement is essential, because the demonstration of both a rise and a subsequent fall in the activities of these enzymes increases the predictive value of the test for AMI. Single determinations of the enzyme activity are of little help in diagnosis; rather, it is the enzyme changes with time that are most helpful. Rising, then falling, activities of LD1 have almost 100% sen-

sitivity and specificity in the diagnosis of AMI *(52,53)*.

LD1 has been used to assess infarct size in AMI patients by calculating cumulative enzyme release. Reduction of the enzyme activity, which corresponded to a limitation of infarct size after thrombolytic therapy, was seen in patients with ST-elevation in the initial electrocardiogram *(54)*. The disadvantage of using LD is its abundance in erythrocytes. However, free hemoglobin levels can be used to correct LD1 activities contributed by erythrocytes *(54)*.

LD1 appears to be a useful test for the diagnosis of perioperative AMI after coronary bypass surgery from days 2–4 with CK-MB mass being the best marker during the first 48 h *(55)*. Patients undergoing procedures necessitating atriotomies had elevations in LD1/LD2 ratios, but these are less than acute perioperative AMI *(55)*.

Since LD and its isoenzymes are present in all tissues, differential diagnosis of an abnormal LD1 level or an LD1/LD2 flip for AMI must include the conditions described in Table 3. Patients with anemia of different types may have high serum LD owing to hemolysis of the erythrocytes, which contain a high concentration of LD1 (Fig. 1). Hemolyzed serum specimen will cause an elevated LD1. LD1/LD2 ratios are increased in hemolytic anemia principally in patients with reticulocytosis *(56)*. In 85% or more of patients with megaloblastic anemia, LD1 is elevated as a result of destruction of erythrocytes in the bone marrow. The sera of these patients may exhibit LD1 patterns similar to AMI *(57)*.

Abnormal serum LD activities usually are present in myocarditis during the course of active inflammation. LD1 values can be markedly abnormal, and the pattern of enzyme abnormalities mimics AMI *(58)*. This has been observed in one case of infectious myopericarditis where AMI was ruled out on the basis of a normal myocardial

**Table 3
Differential Diagnosis of LD
and LD1 Elevations**

AMI
Anemia
   Hemolytic anemia
   Megaloblastic anemia
   Pernicious anemia
   Intravascular hemolysis
   Sickle anemia
Surgery with blood transfusion
Myocarditis
Pericarditis
Hypothyroidism
Congestive heart failure
Open heart surgery
Renal cortical infarct or ischemia
Glomerulonephritis
Seminoma of testes
Dysgerminoma of ovary
Reye's syndrome
Muscular dystrophy
Polymyositis
Rhadomyolysis
Pulmonary infarction or embolism
Malignant diseases
   Acute leukemia
   Germ cell testicular tumor
   Teratoma
   T-cell lymphoma

have had coronary bypass grafting showed significant elevations of LD and LD1, which mimicked a perioperative AMI (63). Reinfusion of shed blood after coronary artery bypass grafting increases 143% of LD compared to their levels before autotransfusion. Such changes can potentially mimic or mask the presence of perioperative myocardial infarction (64). Patients with Reye's syndrome are believed to have myocardial injury. Increased LD is seen in patients with this disorder (65). In a case of hypothyroidism, enzymatic changes falsely indicated AMI (66).

LD was increased in 87% of patients with pulmonary embolism or infarction (58,64,67). The lung tissue contains high activities of LD3. However, it is not commonly increased after pulmonary embolism. Rather, LD1 is increased, possibly from hemolysis of erythrocytes (64,67). A similar explanation may apply to patients with strokes. LD1, which occurs in the brain, does not normally pass the blood–brain barrier. Its increase in serum probably originates from the hemolysis of red blood cells in the thrombus or in the area of hemorrhage in the brain. In acute renal infarction, elevations of LD1 may also be contributed to by hemolysis (40,50).

The powerful contractions of the intercostal muscles caused by the shock release LD. About 18% of patients given electrical countershock to correct heart rhythm disturbances had slightly elevated enzyme, but LD1 remained normal (68). Trauma to skeletal muscle can lead to increased activities of LD in serum. Increases in LD have been seen as a result of exercise. Extreme physical exertion during a 160-km marathon increased LD as much as 12-fold the upper reference limit in 20 runners of ages 27–63 yr, and a serum LD1 > LD2 has been seen (69). The physical stress probably causes release of enzymes from the heart in the absence of AMI. Serum enzyme changes are

scintigram (30). Heart rhythm disturbances usually do not lead to the release of enzymes into the blood. If tachycardia occurs, CK and LD activities may increase (59). Tachycardia may subject the myocardium to unusual stress. Similarly, congestive heart failure without AMI may lead to release of LD (60). However, in angina pectoris, activities of LD isoenzymes in serum are reportedly normal (61). The two commonly performed procedures of cardiac catheterization and coronary arteriography normally do not produce LD abnormalities. Cardiac catheterization usually is not associated with myocardial injury (62). On the other hand, patients who negligible in patients undergoing exercise stress testing. Small increases in LD5 have been seen, although LD1 is normal *(70)*. Elevated LD1 may also be seen in the muscular dystrophies, myositis, and other condition in which muscle is responding to chronic injury *(57,60,71)*.

Systemic injury invariably increases LD in serum. Even in the state of pregnancy, LD is elevated *(72)*. Overdoses of ethanol, hypnotics, sedatives, tranquilizers, and antidepressants, and exposure to CO can lead to marked increase in serum enzymes; in some patients, toxic effects on the heart can be demonstrated. Alcohol overdose can produce myopathic changes leading to two- to fivefold increases in LD *(73)*. Elevated levels of LD activity are commonly seen in patients with liver diseases. The abnormal increases in LD and LD5 in congestive heart failure probably originate from liver as a result of passive congestion *(23,74)*.

It may be of interest to note that LD has been used to assess acute myocardial ischemia as a cause of death. Necropsy specimens of the pericardial fluid showed that LD activities were greatly increased in cases where morphological evidence of myocardial ischemia was found *(74)*. It was suggested that LD may be used to rule out myocardial infarction in cases where reliable morphological findings are lacking.

Reference Range Concentrations— Diagnostic Cutoff Limits

The reference values for total LD activity in serum vary considerably, depending on the direction of the enzyme reaction, the type of method used, and the assay conditions. For the pyruvate-to-lactate reaction at pH 7.4 and 30°C, a range of 95–200 U/L is reported *(75)*. Using the assay parameters developed by the Committee on Enzymes of the Scandinavian Society for Clinical Chemistry and Clinical Physiology, the values ranged from 200–380 U/L (at 37°C) *(76)*.

For the lactate-to-pyruvate reaction at pH 8.8–9.0 and 30°C, a range of 35–88 U/L represents the generally accepted values.

Reference ranges for LD isoenzymes by electrophoresis has been reviewed *(77)*. The values are method- and population-dependent *(58,78)*. Using an agarose gel electrophoresis technique with fluorometric quantitation of generated NADH, a range, as percent of total LD activity, for a healthy population (n = 250) was reported: LD1, 14–26; LD2, 29–39; LD3, 20–26; LD4, 8–16; LD5, 6–16. The LD1/LD2 ratio was 0.45–0.74. A cellulose acetate method using nitroblue tetrazolium staining produced a reference range (as percent of total LD): LD1, 27–35; LD2, 34–44; LD3, 16–22; LD4, 4–8; LD5, 3–7 *(29)*. Ten commercial electrophoresis systems have been reviewed that showed there were slight differences among their reference values, which cover the ranges as percent of total LD: LD1, 14–36; LD2, 25–48; LD3, 12–30; LD4, 2–18; LD5, 2–18 *(27)*.

Although the LD-1/LD2 flip is indicative for AMI, a recommended cutoff value of 0.76 has been made *(45,79)*. In addition to the LD1/LD2 ratio, others found that LD1/LD4 was a better diagnostic test *(80)*. Other parameters of the isoenzymes have been suggested. A reference cutoff of LD1/total LD above 0.4 was found to be efficient in patients up to 5 d after AMI, but not 6–15 d after admission *(41,43)*. The absolute value of LD1 was also implied as the most efficient for diagnosis of AMI *(43)*.

Since serial test results are obtained for the cardiac markers, the differences between two consecutive results would be a sensitive means of detecting myocardial infarction. The use of reference change would include the effects of analytical and biological variations *(81)*. A statistical method has been developed for the calculation of reference changes from routine patient data *(82)*. For total LD activity as determined by the Scandinavian-recommended assay, a reference change limit was found to be −86–85 U/L; for LD1, the limit was −19–15 U/L. This concept may be useful in establishing reference change limits for a local population *(83)*.

Clinical Sensitivity and Specificity

As shown earlier, the tissue distribution of LD is much wider than other cardiac markers; not only does very high LD1 activity present in the heart, but it also occurs in erythrocytes and renal cortex. Measurement of serum LD1 is a useful test, but is less specific than CK-MB for AMI, and is mostly employed in patients with delayed admission after a cardiac event and for confirmatory purposes where there are equivocal or difficult to interpret findings. LD1 is more effective the second day after admission *(84)*.

The sensitivity and specificity of LD and its isoenzymes for the diagnosis of AMI depend on the methodology of the test, the parameters used for the assessment of AMI, the time specimen is collected, and the patient population under investigation. A collection of the maximum diagnostic efficacy from various studies is tabulated in Table 4. Absolute LD activity has a relative low sensitivity and specificity *(105,108)*. The clinical sensitivity of LD1 is about 90% with a specificity of 90–99% *(30,42,84,103)*. The test sensitivity may be further increased by using the LD1/LD2 ratio *(30,52, 85,104,106,107)*. About 80% of all AMIs showed a flipped ratio, i.e., LD1 > LD2. However, it may be more useful to use, as a diagnostic index, elevations of the LD1/LD2 ratio above the laboratory's reference range, since the frequency of a flipped ratio in AMI tends to be method-dependent *(78)*. The test may have greater sensitivity at the expense of specificity for AMI when an LD1/LD2 cutoff ratio of 0.76 or more is used *(79)*.

A common cause of false-positive results with LD1 or LD1/LD2 values is the presence of hemolysis. AMI and hemolysis produce exactly the same effect. Therefore, the finding is meaningful only if the possibility of hemolysis can be ruled out. Usually it can, but the presence of a prosthetic heart valve, which can cause hemolysis, should always be considered.

Serial determinations of the isoenzymes greatly improved sensitivity and specificity *(52,53)*. In one study, a single determination of LD1/LD2 at 48 h after admission had a sensitivity of 86.1% and a specificity of 96.6%, whereas serial determinations at 24, 48, and 72 h after admission had a sensitivity of 100%, although the specificity remained the same *(52)*. The diagnostic efficiency is even better when compared to the single test done at other times.

Diagnostic Utilization for Other Diseases

Various other pathophysiological conditions in addition to AMI cause elevations of LD and its isoenzymes in serum and other body fluids. Analysis of these specimens may provide diagnostic information about these disease states. Total LD activity and the ratio of LD5 to LD1 have been shown to be elevated in blood and vitreous humor in patients with retinoblastoma *(86)*. LD1 was found to be increased in a case of glucagonoma *(87)*. Further studies will be needed to document if this is a widespread phenomenon. Since the liver has a high concentration of LD5, it has been suggested that LD5/LD2 may be useful for monitoring graft function and survival in liver transplantation *(88)*.

Serum LD and its isoenzymes have been reported to be markers in cancer. Historically, total LD measurement has been considered unreliable as a cancer marker, being elevated in 65–70% of patients with carcinomas metastatic to the liver, but only in 20–60% of those without hepatic metastases *(89)*. Isoenzymes could be more useful. Efforts have been made to relate LD isoen-

Table 4
Sensitivity and Specificity of LD and Isoenzymes

Patient: total/AMI	Method	Parameter	% Sensitivity	% Specificity	Ref.
61/27	Electrophoresis	LD1	91	—	*103*
328/91	Electrophoresis	LD1 > LD2	90	95	*85*
94/46	Electrophoresis	LD1 > LD2	78	99	*104*
201/87	Reaction rate	LD	91	80	*84*
201/87	Chromatography	LD1	86	90	*84*
401/192	Enzymatic	LD	97	81	*105*
98/44	Electrophoresis	LD1 > LD2	70	94	*106*
228/101	Electrophoresis	LD1/LD2 > 0.76	100	91	*79*
71/28	Electrophoresis	LD1 > LD2	61	98	*107*
67/29	Reaction rate	LD	100	39	*108*
194/87	Inhibition	LD1	89	95	*42*
194/87	Inhibition	LD1/LD	71	98	*42*
230/180	Electrophoresis	LD1/LD2 > 0.76	91	87	*52*
230/180	Electrophoresis	LD1 > LD2	86	97	*52*
230/180	Electrophoresis	LD1/LD2 > 0.76 (serial)	100	80	*52*
230/180	Electrophoresis	LD1 > LD2 (serial)	100	97	*52*
229/40	Inhibition	LD1/LD > 0.4	100	95	*41*
82/54	Immunochemical	LD1	94	96	*33*
82/54	Electrophoresis	LD1 > LD2	87	96	*33*
100/47	Chromatography	LD1/LD-2 > 0.76	96	97	*31*
120/80	Electrophoresis	LD1	98	98	*43*
120/80	Electrophoresis	LD1 > LD2	98	98	*43*
120/80	Electrophoresis	LD1/LD > 0.4	96	88	*43*
65/26	Immochemistry	LD1	96	97	*34*

zyme patterns to various malignancies. In one study, the ratio of LD4 to LD1 was 9.72 in normal colonic tissue, and 1.67 in colon carcinoma *(90)*. A retrospective evaluation of surgical specimens indicated that the patients with colorectal cancer had a mean LD4 to LD1 ratio of <1. The LD1/LD2 flipped pattern has also been reported in ovarian and germ cell tumors, and LD1 has been found in serum of patients with advanced testicular cancer *(91)*. In patients with metastatic testicular germ cell tumors, LD1 had an overall predictive value regarding treatment response of 80% and total LD 64% *(92)*. The serum LD3 level is elevated in more than 90% of patients with active chronic granulocytic leukemia (CGL), but was essentially normal in patients who are in remission *(93)*. Thus, LD3 may be a useful diagnostic marker in CGL and may have a role in monitoring changes in clinical status.

Total LD level in other body fluids has also been investigated. In cerebrospinal fluid, LD5 has been found to be helpful in separating leptomeningeal carcinomatosis from infection or primary cerebral tumors. In the absence of acute bacterial meningitis or other processes associated with a polymorphonuclear pleocytosis, an LD5 fraction >10% suggests leptomeningeal malignancy, and a percentage of more than 15% strongly supports that diagnosis *(89)* Cerebrospinal fluid LD5 is prominently elevated in metastatic tumors, whereas a primary brain tumor demonstrated an increase in all fractions. Viral encephalitis revealed an increase in the first three isoenzymes and bacterial meningitis, the last two. Elevation of the first three fractions was usually owing to brain tissue damage or hemorrhage, whereas the last two were related to anaerobic metabolism in the central nervous system (CNS) or to granulocytic infiltration. Thus, LD isoenzymes may be helpful in differential diagnosis of various CNS disorders (94).

Total LD activity in peritoneal, pleural, and other fluids has been used to assist the determination of whether these fluids are transudates or exudates. A fluid to serum ratio >0.6 is taken as evidence of an exudate, since LD is liberated from the cells into the fluids as a result of infection or malignancy.

LD-C4 or LD-X is a specific cell isoenzyme of spermatogenesis and spermatozoa of humans and animals. Studies in semen showed a positive trend of LD-X to changes in sperm density and becomes absent in obstructive and vasectomized azoospermia. LD-X may be diagnostically useful for germ cell aplasia (95). The LD-C4/sperm ratio may be a useful marker for assessing the status of the seminiferous epithelium and for making a differential diagnosis in men with low sperm count (10).

FUTURE DEVELOPMENTS

The rise in serum total LD and LD1 begins at 8–12 h after myocardial cell damage, peaks at 24–72 h, and returns to baseline by 8–14 d (30,45,48). Serial samples from a suspected AMI patient are generally taken at approx 10-h intervals for 1–2 d. The benefit of using LD1 over CK-MB would be in those instances where patient presentation to the hospital is delayed more than 24 h following the acute episode and where CK levels may have already returned to normal. Because of the widespread distribution of LD, elevated levels of LD occur in a variety of conditions, making the measurement of LD a nonspecific test for AMI (96,97). The significance of an LD flip is equivocal without a concurrent increase in total LD. The most sensitive and specific marker is the LD1/total LD ratio (34). However, LD5 is frequently elevated as a result of liver congestion at the late period of heart dysfunction. In these circumstances, percent LD1/total LD may result in false negative (98). The measurement of absolute LD1 and LD1/total LD ratio are more convenient and rapid with shorter turnaround times because of the automation of the test using chemical inhibition methods on a variety of chemistry analyzers. Measurement of the LD1/LD2 ratio requires the more tedious, time-consuming, and expensive electrophoresis method.

Measuring LD1 on all patients regardless of total LD activity is unnecessary, since one study showed that LD1 played a confirmatory role in only 1 of 44 patients (99). This observation confirms the claim by others (100) that routine use of LD and its isoenzymes was of no use in most patients. A more effective approach would be to measure LD1 only if total CK was abnormal, only if CK-MB were negative, and only if total LD was abnormal (99) and in late presentations (>48 h) (99,100).

Recent availability of commercial cardiac troponin T (cTnT) and I (cTnI) assays has provided an additional choice of cardiac markers. These recent tests have been deemed cardiospecific in assessing heart muscle damage by numerous studies as elaborated elsewhere in this volume. CTnI can remain elevated 5–9 d, whereas cTnT about 2 wk after an AMI. Thus, the cardiac troponin isoforms cover the same diagnostic time window for AMI as CK, CK-MB, LD, and LD1. With reductions in costs and acceptance by cardiologists, these tests will eventually replace LD and LD1 for AMI diagnosis, and the application of LD and its isoenzymes will be directed to other diseases *(101,102)*.

ABBREVIATIONS

AMI, Acute myocardial infarction; CGL, chronic granulocytic leukemia; CK, creatine kinase; CNS, central nervous system; cTnI, T, cardiac troponins I and T; DEAE, diethylaminoethyl; GSCN, guanidinium thiocyanate; HD, hexanediol; HBDH, α-hydroxybutyrate dehydrogenase; IFCC, International Federation of Clinical Chemistry; kDa, kilodaltons; LD, lactate dehydrogenase; NAD(H), nicotinamide, adenine dinucleotide (reduced); NADP (H), nicotinamide adenine dinudeotide phosphate (reduced).

REFERENCES

1. Schwert GW and Winer AD (1963) Lactate dehydrogenase. In: The Enzymes, vol. 7, Boyer PD, Lardy HA, and Myrback K, eds. Press, New York, Academic, pp. 127–148.
2. Everse J and Kaplan NO (1973) Lactate dehydrogenase. Structure and function. Adv. Enzymol. 61–133.
3. Holbrook JJ, Liljas A, Steindel SJ, and Rossmann MG (1975) Lactate dehydrogenase. In: The Enzymes, 3rd ed., vol 11, Boyer PD, ed., New York, Academic, pp. 191–292.
4. Hakala MT, Glaid AJ, and Schwert GW (1956) Lactate dehydrogenase. II. Variation of kinetic and equilibrium constants with temperature. J. Biol. Chem. 221:191–209.
5. McComb RB (1983) The measurement of lactate dehydrogenase. In Clinical and Analytical Concepts in Enzymology, Homburger, HA, ed., Skokie, IL, College of American Pathologists, pp. 157–171.
6. Gay RS, McComb RB, and Bowers GN Jr (1968) Optimum reaction conditions for human lactate dehydrogenase isoenzyme as they affect total lactate dehydrogenase activity. Clin. Chem. 14:740–747.
7. Prochazka B and Wachsmuth ED (1972) Isozyme pattern of lactate dehydrogenase, creatine phosphokinase, phosphoglucomutase and aldolase of guinea pig tissue during ontogeny. J. Exp. Zool. 182:201–209.
8. Virji N and Naz RK (1995) The role of lactate dehydrogenase C_4 in testicular function and infertility. Int. J. Androl. 18:1–7.
9. Stambaugh R and Buckley J (1967) The enzymic and molecular nature of the lactate dehydrogenase subbands and X_4 isoenzyme. J. Biol. Chem. 242:4053–4059.
10. Taylor SS, Allison WS, and Kaplan NO (1975) The amino acid sequence of the tryptic peptides isolated from dogfish M_4 lactate dehydrogenase. J. Biol. Chem. 250: 8740–8747.
11. Emes AV, Gallimore MJ, Hodson AW, and Latner AL (1974) The preparation of crystalline human L-lactate-nicotinamide adenine dinucleotide oxidoreductase isoenzyme 1 involving preparative polyacrylamide gel electrophoresis. Biochem. J. 143:453–460.
12. Elliot BA, Jepson EM, and Wilkinson JH (1962) Serum alpha-hydroxybutyrate dehydrogenase: A new test with improved specificity for myocardial lesions. Clin. Sci. 23:305–316.
13. Wong SS and Wong L-JC (1983) A one-step PMR determination of hydrogen transfer stereospecificity of $NADP^+$-linked oxidoreductases. Int. J. Biochem. 15:147–150.
14. Latner AL and Skillen AW (1968) Isozymes in biology and medicine. New York, Academic.
15. Busch H and Nair PV (1957) Inhibition of lactic acid dehydrogenase by fluoropyruvic acid. J. Biol. Chem. 229:377–387.
16. Demetriou JA, Drewes PA, and Gin JB (1974) Enzymes. In: Clinical chemistry principles and technics, 2nd ed., Henry RJ, Cannon DC, and Winkleman JW, eds. Hagerstown MD, Harper and Row, pp. 815–1001.
17. Shirahase Y, Watazu Y, Kaneda N, Uji Y, Okabe H, and Karmen A (1992) Specific assay of serum lactate dehydrogenase isoenzyme 1 by proteolysis with alpha-chymotrypsin and protein denaturation. Clin. Chem. 38:2193–2196.
18. Panteghini M, Bonora R, and Pagani F (1990) Evaluation of a new commercial assay kit for quantification of isoenzyme 1 in serum. J. Clin. Chem. Clin. Biochem. 28: 545–548.
19. Tanishima K, Hayashi M, Matsushima M, and Mochikawa Y (1985) Activity of lactate

dehydrogenase isoenzymes LD$_1$ and LD$_2$ in serum as determined by using an inhibitor of the M-subunit. Clin. Chem. 31:1175–1177.

20. Onigbinde TA, Wu AHB, Wu Y-S, Simmons MJ, and Wong SS (1992) Mechanism of differential inhibition of lactate dehydrogenase isoenzymes in the BMC LD1 assay. Clin. Biochem. 25:425–429.

21. Dixon M and Webb EC (1964) Enzymes, 2nd ed., New York, Academic.

22. Lott JA and Nemesanszky E (1986) Lactate dehydrogenase (LD). In: Clinical enzymology. A case-oriented approach, Lott JA and Wolf PL., eds. New York, Field and Rich/Year Book, pp. 213–244.

23. Lott JA and Turner K (1982) Lactate dehydrogenase in serum. In: Selected methods for the small clinical chemistry laboratory, Meites S and Faulkner W, eds. Washington, DC, American Association for Clinical Chemistry, p. 271.

24. Bais R and Philcox M (1994) Approved recommendation on IFCC methods for the measurement of catalytic concentration of enzymes. Part 8. IFCC method for lactate dehydrogenase (L-lactate: NAD$^+$ Oxidoreductase, EC 1.1.1.27). International Federation of Clinical Chemistry (IFCC). Eur. J. Clin. Chem. Clin. Biochem. 32:639–655.

25. Lorentz K, Kauke R, and Schmidt E (1993) Recommendation for the Determination of the catalytic concentration of lactate dehydrogenase at 37°C. Eur. J. Clin. Chem. Clin. Biochem. 31:897–899.

26. Marshall T, Williams J, and Williams KM (1991) Electrophoresis of serum isoenzymes and proteins following acute myocardial infarction. J. Chromatogr. 569:323–345.

27. Moses GC, Ross ML, and Henderson AR (1988) Ten electrophoretic methods compared with a selected method for quantifying lactate dehydrogenase isoenzymes in serum. Clin. Chem. 34:1885–1890.

28. Van der Helm JJ, Zondag HA, Hartog HAP, and Van der Kooi MW (1962) Lactate dehydrogenase isoenzymes in myocardial infarction. Clin. Chim. Acta. 7:540–549.

29. McKenzie D and Henderson AR (1983) Electrophoresis of lactate dehydrogenase isoenzymes. Selected Methods of Clin. Chem. 10:58–67.

30. Lott JA and Stang JM (1980) Serum enzyme and isoenzymes in the diagnosis and differential diagnosis of myocardial ischemia and necrosis. Clin. Chem. 26:1241–1250.

31. Vasudevan G, Mercer DW, and Varat MA (1978) Lactate dehydrogenase isoenzyme determination in the diagnosis of acute myocardial infarction. Circulation 57:1055–1057.

32. Otto A and Birkenmeier G (1993) Recognition and separation of isoenzymes by metal chelates. Immobilized metal ion affinity partitioning of lactate dehydrogenase isoenzymes. J. Chromatogr. 644:25–33.

33. Usategui-Gomez M, Wicks RW, and Warshaw M (1979) Immunochemical determination of the heart isoenzyme of lactate dehydrogenase (LDH$_1$) in human serum. Clin. Chem. 25:729–734.

34. Bruns DE, Emerson JC, Intemann S, Berthoff R, Hille KE, and Savory J (1981) Lactate dehydrogenase isoenzyme-1: changes during the first day after acute myocardial infarction. Clin. Chem. 27:1821–1823.

35. Gordesky SE and Winsten S (1982) LD-1/LD ratio as a diagnostic determinant for myocardial infarction. Clin. Chem. 28:1239.

36. Emerson PM and WIlkinson JH (1965) Urea and oxalate inhibition of the serum lactate dehydrogenase. J. Clin. Pathol. 18:803–807.

37. Scharer KA, Karcher RE, Epstein E, and Kiechle FL (1989) Comparison of agarose gel electrophoresis and a chaotropic method for lactate dehydrogenase isoenzyme-1. Clin. Chem. 35:2250.

38. Paz JM, Garcia A, Gonzales M, Trevino M, Tutor JC, Jaquet M, and Rodringuez-Segade S (1990) Evaluation of determination of lactate dehydrogenase isoenzyme 1 by chemical inhibition with perchlorate or with 1,6-hexanediol. Clin. Chem. 36:355–358.

39. Shamberger RJ (1987) Lactate dehydrogenase isoenzyme 1 as determined by inhibition with 1,6-hexanediol and by two other methods in patients with myocardial infarction or cardiac-bypass surgery. Clin. Chem. 33:589–591.

40. Lazarus EF and Kapke GF (1991) Use of chemical denaturation for centrifugal analyzer determination of lactate dehydrogenase 1 [Letter]. Clin. Chem. 37:1464.

41. Onigbinde TA, Wu AHB, Johnson M, Wu Y-S, Collinsworth WL, and Simmons MJ (1990) Clinical evaluation of an automated chemical inhibition assay for lactate dehydrogenase isoenzyme 1. Clin. Chem. 36: 1819–1822.

42. Painter PC, Van Meter S, Dabbs RL, and Clement GE (1994) Analytical evaluation and comparison of DuPont aca lactate dehydrogenase-1 (LD1) isoenzyme assay diagnostic efficiency for acute myocardial infarction detection with other LD1 methods and aca CK-MB. A two-site study. Angiology 45:585–595.

43. Rotenberg Z, Davidson E, Weinberger I, Fuchs J, Sperling O, and Agmon J (1988) The efficiency of lactate dehydrogenase isoenzyme determination for the diagnosis of acute myocardial infarction. Arch. Pathol. Lab. Med. 112:895–897.

44. Batsakis JG and Briere RO (1967) Interpretative Enzymology, Springfield, IL, American Society of Clinical Pathology.

45. Leung FY and Handerson AR (1979) Thin-layer agarose electrophoresis of lactate dehydrogenase isoenzymes in serum: A note on the method of reporting and on the lactate dehydrogenase isoenzyme-1/isoenzyme-2 ratio in acute myocardial infarction. Clin. Chem. 25:209–211.

46. Blomberg DJ, Kimber WD, and Burke MD (1975) Creatine kinase isoenzymes. Predictive value in the early diagnosis of acute myocardial infarction. Am. J. Med. 59:464–469.

47. Smith DA, Leung FY, Jablonsky G, and Henderson AR (1987) Determination, by radioimmunoassay, of the mass of lactate dehydrogenase isoenzyme 1 in human serum and of its rate of removal from serum after a myocardial infarction. Clin. Chem. 33: 1863–1868.

48. Ellis AK (1991) Serum protein measurements and the diagnosis of acute myocardial infarction. Circulation 83:1107–1109.

49. Roe CR (1977) Diagnosis of myocardial infarction by serum isoenzyme analysis. Ann. Clin. Lab. Sci. 7:201–209.

50. Lott JA (1984) Serum enzyme determinations in the diagnosis of acute myocardial infarction. An update. Human Pathol. 15:706–716.

51. Galen RS and Gambino SR (1975) Beyond normality: the predicative value and efficiency of medical diagnosis. New York, John Wiley.

52. Rotenberg Z, Weinberger I, Davidson E, Fuchs J, Sperling O, and Agmon J (1988) Does serial determination of lactate dehydrogenase isoenzyme 1 and 2 ratios contribute to the diagnosis of acute myocardial infarction? Clin. Chem. 34:1506–1507.

53. Ruzich RS (1992) Cardiac enzymes. How to use serial determinations to confirm acute myocardial infarction. Postgrad. Med. 92(7):85–89.

54. Vermeer F and Van der Laarse A (1993) Cumulative enzyme release as a measure of infarct size in patients with acute myocardial infarction receiving thrombolytic therapy. Arch. Mal. Coeur. Vaiss. 4:25–28.

55. Graeber GM, Shawl FA, Head HD, Wolf RE, Burge JR, Cafferty PJ, Lough FC, and Zajtchuk R (1986) Changes in serum creatine kinase and lactate dehydrogenase caused by acute perioperative myocardial infarction and by transatrial cardiac surgical procedures. J. Thorac. Cardiol. Surg. 92: 63–72.

56. Kazmierczak SC, Castellani WJ, van Lente F, Hodges ED, and Udis B (1990) Effect of reticulocytosis on lactate dehydrogenase isoenzyme distribution in serum. In vivo and in vitro studies. Clin. Chem. 36:1638–1641.

57. Zimmerman HJ and Henry JB (1979) Clinical enzymology. In: Clinical diagnosis and management by laboratory methods, Henry JB, ed., Philadelphia, Saunders, p. 368.

58. Cohen L, Djordjevich J, and Jacobsen, S (1966) The contribution of isoenzymes of serum lactic dehydrogenase (LD) to the diagnosis of specific organ injury. Med. Clin. North Am. 50:193–209.

59. Runde I and Dale J (1966) Serum enzymes in acute tachycardia. Acta. Med. Scand. 179:535–541.

60. Glick JH (1969) Serum lactate dehydrogenase isoenzymes and total lactate dehydrogenase values in health and disease, and clinical evaluation of these tests by means of discriminant analysis. Am. J. Clin. Pathol. 52:320–326.

61. Auvinen S (1974) Evaluation of serum enzyme tests in the diagnosis of acute myocardial infarction. Acta. Med. Scand. Suppl. 539:7–62.

62. Michie DD, Conley MA, Carretta RF, and Booth RN (1970) Serum enzyme changes following cardiac catheterization with and without selective coronary arteriography. Am. J. Med. Sci. 260:11–20.

63. Kutsal A, Saydam GS, Yucel D, and Balk M (1991) Changes in the serum levels of CK-MB, LD, LD1, SGOT and myoglobin due to cardiac surgery. J. Cardiovasc. Surg. 32:516–522.

64. Trujillo NP, Nutter D, and Evans JM (1967) The isoenzymes of lactic dehydrogenase. II. Pulmonary embolism, liver disease, the postoperative state and other medical conditions. Arch. Intern. Med. 119:333–344.

65. Forman DT, Kieffer H, and Grayson SH (1977) Serum creatine kinase inhibition in Reye's syndrome. Clin. Chem. 23: 1364–1365.

66. Minutiello L (1993) The enzymatic and electrocardiographic changes falsely indicative of an acute myocardial infarct during hypothyroidism [Italian]. Minerva Cardioangiol. 41:597–602.

67. Konttinen A, Somer H, and Auvinen S (1974) Serum enzymes and isoenzymes, extrapulmonary sources in acute pulmonary embolism. Arch. Intern. Med. 133:243–246.

68. Reiffel JA, McCarthy DM, and Leahey EB Jr (1979) Does DC cardioversion affect isoenzyme recognition of myocardial infarction? Am. Heart J. 97:810–811.

69. Kielblock AJ, Manjoo M, Booyens J, and Katzeff IE (1979) Creatine phosphokinase and lactate dehydrogenase levels after ultra long-distance running. S. Afr. Med. J. 55:1061–1064.

70. Wolfson S, Rose LI, Brousser JE, Parisi AF, Acosta AE, Cooper KH, and Schechter E (1972) Serum enzyme levels during exercise in patients with coronary heart disease: effects of training. Am. Heart J. 84:478–483.

71. Wieme RJ and Herpol JE (1962) Origin of the lactate dehydrogenase isoenzyme pattern found in the serum of patients having primary muscular dystrophy. Nature 194:287–289.

72. Cohen L, Block J, and Djordjevich J (1967) Sex related differences in isoenzymes of

serum lactic dehydrogenase (LDH). Proc. Soc. Exp. Biol. Med. 126:55–62.

73. Spector R, Choudhury A, Cancilla P, and Lakin R (1979) Alcohol myopathy. Diagnosis by alcohol challenge. J. Am. Med. Assoc. 242:1648–1649.

74. Perez-Carceles MD, Osuna E, Vieira DN, Martinez A, and Luna A (1995) Biochemical assessment of acute myocardial ischaemia. J. Clin. Pathol. 48:124–128.

75. Tietz NW, and Finley PR, eds. (1983) Clinical guide to laboratory tests. Philadelphia, Saunders.

76. Scandinavian Society for Clinical Chemistry and Clinical Physiology (1974) Recommended methods for the determination of four enzymes in blood. Scand. J. Clin. Lab. Invest. 33:291–306.

77. DiGiorgio J (1971) Determination of serum lactic dehydrogenase isoenzymes by use of the "diagnostest" cellulose acetate electrophoresis system. Clin. Chem. 17:326–331.

78. Dietz AA, Lubrano T, and Rubinstein HM (1972) LDH isoenzymes. Stand Methods Clin. Chem. 7:49–61.

79. Jablonsky G, Leung FY, and Henderson AR (1985) Changes in the ratio of lactate dehydrogenase isoenzymes 1 and 2 during the first day after acute myocardial infarction. Clin. Chem. 31:1621–1624.

80. Loughlin JF, Krijnen PM, Jablonsky G, Leung FY, and Henderson AR (1988) Diagnostic efficiency of four lactate dehydrogenase isoenzyme-1 ratios in serum after myocardial infarction. Clin. Chem. 34: 1960–1965.

81. Harris EK and Yasaka T (1983) On the calculation of a "reference change" for comparing two consecutive measurements. Clin. Chem. 29:25–30.

82. Kairisto V, Virtanen A, Uusipaikka E, Voipio-Pulkki LM, Nanto V, Peltola O, and Irjala K (1993) Method for determining referene changes from patient's serial data: examples of cardiac enzymes. Clin. Chem. 39:2298–2304.

83. Magid E, Hyltoft, Petersen P, and Christensen M (1992) A note on the theory of reference changes. Scan. J. Clin. Lab. Invest. 52(Suppl 208):95–101.

84. Kraft J, Aastrup H, and Schroder P (1978) Diagnostic value for acute myocardial infarc-

tion of creatine kinase and lactate dehydrogenase isoenzymes compared with total enzymes. Acta. Med. Scand. 203:167–174.

85. Wagner GS, Roe CR, Limbird LL, Rosti RR, and Wallace AG (1973) The importance of identification of the myocardial specific isoenzyme of creatine phosphokinase (MB form) in the diagnosis of acute myocardial infarction. Circulation 47:263–269.

86. Rehurek J and Snopkova J (1995) Lactate dehydrogenase activity in the diagnosis of retinoblastoma. (Czech). Cesk. Oftalmol. 51:14–18.

87. Kanowski D and Clague A (1994) Increased lactate dehydrogenase isoenzyme-1 in a case of glucagonoma [Letter]. Clin. Chem. 40:158–159.

88. Rodrigue F, Boyer O, Feillet F, and Lemonnier A (1995) Lactate dehydrogenase isoenzyme LD5/LD2 ratio as an indicator of early graft function and complications following pediatric orthotopic liver transplantation. Transplant Proc. 27:1871–1874.

89. Schwartz MK (1978) Enzymes in cancer. Clin. Chem. 19:10–22.

90. Langvad F and Jemec B (1975) Prediction of local recurrence in colorectal carcinoma: an LDH isoenzymatic assay. Br. J. Cancer 35:661–664.

91. Liu F, Fritsche HA, Trujillo JM, and Samuels ML (1982) Serum lactate dehydrogenase isoenzyme 1 in patients with advanced testicular cancer. Am. J. Clin. Pathol. 78:178–183.

92. Seronie-Vivien S, Favre G, Chevreau C, and Soula C (1992) Abnormal lactate dehydrogenase isoenzyme pattern in serum of a patient with a testicular tumor [Letter]. Clin. Chem. 38:2354–2355.

93. Buchsbaum RM, Liu FJ, and Trujillo JM (1991) Serum lactate dehydrogenase-3 (LD-3) isoenzyme in chronic granulocytic leukemia. Am. J. Clin. Pathol. 96:464–469.

94. Fleisher M, Wasserstrom W, Schold S, Schwartz MK, and Posner J (1981) Lactic dehydrogenase isoenzymes in the cerebrospinal fluid of patients with systemic cancer. Cancer 41:105–107.

95. Verma PK, Singh JN, and Quadros M (1993) LDH-X in azoospermia: A new diagnostic alternative to vasography and testicul biopsy. Indian J. Med. Sci. 47:204–207.

96. Wong SS and Huie R (1995) Comparison of Trace and BMC LD-1 isoenzyme reagents on DuPont Dimension AR and Hitachi 717 analyzers. Clin. Chem. 41:S177.

97. Sandstad JS, McKenna RW, and Keffer JH, eds. (1992) Handbook of clinical pathology. Chicago, American Society of Clinical Pathology Press, pp. 69–72.

98. Levinson SS and Hobbs GA (1994) Usefulness of various lactate deydrogenase isoenzyme 1 profiles after myocardial infarction. Ann. Clin. Lab. Sci. 24:364–370.

99. Lum G (1988) Evaluation of a protocol for lactate dehydrogenase (LD) isoenzymes. Am. J. Clin. Pathol. 90:613–617.

100. Reis GJ, Kaufman HW, Horowitz GL, and Pasternak RC (1988) Usefulness of lactate dehydrogenase and lactate dehydrogenase isoenzymes for diagnosis of acute myocardial infarction. Am. J. Card. 61:754–758.

101. Jaff AS, Landt Y, Parvin AC, Abendschein DR, Geltman EM, and Ladenson JH (1996) Comparative sensitivity of cardiac troponin I and lactate dehydrogenase isoenzymes for diagnosis of acute myocardial infarction. Clin. Chem. 42:1770–1776.

102. Martins JT, Li DJ, Baskin LB, Jialal I, and Keffer JH (1996) Comparison of cardiac troponin I and lactate dehydrogenase isoenzymes for the late diagnosis of myocardial injury. Am. J. Clin. Pathol. 106:705–708.

103. Konttinen A and Somer H (1973) Specifity of serum creatine kinase isoenzyme in diagnosis of acute myocardial infarction. Br. Med. J. 1:386–389.

104. Galen RS, Reiffel JA, and Gambino SR (1975) Diagnosis of acute myocardial infarction. Relative efficiency of serum enzyme and isoenzyme measurements. J. Am. Med. Assoc. 232:145–147.

105. Grande P, Christianseim C, and Pedersen A (1978) Creatine kinase MB isoenzyme in diagnosis of acute myocardial infarction. Acta. Med. Scand. Suppl. 623:48–52.

106. Gann D, Cabello B, DiBella J, Rywlin AM, and Samet P (1978) Optimal enzyme test combination for diagnosis of acute

myocardial infarction. South Med. J. 71: 1459–1462.

107. Obzansky D and Lott JA (1980) Clinical evaluation of an immunoinhibition procedure for creatine kinase MB. Clin. Chem. 26:150–152.

108. Strauss HD and Roberts R (1980) Plasma creatine kinase activity and other conventional enzymes. Arch. Intern. Med. 140:336–339.

Part III
Structural Markers

Biochemistry and Molecular Biology of Troponins I and T

Kenneth J. Dean

INTRODUCTION

Troponins I (TnI) and T (TnT) were first recognized as a serum markers of myocardial injury in the late 1970s and 1980s, respectively *(1,2)*, but the proteins of the troponin complex are believed to be ancient: appearing some 250 million years ago, before the divergence of avian and mammalian lines *(3)*. An epitope on cardiac troponin T (cTnT,* a 17-residue peptide) has been identified that has been conserved across vertebrate phyla *(4)*, and major portions of the carboxy-terminal region of TnI are conserved across avian and mammalian species *(5)*. Studies of alternative RNA splicing of exons, one of the mechanism underlying the expression of different TnT isoforms in various striated muscle types, have revealed this to be common to both birds and mammals *(6)*.

In 1965, the discovery of "a new protein factor promoting aggregation of tropomyosin" was made *(7)*, which was later termed troponin *(8)*. In 1968, it was determined that troponin is a complex of at least two different protein factors: a calcium-sensitizing factor and a factor that inhibited ATPase activity *(9)*. Troponin was not described as having three components until 1971, when purified troponin was separated into factors I (40 kDa), II (22 kDa), and III (17 kDa) by SDS gel electrophoresis *(10)*. The third troponin factor appeared to confer both the inhibitory activity and the calcium-sensitizing activity of the troponin complex to the ATPase activity of actinomycin in the presence of tropomyosin *(11,12)*. The nomenclature "troponin C (TnC), troponin I, and troponin T," for the three constituents of the troponin complex was coined in 1973, based on their functional properties ("C" for calcium binding, "I" for inhibitory, and "T" for tropomyosin binding) *(13)*.

BIOCHEMISTRY AND MOLECULAR BIOLOGY OF TNI AND TNT

Location and Physiologic Role

The troponin complex is found on the thin filaments within the sarcomere of all types of striated muscle (fast, slow, and cardiac), where it regulates calcium-mediated muscle contraction. It is not found in smooth muscle, where calmodulin regulates muscle contraction *(14,15)*. The minimal structural unit of the striated muscle thin filament

---

*See p. 200 for list of abbreviations used in this chapter.

From: Cardiac Markers *Edited by:* Alan H. B. Wu
© *Humana Press Inc., Totowa, NJ*

consists of seven actin monomers bridged by a single troponin–tropomyosin complex *(16,17)*. The complex is located redundantly along the thin filament strands at intervals of 3850 nm. It is about 2650 nm long, with a globular region that has a diameter of about 1000 nm and an extended, rod-like tail that is about 1600 nm long and about 200 nm wide *(18)*. The globular head is made up of dumbbell-shaped TnC, globular TnI, and the carboxy-terminal region of TnT. The amino-terminal portion of TnT makes up the rod-like tail, as shown in Fig. 1.

The cTnT content in normal human ventricular myocardium is about 10.8 mg/g wet wt, compared to 1.4 mg/g wet wt for creatine kinase (CK-MB) and 23.6 mg/g wet wt for myoglobin *(19)*. cTnT is found in two intracellular pools: a free cytosolic pool and a bound myofibrillar pool. Only 6–8% of cTnT is found in the cytosolic pool, compared to 100% of CK-MB and myoglobin *(19,20)*. Cytosolic cTnT does not appear to be degraded, but has the same apparent molecular weight and immunoreactivity as myofibrillar cTnT *(20)*. The origin of this cytosolic cTnT is not clear. Protein turnover studies do not support the existence of an unbound intracellular TnT pool *(21)*. Immunohistochemical studies on the disruption of contractile protein structures brought about by ischemia in explanted human myocardium in vitro showed that staining patterns for TnT begin to change after only 10 min of ischemia, with loss of any recognizable pattern after 20 min *(22)*. With complete coronary occlusion, cell necrosis will begin after about 20 min *(23)*. Perhaps cTnT detected in the cytosol *(19,20)* had been released from myofibrils as the result of ischemic injury to the donor organs, and is not normally found in the cytosol.

The cardiac troponin I (cTnI) content of human myocardium is 4.0–6.0 mg/g wet wt, with 2.8–4.1% found in the cytosol *(24,25)*. Protein turnover studies support the pres-

ence of a precursor pool of unassembled cTnI. The half-life of cTnI in rat myocardium is 3.2 d, compared to 3.5 d for cTnT and 5.3 d for cTnC, but the mechanism for differential turnover of these proteins is not known *(21)*. The half-life of cTnT in serum is 120 min *(20)*. However, the half-life of cTnI in serum has not been reported. CTnI found in serum is a heterogeneous mixture of intact and fragmented cTnI, and cTnI complexed to cTnC and cTnI *(26–28)*. The N-terminal region of cTnI is reported to be labile in serum *(29)*, which may be owing to proteolysis at cysteine 80 (cysteine 81 in rat cTnI) *(30)*. The identification of cTnI–cTnC complexes in serum is not surprising, since TnI is known to be stabilized by TnC in the presence of Mg^{2+} or Ca^{2+} ions, which is the basis for a patent *(31)*. Proteolytic degradation of TnI may account for the shortened period of cTnI elevation in serum following AMI compared to cTnT *(26,32)*, and for differences in performance between commercial cTnI assays *(29)*. cTnI binding to cTnC may also cause interference in some commercial cTnI assays *(33)*.

Troponin's mechanism of control involves the inhibition of an otherwise strong and favorable interaction between actin and myosin, a characteristic common to systems where a quick, concerted, and highly sensitive response to a stimulus is necessary *(15)*. The inhibitory element within the troponin complex is TnI, which binds to actin–tropomyosin to inhibit actomyosin Mg^{2+}-ATPase in the absence of intracellular calcium. Calcium binding to TnC results in a conformational change that exposes a hydrophobic pocket on TnC, which has increased affinity for TnI and causes it to move away from binding sites on actin–tropomyosin, thereby relieving the inhibition *(15,34)*. TnT is not an enzyme, but serves as a binding protein to attach the troponin complex to tropomyosin and as a signal amplifier. TnT:

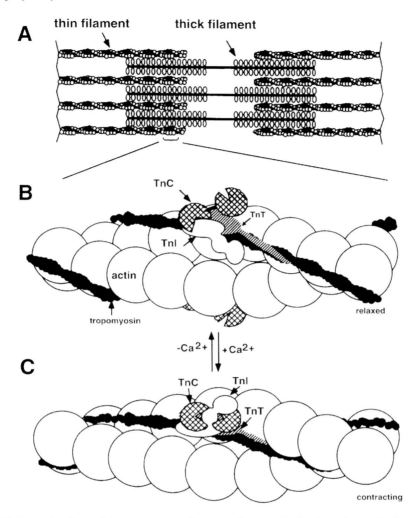

Fig. 1. (A) Organization of the sacromere showing the interdigitation of myosin-based thick filaments and actin-based thin filaments. During muscle contraction, these filaments use the energy of ATP hydrolysis to slide past one another and/or to generate tension along the fiber axis. This interaction is controlled by levels of intracellular Ca^{2+}. **(B)** Model of the troponin–tropomyosin–actin interaction in the absence of Ca^{2+}. **(C)** Ca^{2+} binding to troponin leads to a conformational change in the troponin complex. (Adapted from ref. *15*, and used with permission.)

1. Transmits the inhibitory effect of TnI in the absence of calcium to all of the actin units associated with that troponin–tropomyosin complex;
2. Transmits the relief of inhibition, in the presence of calcium, to the actin monomers associated with that complex; and
3. Stimulates actomyosin Mg^{2+}-ATPase activity *(15,35)*.

The carboxy-terminal portion of TnT, located at the globular head of the troponin complex, contains binding sites for troponin C *(3,15,36)*, TnI *(3,15)*, and the midsection of tropomyosin *(15,16,18)*. TnT has extensive interactions with polymeric tropomyosin, covering about a third of the monomeric molecular length of the latter over its central and carboxy-terminal regions. The amino-terminal portion of TnT, located at the end of the rod-like tail of the troponin complex, is thought to promote the head-to-tail (carboxy-terminus to amino-terminus) polymerization of tropomyosin by overlapping with and forming ternary complexes with the carboxy- and amino-terminal peptides of sequential tropomyosin molecules (15,16). In addition, phosphorylation of TnT, particularly the highly conserved serine residue at the amino-terminus, may play a role in regulation of ATPase activity (37). However, this is not well understood at the present time (38).

TnI binds to actin, tropomyosin, TnT, and TnC (15,34). As previously stated, TnI is not an enzyme, but an inhibitor of actomyosin Mg^{2+}-ATPase. The stoichiometry of this inhibition is significant, since it describes signal amplification in muscle contraction. In the absence of tropomyosin, TnT, and TnC, inhibition of actomyocin Mg^{2+}-ATPase activity by TnI is independent of Ca^{2+} and one TnI molecule per actin monomer is required. In the presence of TnT, TnC, and tropomyosin, the amount of TnI needed for inhibition is reduced and dependence on Ca^{2+} is restored (34). A single troponin–tropomyosin complex presumably inhibits seven actin monomers interactions with myosin. The carboxy-terminal half of TnI (residues 103–182 in rabbit fast skeletal TnI) is necessary for full inhibition of actomyocin Mg^{2+}-ATPase by the troponin complex. TnI has two binding sites for dumbbell-shaped TnC, at both the amino- and carboxy-termini of TnI. TnT binds to an adjacent region near the amino-terminus of TnI (15). There are multiple sites for phosphorylation of TnI, which plays an important role in regulating Ca^{2+} sensitivity and actomyosin Mg^{2+}-ATPase activity (39). Protein kinase A phosphorylates serines 23 and 24 of cTnI in response to adrenaline, reducing the Ca^{2+} sensitivity of troponin-regulated

actomyosin Mg^{2+}-ATPase (40). TnI can also be phosphorylated by protein kinase C, resulting in a reduction of Ca^{2+}-stimulated actomyosin Mg^{2+}-ATPase activity (37,41).

Genetics, Molecular Biology, and Structure

The TnT and TnI found in different types of adult striated muscles (fast, slow, and cardiac) have different (unphosphorylated) calculated molecular weights (30.062, 30.549, and 34.566 kDa, respectively, for TnT; 21.190, 21.637, and 23,980 kDa, respectively, for TnI) and regions with amino acid sequences that are unique to that muscle type. These different forms of TnT and TnI are termed "isoforms." The amino acid sequences of the principal adult TnT isoforms are compared in Fig. 2, and TnI isoforms in Fig. 3. There are 125 amino acid sequence differences (56.6% homology) between adult fast skeletal muscle and cardiac TnT isoforms and 120 amino acid sequence differences (58.3% homology) between adult slow skeletal muscle and cTnT isoforms. There are 123 amino acid sequence differences (41.4% homology) between adult fast skeletal muscle and cTnI isoforms, and there are 113 amino acid sequence differences (46.2% homology) between adult slow skeletal muscle and cTnI isoforms. The existence of muscle-specific isoforms are common among the contractile proteins (48–51). This is owing, in part, to different genes encoding TnT and TnI in different types of striated muscles. A single gene encoding the human cardiac isoform of TnT is carried on chromosome 1q32 (43,52,53), the human slow skeletal TnT isoform on chromosome 19q13.4 (54,55), and the gene encoding the fast skeletal TnT isoform was recently identified on chromosome 11p15.5 (56). The gene encoding human cTnI is carried on chromosome 19q13.3 (57), and human slow skeletal TnI isoform on chromosome 1q12 (58). The location of

```
Fast Sktl   M S D · E E V E Q V E E Q Y E E E E E A Q E E E E V · · · Q E│D T A E E D A E│    35
Slow Sktl   M S D T E E Q E · · · · · Y E E E · · · Q P E E E A A E E E E E · · · · · ·        24
Cardiac     M S D I E E V · · V E E · Y E E E E · · · Q E E A · A V E E Q E│E A A E E D A E│    33
                                                                          a

Fast Sktl   · · · · · · · · · · · · · · · · · · · · · · · · · · · · E E K A R P K · · · ·      42
Slow Sktl   · · · · · · · · · · · · · · · · · · · · · · · · · · E E E · · R P K P S R P        34
Cardiac     A E A E T E E T R A E E D E E E E E A K E A E D G P M E E S K · · P K P · R S      69

Fast Sktl   · · · · L T A P K I P E G E K V D F D D I Q K K R Q N K D L M E L Q A L I D S      77
Slow Sktl   V V P P L I P P K I P E G E R V D F D D I H R K R M E K D L L E L Q T L I D V      73
Cardiac   │F M P N L V P P K I│P D G E R V D F D D I H R K R M E K D L N E L Q A L I E A      108
           b

Fast Sktl   H F E A R K K E E E E L V A L K E R I E K R R A E R A E Q Q R I R A E K E R E      116
Slow Sktl   H F E Q R K K E E E E L V A L K E R I E R R R S E R A E Q Q R F R T E K E R E      112
Cardiac     H F E N R K K E E E E L V S L K D R I E R R R A E R A E Q Q R I R N E R E K E      147

Fast Sktl   R Q N R L A E E K A R R E E E D A K R R A E D D L K K K K A L S S M G A N Y S      155
Slow Sktl   R Q A K L A E E K M R K E E E E A K K R A E D D A K K K K V L S N M G A H F G      151
Cardiac     R Q N R L A E E R A R R E E E E N R R K A E D E A R K K K A L S N M · M H F G      185

Fast Sktl   S Y L A K · A D Q · · K R G K K Q T A R E M K K K I L A E R R K P L N I D H L      191
Slow Sktl   G Y L V K · A E Q · · K R G K R Q T G R E M K V R I L S E R K K P L D I D Y M      187
Cardiac     G Y I Q K Q A Q T E R K S G K R Q T E R E K K K K I L A E R R K V L A I D H L      224

Fast Sktl   G E D K L R D K A K E L W E T L H Q L E I D K F E F G E K L K R Q K Y D            227
Slow Sktl   G E E Q L R E K A Q E L S D W I H Q L E S E K F D L M A K L K Q Q K Y E            223
Cardiac     N E D Q L R E K A K E L W Q T I Y N L E A E K F D L Q E K F K Q Q K Y E            260

            β -sequence (human fetal)                c
           │I · T T L R S R I D Q A Q K H│

            α -sequence (rabbit = rat)               c
Fast Sktl  │I M N V · R A R V E M L A K F│S K K A G T P A K G K V G G R W K                    258
Slow Sktl   I · N V L Y N R I S H A Q K F R K G A G · · · K G R V G G R W K                    251
Cardiac     I · N V L R N R I N D N Q K V S K T R G · · · K A K V T G R W K                    288
```

Fig. 2. Alignment of the principal adult human TnT amino acid sequences from fast skeletal muscle (Fast Sktl) *(3)*, slow skeletal muscle (Slow Sktl) *(42)*, and myocardium (Cardiac) *(43)*. The single-letter amino acid code is used and (*) indicates no corresponding amino acid. (a) A human fetal exon encoding the sequence DTAEEDAE has been reported to be similar to these sequences in both adult fast sktl and adult cTnT *(44)*. (b) This epitope is conserved across phyla *(4)*. (c) This amino acid sequence corresponds to fetal TnTf exon 17 (β-exon) *(3)*, and the amino acid sequence corresponding to adult TnTf exon (16 α-exon) in adult rat and rabbit is expected to be conserved in adult human fast sktl TnT.

the human fast skeletal TnI gene has not been described. It has also been reported that mutations in the cTnT gene account for about 15% of cases of familial hypertrophic cardiomyopathy *(52,59)*.

Within the various striated muscles, further diversity of troponin T isoforms arise from alternative splicing of the RNA transcripts of the respective gene *(3,42,44, 53,60–63)*, as shown in Fig. 4. In fast skeletal muscle, for example, it has been suggested that there are 64 possible 5′-alternatively spliced mRNA variants, but few are actually found as protein isoforms or full-length cDNA *(3,42,44,64)*. The expression of different exons appears to be under strict control, varying as a function of both developmental stage and health or injury. For example, the expression of exons 16 and 17 (α- and β-exons) of fast skeletal muscle troponin T (TnTf) is developmentally regulated and mutually exclusive *(3,60)*. Exon 16 is expressed in adult muscle as the α-TnTf isoform, and exon 17 is expressed in fetal muscle as β-TnTf, with a different peptide appearing near the carboxy-terminus (*see* Figs. 2 and 4). Isoforms, like β-TnTf, that are expressed during development, but

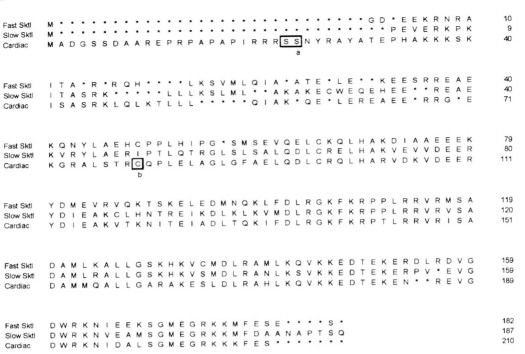

Fig. 3. Alignment of adult human TnI amino acid sequences from fast skeletal muscle (Fast Sktl) *(45)*, slow skeletal muscle (Slow Sktl) *(46)*, and myocardium (Cardiac) *(47)*. The single-letter amino acid code is used, and (*) indicates no corresponding amino acid. (a) These amino acids are phosphorylated by protein kinase A in response to adrenaline *(40)*. (b) Site of cTnI cleavage by endogenous proteases *(30)*.

do not normally appear in adult muscle could be termed "oncoforms." In rabbit, a total of only five fetal TnTf isoforms have been reported to date *(44)*, arising from variations in the expression of 5′-exons producing different amino-terminal peptide sequences. The expression of particular exons does not appear to be under unique control only for TnT: specific combinations of TnT, tropomyosin, and α-actinin isoforms are coexpressed during development and in adult fast skeletal muscle *(64)*. It has been suggested that neural stimulation *(65)*, thyroid hormone, or various growth factors could be the secondary messengers that trigger these changes in isoform expression *(66)*.

Several investigators have reported differences in the functional properties of TnT isoforms found in bovine *(67)* and rabbit myocardium *(68)*, and rabbit fast skeletal muscle *(66,69)*. There are two isoforms of cTnT in adult bovine heart, and one of these requires less calcium to activate ATPase activity in reconstituted myofibril preparations *(67)*. Developmental changes in the calcium sensitivity of myofibrillar ATPase in rabbit myocardium correlates with changes in the cTnT isoform composition *(68,69)*. Five isoforms have been identified in human heart, with differential expression during development, although 36 alternative splicing isoforms are theoretically possible *(53,62,63,70)*. The expression of one of the fetal isoforms has to be upregulated in adult patients with heart failure *(62,63,71,72)*. Heart failure is also associated with reduced calcium-sensitive ATPase activity *(71,73)*. Furthermore, studies in rats indicate that

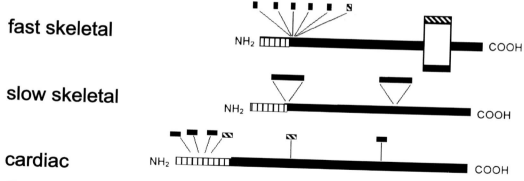

Fig. 4. Schematic comparing alternative exon splicing patterns of the three TnT genes *(42,44,53,61)*. The variable regions at the amino-terminus are shown in vertical stripes, and the highly conserved regions are shown in solid black. Exons are shown as branches, with adult exons in black and fetal exons in hatch.

cardiac hypertrophy is associated with an adult-to-fetal isoform transition of myosin, α-actin, and tropomyosin *(74)*. These findings suggest that a general mechanism for selection of exon expression may be involved in the expression of these isoforms, similar to that described during ontogeny.

The TnI isoforms do not appear to undergo alternative splicing of RNA transcripts of the respective genes.

Ontogeny and Isoform Switching

The heterogeneity of TnT isoforms in normal developing fetal muscles is further complicated by the simultaneous expression of isoforms from the three TnT genes *(50)*, which are not seen in normal adult muscles. In humans, five cTnT isoforms are expressed in fetal cardiac muscle, but neither fast nor slow skeletal muscle isoforms are expressed *(53,62,63,70)*. In human fetal skeletal muscle, fetal cTnT isoforms are transiently expressed at both the transcriptional *(50,70)* and translational levels *(42,75)*. No fetal or adult cTnT isoforms have been detected in adult skeletal muscle *(62)*, although traces of fetal cardiac mRNA have been found *(70)*. Similar findings have been reported in chicken *(76,77)*, mouse *(78)*, rat *(50,65,75)*,

and rabbit *(4)*. The proportion of human fetal skeletal TnT that is made up of fetal cTnT is low, with a predominance of TnTf isoforms *(50,62)*. This is unlike fetal skeletal TnT expression in rat, where cTnT makes up about 30% of the total, and there is a predominance of slow skeletal TnT isoforms *(50)*. These findings are consistent with the origination of cardiac and skeletal muscles from different precursor cells of the developing embryo *(79)*. The mixture of isoforms in the early differentiation program may favor the efficient formation of new sarcomeres, and that the acquisition of "structure" precedes the acquisition of function during muscle development *(50)*.

The unique mixture of TnT isoforms found in fetal skeletal muscle has fueled great interest in TnT isoform expression in regenerating skeletal muscle *(50,65,80)*. cTnT mRNA was found together with fast and slow skeletal muscle TnT isoforms in both fast and slow adult rat skeletal muscle regenerating following surgical or myotoxic injury. The proportions of each isoform found did not vary as a function of the regenerating muscle type (fast or slow), and corresponded to the proportions seen in fetal skeletal muscle *(50)*. Immunohistochemical investigations of slow adult rat skeletal muscle following freezing injury or denervation yielded similar findings *(65)*. An immunohistochemical study was also carried out in normal and diseased adult human muscles, but the results were inconclusive, because the polyclonal goat anti-cTnT antibodies used were directed against an amino-terminal peptide of cTnT of amino acid residues 3–15 *(80)*. Unlike cTnI, in which the first 31 amino-terminal residues are unique to the cardiac isoform, the first 33 amino-terminal residues of cTnT have some homology with adult TnTf and slow skeletal muscle TnT isoforms (*see* Figs. 2 and 3). However, a peptide with 28 amino acid residues unique to cTnT is found following the first 33 amino-terminal residues. The clinical implications of the expression of cTnT in regenerating skeletal muscle in humans is discussed in the next chapter.

Heterogeneity of TnI isoform expression in fetal muscle development is also seen *(46,81,82)*. The slow skeletal muscle isoform of TnI is the predominant isoform in fetal striated muscle *(46)*. Slow skeletal TnI in early fetal fast skeletal muscle is replaced with fast skeletal TnI during later fetal development *(83)*. Only slow skeletal TnI is found in adult slow-twitch skeletal muscle, only fast skeletal TnI is found in adult fast-twitch skeletal muscle, and cTnI is not found in either *(84)*. Slow skeletal TnI is present in newborn human myocardium for up to 33 wk of postnatal development, but is undetectable by 9 mo. CTnI is detectable in fetal myocardium throughout development, but the transition to exclusive expression of cTnI in myocardium does not occur until after birth *(81,85)*. There has been great interest in the possible re-expression of slow skeletal TnI in diseased myocardium *(86)*. Slow skeletal TnI has not been detected in adult human myocardium from patients with cardiomyopathy *(58)* or end-stage heart failure *(81)* using Northern blot hybridization with slow-twitch TnI cDNA to probe diseased myocardium.

ABBREVIATIONS

CK, creatine kinase; cTnI, T, C, cardiac troponins I, T, and C; kDa, kilodaltons; TnTf, fast skeletal TnT.

ACKNOWLEDGMENTS

The author gratefully acknowledges the assistance of Stephen D. Cunningham, Boehringer Mannheim Corp., who provided invaluable information and literature searches.

REFERENCES

1. Katus HA, Remppis A, Looser S, Hallermeier K, Scheffold T, and Kubler W (1989) Enzyme linked immunoassay of cardiac troponin T for the detection of acute myocardial infarction in patients. J. Mol. Cell. Cardiol. 21:1349–1353.
2. Cummins P, McGurk B, Littler WA (1979) Possible diagnostic use of cardiac specific contractile proteins in assessing cardiac damage. Clin. Sci. 56:30.
3. Wu Q-L, Jha PK, Raychowdhury MK, Du Y, Leavis PC, and Sarkars S (1994) Isolation and characterization of human fast skeletal β troponin T cDNA: comparative sequence analysis of isoforms and insight into the evolution of members of multigene family. DNA Cell Biol. 13:217–223.
4. Malouf NN, McMahon D, Oakeley AE, and Anderson PA (1992) A cardiac troponin T epitope conserved across phyla. J. Biol. Chem. 267:9269–9274.
5. Wu Q-L, Raychowdhury MK, Du Y, Jha PK, Leavis PC, and Sarkar S (1993) Characterization of a rabbit fast skeletal troponin I cDNA: a comparative sequence analysis of vertebrate isoforms and tissue-specific expression of a single copy gene. J. DNA Sequencing and Mapping 4:113–121.
6. Breitbart RE, Andreadis A, and Nadal-Ginart B (1987) Alternative splicing: a ubiquitous mechanism for the generation of multiple protein isoforms from single genes. Ann. Rev. Biochem. 56:467–495.
7. Ebashi S and Kodama A (1965) A new protein factor promoting aggregation of

tropomyosin. J. Biochem. (Tokyo) 58: 107–108.

8. Ebashi S and Kodama A (1966) Interaction of troponin with f-actin in the presence of tropomyosin. J. Biochem. (Tokyo) 59: 425–426.

9. Hartshorne DJ and Mueller H (1968) Fractionation of troponin into two distinct proteins. Biochem. Biophys. Res. Commun. 31:647–653.

10. Ebashi S, Wakabayashi T, and Ebashi F (1971) Troponin and its components. J. Biochem. (Tokyo) 69:441–445.

11. Greaser ML and Gergely J (1971) Reconstitution of troponin activity from three protein components. J. Biol. Chem. 246: 4226–4233.

12. Staprans I, Takahashi H, Russell MP, and Watanabe S (1972) Skeletal and cardiac troponins and their components. J. Biochem. (Tokyo) 72:723–735.

13. Greaser M and Gergely J (1973) Purification and properties of the components from troponin. J. Biol. Chem. 248:2125–2133.

14. Katus HA, Scheffold T, Remppis A, and Zehlein J (1992) Proteins of the troponin complex. Lab Med. 23:311–317.

15. Farah CS and Reinach FC (1995) The troponin complex and regulation of muscle contraction. FASEB J. 9:755–767.

16. Heeley DH, Golkosinska K, and Smillie LB (1987) The effects of troponin T fragments T1 and T2 on the binding of nonpolymerizable tropomyosin to f-actin in the presence and absence of troponin I and troponin C. J. Biol. Chem. 262:9971–9978.

17. Geeves MA and Lehrer SS (1994) Troponin increases the size of the tropomyosin-actin cooperative unit of the regulatory switch of the muscle thin filament [Abstract]. Biophys. J. 66:A309.

18. Flicker PF, Phillips GN Jr, and Cohen C (1982) Troponin and its interactions with tropomyosin: an electron microscope study. J. Mol. Biol. 162:495–501.

19. Voss EM, Sharkey SW, Gernert AE, Murakami MM, Johnston RB, Hsieh CC, and Apple FS (1995) Human and canine cardiac troponin T and creatine kinase-MB distribution in normal and diseased myocardium: infarct sizing using serum profiles. Arch. Pathol. Lab. Med. 119:799–806.

20. Katus HG, Remppis A, and Scheffold T (1991) Intracellular compartmentation of cardiac troponin T and its release kinetics in patients with reperfused and nonreperfused myocardial infarction. Am. J. Cardiol. 67:1360–1367.

21. Martin AF (1981) Turnover of cardiac troponin subunits. J. Biol. Chem. 256:964–968.

22. Hein S, Scheffold T, and Schaper J (1995) Ischemia induces early changes to cytoskeletal and contractile proteins in diseased human myocardium. J. Thorac. Cardiovasc. Surg. 110:89–98.

23. Guth BD, Schulz R, and Heusch G (1993) Time course and mechanisms of contractile dysfunction during acute myocardial ischemia. Circulation 87(Suppl.):IV35–IV42.

24. Adams JE III, Schechtman KB, Landt Y, Ladenson JH, and Jaffe AS (1994) Comparable detection of acute myocardial infarction by creatine kinase MB Isoenzyme and cardiac troponin I. Clin. Chem. 40: 1291–1295.

25. Mair J, Genser N, Morandell D, Maier J, Mair P, Lechleitner P, Calzolari C, Larue C, Ambach E, Dienstl F, Pan B, and Puschendorf B (1996) Cardiac troponin I in the diagnosis of myocardial injury and infarction. Clin. Chim. Acta 245:19–38.

26. Lavigne L, Waskiewicz S, Pervaiz G, Fagan G, and Whiteley G (1996) Investigation of serum troponin I heterogeneity and complexation to troponin T [Abstract]. Clin. Chem. 42:S312.

27. Katrukha A, Petterson K, Lovgren T, Mitrunen K, Beresnikova A, Bulargina T, Esakova T, and Severina M (1996) Cardiac troponin I-cardiac troponin C complex in serum of patients with acute myocardial infarction [Abstract]. Proc. XVI Int. Cong. Clin. Chem. 221.

28. Feng YJ, Moore RE, and Wu AHB (1997) Identification and analysis of cardiac troponin complexes in blood by gel filtration chromatography [Abstract]. Clin. Chem. 43: S159.

29. Waskiewicz D, Sahaney J, Lavigne L, Fagan G, and Whiteley G (1996) Sample stability differences among troponin I kits [Abstract]. Clin. Chem. 42:S311.

30. Krudy GA, Kleerekoper Q, Guo X, Howarth JW, Solaro RJ, and Rosvear PR (1994)

NMR studies delineating spatial relationships within the cardiac troponin I-troponin C complex. J. Biol. Chem. 269:23,731–23,735.

31. LaRue C and Marquet P-Y (1996) Stabilized composition of troponin. UK Patent Office, GB 2 275 774.

32. Zehelein J, Schroeder A, Kraus O and Brown B (1995) Release kinetics of troponin T and troponin I in patients with acute myocardial infarction [abstract]. Circulation 92(Suppl.):I–678.

33. Katrukha A, Petterson K, Lovgren T, Mitrunen K, and Mykkanen P (1996) Cardiac troponin C influences the binding of monoclonal antibodies to cardiac troponin I (abstract). Proc. XVI Int. Cong. Clin. Chem. 221.

34. Zot AS and Potter JD (1987) Structural aspects of troponin-tropomyosin regulation of skeletal muscle contraction. Ann. Rev. Biophys. Chem. 16:535–559.

35. Potter JD, Sheng Z, Pan B-S, and Zhao J (1995) A direct regulatory role for troponin T and a dual role for troponin C in the Ca^{+2} regulation of muscle contraction. J. Biol. Chem. 270:2557–2562.

36. Lin T-I, Mayadevi M, and Dowben RM (1993) Modulation of troponin-C binding to troponin T by Ca^{+2}, probed by fluorescence. J. Chin. Chem. Soc. 40:607–619

37. Karczewski P, Bartel S, and Krause E-G (1993) Protein phosphorylation in the regulation of cardiac contractility and vascular smooth muscle tone. Curr. Opinion Nephrol. Hypertens. 2:33–40.

38. Gusev NB, Barskaya NV, Verin AD, Duzhenkova IV, Khuchua ZA, and Zheltova AO (1983) Some properties of cardiac troponin T structure. Biochem. J. 213:123–129.

39. Kitsis RN and Scheuer J (1996) Functional significance of alterations in cardiac contractile protein isoforms. Clin. Cardiol. 19:9–18.

40. Quirk PG, Patchell VB, Gao Y, Levine BA, and Perry SV (1995) Sequential phosphorylation of adjacent serine residues on the N-terminal region of cardiac troponin-I: structure-activity implications of ordered phosphorylation. FEBS Lett. 370:175–178.

41. Venema RC and Kuo JF (1993) Protein kinase C-mediated phosphorylation of troponin I and C-protein in isolated myocar-dial cells is associated with inhibition of myofibrillar actomyosin MgATPase. J. Biol. Chem. 268:2705–2711.

42. Gahlmann R, Troutt AB, Wade RP, Gunning P, and Ledes L (1987) Alternative splicing generates variants in important functional domains of human slow skeletal troponin T. J. Biol. Chem. 262:16,122–16,126.

43. Townsend PJ, Farza H, MacGeoch C, Spurr KNK, Wade R, Gahlamann R, Yocoub M, and Barton PJ (1994) Human cardiac troponin T: identification of fetal isoforms and assignment of the TNNT2 locus to chromosome 1q. Genomics 21:311–316

44. Briggs MM, Maready M, Schmidt JM, and Schachat F (1994) Identification of a fetal exon in the human fast troponin T gene. FEBS Lett. 350:37–40.

45. Zhu L, Perez-Alvarado G, and Wade R (1994) Sequencing of a cDNA encoding the human fast-twitch skeletal muscle isoform of troponin I. Biochim. Biophys. Acta 1217:338–340.

46. Corin SJ, Juhasz O, Zhu L, Conley P, Keded L, and Wade R (1994) Structure and expression of the human slow twitch skeletal muscle troponin I gene. J. Biol. Chem. 269:10,651–10,659.

47. Vallins WJ, Brand NJ, Dabhade N, Butler-Browne G, Yacoub MH, and Barton PJ (1990) Molecular Cloning of human cardiac troponin I using polymerase chain reaction. FEBS Lett. 270:57–61.

48. Ordahl CP (1986) The skeletal and cardiac α-actin genes are coexpressed in early embryonic striated muscle. Dev. Biol. 117: 488–492.

49. Seidel U, Bober E, Winter B, Lenz S, Lohse P, and Arnold HH (1987) The complete nucleotide sequences of cDNA clones coding for human myosin light chains 1 and 3. Nucleic Acids Res. 15:4989.

50. Sutherland CJ, Esser KA, Elsom VL, Gordon ML, and Hardeman EC (1993) Identification of a program of contractile protein gene expression initiated upon skeletal muscle differentiation. Dev. Dynam. 196:25–36.

51. Dhoot GK, Frearson N, and Perry SV (1979) Polymorphic forms of troponin T and troponin C and their localization in striated muscle cell types. Exp. Cell Res. 122: 339–350.

52. Thierfelder L, Watkins H, MacRae C, Lamas R, McKenna W, Vosberg JP, Seidman JG, and Seidman CE (1994) α-Tropomyosin and cardiac troponin T mutations cause familial hypertrophic cardiomyopathy: a disease of the sarcomere. Cell 77:701–712.

53. Mesnard L, Logeart D, Taviaux S, Diriong S, Mercadier JJ, and Samson F (1995) Human cardiac troponin T: cloning and expression of new isoforms in the normal and failing heart. Circ. Res. 76:687–692.

54. Samson F, Lee JE, Hung WY, Potter JG, Herbstreith M, Roses AD, and Gilbert JR (1990) Isolation and localization of a slow troponin (TnT) gene on chromosome 19 by subtraction hybridization of a cDNA muscle library using myotonic dystrophy muscle cDNA. J. Neurosci. Res. 27:441–451.

55. Samson F, De Jong PJ, Trask BJ, Koza-Taylor P, Speer MC, Potter T, Roses AD, and Gilbert JR (1992) Assignment of the human slow skeletal troponin T gene to 19q13. 4 using somatic cell hybrids and fluorescence in situ hybridization analysis. Genomics 13:1374–1375.

56. Mao C, Baumgartner AP, Jha PK, Huang TH-M, and Sarkar S (1996) Assignment of the human fast skeletal troponin T gene (TNNT3) to chromosome 11p15. 5: evidence for the presence of 11pter in a mono-chromosome 9 somatic cell hybrid in NIGMS mapping panel 2. Genomics 31:385–388.

57. Bermingham N, Hernandez D, Balfour A, Gilmour F, Martin JE, and Fisher EMC (1995) Mapping TNNC1, the gene that encodes cardiac troponin I in human and the mouse. Genomics 30:620–622.

58. Wade R, Eddy R, Shows TB, and Kedes L (1990) cDNA sequence, tissue-specific expression, and chromosomal mapping of the human slow-twitch skeletal muscle isoform of troponin I. Genomics 7:346–357.

59. Watkins H, McKenna WJ, Thierfelder L, Suk HJ, Anan R, O'Donoghue A, Spirito P, Matsumori A, Moravec CS, Seidman JG, and Seidman CE (1995) Mutations in the genes for cardiac troponin T and α-tropomyosin in hypertrophic cardiomy-opathy. N. Engl. J. Med. 332:1058–1064.

60. Medford RM, Nguyen HT, Destree AT, Summers E, and Nadal-Ginard B (1984) A novel mechanism of alternative RNA splicing for the developmentally regulated generation of troponin T isoforms from a single gene. Cell 38:409–421.

61. Townsend PJ, Barton PJ, Yacoub MH, and Farza H (1995) Molecular cloning of human cardiac troponin T isoforms: expression in developing and failing heart J. Mol. Cell Cardiol. 27:2223–2236.

62. Anderson PAW, Malouf NN, Oakeley AE, Pagani ED, and Allen PD (1991) Troponin T isoform expression in humans: a comparison among normal and failing adult heart, fetal heart, and adult and fetal skeletal muscle. Circ. Res. 69:1226–1233.

63. Anderson PAW, Greig A, Mark TM, Malouf NN, Oakeley AE, Ungerleider RM, Allen PD, and Kay BK (1995) Molecular basis of human cardiac troponin T isoforms expressed in the developing, adult, and fail-ing heart. Circ. Res. 76:681–686.

64. Briggs MM, McGinnis HD, and Schachat F (1990) Transitions from fetal to fast troponin T isoforms are coordinated with changes in tropomyosin and α-actinin isoforms in developing rabbit skeletal muscle. Dev. Biol. 140:253–260.

65. Saggin L, Gorza L, Ausoni S, and Schiaffino S (1990) Cardiac troponin T in developing, regenerating and denervated rat skeletal muscle. Development 110:547–554.

66. Nadal-Ginard B and Mahdavi V (1989) Mol-ecular basis of cardiac performance. J. Clin. Invest. 84:1693–1700.

67. Tobacman LS and Lee R (1987) Isolation and functional comparison of bovine cardiac troponin T isoforms. J. Biol. Chem. 262: 4059–4064.

68. McAuliffe JJ, Gao L, and Solaro RJ (1990) Changes in myofibrillar activation and tro-ponin C Ca^{+2} binding associated with tro-ponin T isoform switching in developing rabbit heart. Circ. Res. 66:1204–1216.

69. Schachat FH, Diamond MS, and Brandt PW (1987) Effect of different troponin T-tropomyosin combinations on thin fila-ment activation. J. Mol. Biol. 198:551–554.

70. Mesnard L, Samson F, Espinasse I, Durand J, Neveux JY, and Mercadier JJ (1993) Mol-ecular cloning and developmental expres-sion of human cardiac troponin T. FEBS Lett. 328:139–144.

71. Solaro RJ, Powers FM, Gao L, and Gwathmey JK (1993) Control of myofilament activation in heart-failure. Circulation 87 (Suppl.):38–42.

72. Saba Z, Nassar R, Ungerleider RM, Oakeley AE, and Anderson PAW (1996) Cardiac troponin T isoform expression correlates with pathophysiological descriptors in patients who underwent corrective surgery for congenital heart disease. Circulation 94: 472–476.

73. Meyer M, Schillinger W, Pieske B, Holubarsch C, Heimnamm C, Posival H, Kuwajimia G, Mikoshiba K, Just H, and Hasenfuss G (1995) Alterations of sarcoplasmic reticulum proteins in failing human dilated cardiomyopathy. Circulation 92:778–784.

74. Isumo S, Nadal-Ginard B, and Mahdavi V (1988) Protooncogene induction and reprogramming of cardiac gene expression produced by pressure overload. Proc. Natl. Acad. Sci. USA 85:339–343.

75. Sabry MA and Dhoot GK (1991) Identification of and pattern of transitions of cardiac, adult slow and slow skeletal muscle-like embryonic isoforms of troponin T in developing rat and human skeletal muscles. J. Musc. Res. Cell Motil. 12:262–270.

76. Toyota N and Shimada Y (1981) Differentiation of troponin in cardiac and skeletal muscles in chicken embryos as studied by immunofluorescence microscopy. J. Cell Biol. 91:497–504.

77. Cooper TA and Ordahl CP (1984) A single troponin T gene regulated by different programs in cardiac and skeletal muscle development. Science 226:979–982.

78. McAuliffe JJ, Roulier E, Aronow B, and White D (1994) Delineation of the cardiac troponin T expression pattern during murine development [Abstract]. J. Cell Biochem. 18D (Suppl.):519.

79. Mar JH, Iannello RC, and Ordahl CP (1992) Cardiac troponin T gene expression in muscle. Symp. Soc. Exp. Biol. (Engl.) 46: 237–249.

80. Bodor GS, Porterfield D, Voss E, Kelly J, Smith S, and Apple FS (1995) Cardiac troponin-T composition in normal and regenerating human skeletal muscle [Abstract]. Clin. Chem. 41:S148.

81. Sasse S, Brand NJ, Kyprianou P, Dhoot GK, Wade R, Arai M, Periasamy M, Yacoub MH, and Barton PJ (1993) Troponin I gene expression during human cardiac development and in end-stage heart failure. Circ. Res. 72:932–938.

82. Bhavsar PK, Brand NJ, Yacoub MH, and Barton PJR (1996) Isolation and characterization of the human cardiac troponin I gene (TNNI3). Genomics 35:11–23.

83. Krishan K and Dhoot GK (1996) Changes in some troponin and insulin-like growth factor messenger ribonucleic acids in regenerating and denervated skeletal muscles. J. Muscle Res. Cell Motil. 17:513–521.

84. Bodor GS, Porter S, Landt Y, and Ladenson JH (1992) Development of monoclonal antibodies for an assay of cardiac troponin-I and preliminary results in suspected cases of myocardial infarction. Clin. Chem. 38: 2203–2214.

85. Bhavsar PK, Dhoot GK, Cumming DVE et al. (1991) Developmental expression of troponin I isoforms in fetal human heart. FEBS Lett. 292:5–8.

86. Hunkler NM and Murphy AM (1990) cDNA sequence of human cardiac troponin I (cTnI) and expression of TnI isoforms in diseased hearts (Abstract). Circulation 82(Suppl.): III–188.

Cardiac Troponin T as a Marker of Myocardial Injury

Kenneth J. Dean

INTRODUCTION

Contractile proteins have been of interest as potential markers of myocardial injury since the late 1970s, when they were found to have unique isoforms in various striated muscle types (fast, slow, and cardiac) *(1,2)*. Markers unique to the myocardium offer advantages over markers that are universally found in skeletal muscle (e.g., myoglobin and total creatine kinase [CK]*), or are enriched in myocardium, but are not unique to that muscle (e.g., CK-MB$_2$ isoform). Truly cardiac-specific markers should be very low or undetectable in circulating blood. The upper limit of normal for such markers reflects in part the imprecision of a particular analyzer at very low concentrations. There should be no population variations in normal range concentrations because of gender (muscle mass), lifestyle, or (noncardiac) state of health, as are seen with markers that are not cardiac-specific. It should be possible to diagnose injuries involving smaller amounts of myocardium than can be diagnosed with markers having normal circulating levels with noncardiac origins. This is because the uncertainty created by a low signal-to-noise ratio (SNR) in the vicinity of the clinical cutoff or discriminator concentration of the marker should be shifted to a much lower concentration. Finally, myocardial injury (or the absence of injury) should be easily discerned, even in the presence of concomitant skeletal muscle injury or disease. An immunoassay for cardiac troponin T (cTnT) was first reported in 1989 *(3)*, and the singularity of this cTnT immunoassay was the basis for a European patent *(4)*.

ASSAYS

Formats

The first assay described for cTnT was a research-based enzyme-linked immunosorbent assay (ELISA) that utilized goat anti-human cTnT antiserum immobilized on polyvinylchloride (PVC) test tubes as the capture antibody and mouse monoclonal antihuman cTnT antibody labeled with horseradish peroxidase *(3)*. The assay had 1–2% crossreactivity with skeletal TnT (sTnT) and a detection limit of 0.25–0.5 ng/mL *(5)*.

The first-generation commercial assay (CARDIAC T® ELISA TnT) used a biotin-labeled mouse monoclonal anti-cTnT antibody in place of goat antiserum and streptavidin immobilized on PVC test tubes *(6)*. This monoclonal antibody (MAb) had no detectable crossreactivity with sTnT producing an assay that had overall crossreac-

---

*See p. 220 for list of abbreviations used in this chapter.

From: Cardiac Markers Edited by: Alan H. B. Wu
© Humana Press Inc., Totowa, NJ

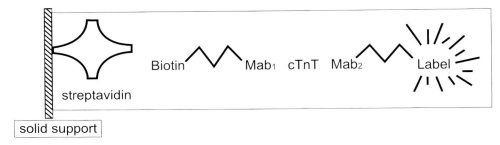

Fig. 1. Block diagram of the BMC cTnT assays.

tivity of 3.6% against sTnT. False elevations could occur owing to nonspecific binding of sTnT to the PVC test tubes *(7)*. This commercial assay had a lower detection limit of 0.04 ng/mL. An improved, second-generation assay (the CARDIAC T® Enzymun-Test® TnT) has since been introduced. The crossreactive MAb was eliminated, and a second cardiac-specific mouse MAb was employed *(8)*. No crossreactivity with sTnT up to 1000 ng/mL (<0.005%) was detected. The lower detection limit for cTnT was 0.02 ng/mL.

A qualitative immunoassay for cTnT was also introduced *(9)*. The test utilized the same two MAb used in the original ELISA assay. However, the labeling of the antibodies was switched to reduce the crossreactivity against sTnT. The crossreactivity of the assay with sTnT was 0.5%. The detection limit and the clinical cutoff concentration were the same because of the qualitative nature of the method; the rapid assay yielded positive results when the cTnT in whole blood was ≥0.2 ng/mL, as measured in serum on the ES 300 *(6)*. Chapter 16 describes this point-of-care assay in more detail.

An improved ultrasensitive CARDIAC T® Rapid Assay using the same MAb that are in the second-generation CARDIAC T® Enzymun-Test® TnT assay is now available. An electrochemiluminescent assay for cTnT *(10)* has been developed (Elecsys® TnT), which utilizes the same pair of MAb used in

the CARDIAC T® Enzymun-Test® TnT method. The detection limit and crossreactivity toward sTnT are 0.01 ng/mL and <0.001%, respectively. The test has a 9-min incubation period. The evolution of cTnT assays is summarized in Table 1 and their general format is shown in Fig. 1.

Normal Range Concentration

The first-generation commercial cTnT assay had 3.6% crossreactivity with sTnT *(6)*, and a normal range of in healthy individuals 0–0.08 ng/mL *(11)*. The second-generation assay had <0.005% crossreactivity with sTnT, and the concentration of cTnT in 99.6% of 4955 noncardiac patients was <0.10 ng/mL *(8)*. The cutoff concentration for the first-generation qualitative CARDIAC T® Rapid Assay was ≥0.2 ng/mL, and the crossreactivity with sTnT was <0.5%. In a study of 100 patients with chest pain suspicious for AMI, 61 of 66 patients who did not fulfill criteria for the diagnosis of AMI yielded negative results *(12)*. The cutoff concentration for the second-generation qualitative Rapid Assay is ≥0.08 ng/mL and the crossreactivity with sTnT is <0.016%. In a study of 136 normal individuals, serum cTnT was <0.05 ng/mL, and negative results were obtained with the Rapid Assay in all cases *(13)*.

Interferences

The use of a biotin–streptavidin capture system to bind the antibody–analyte sand-

Infarct Sizing

The estimation of infarct size following AMI can be useful for subsequent clinical management *(45)*. Imaging procedures, such as ^{201}Tl, are used to estimate infarct size *(46)*, and cardiac markers have also been correlated with infarct size *(47)*. CK-MB peak activity and the late cTnT peak concentration correlated equally well with radionuclide imaging ($r = 0.73$ for each) for the estimation of infarct size in 21 AMI patients (5 anterior and 16 inferior wall AMIs) *(46)*. CK peak activity was weakly correlated with the infarct size estimated by [99m]Tn-sestamibi scintigraphy ($r = 0.56$). Similar correlations between the late cTnT peak concentrations and ^{201}Tl scintigraphy ($r = 0.77$, and $r = 0.75$, respectively) have been reported *(47)*.

Perioperative Myocardiac Infarction (MI)

Diagnosis of a perioperative MI in cardiac and noncardiac surgery poses a unique challenge to the cardiologist. The ECG may exhibit nonspecific ST-segment and T-wave changes, and serum CK, CK-MB, and CK-MB isoform measurements are of little value because of their release from noncardiac tissues injured by the surgery *(48)*. A truly cardiac-specific marker, with low or undetectable serum baseline levels, may provide more accurate diagnosis of perioperative MI in noncardiac surgery patients. Patients undergoing cardiac surgery, on the other hand, are one of those groups where careful consideration of the appropriate clinical cutoff is required. Unlike the baseline levels seen with noncardiac surgery patients, the baseline levels of a cardiac-specific marker will be elevated as a result of surgical injury to the heart, and the accurate diagnosis of further injury to the myocardium by a perioperative MI must take this elevated baseline into account.

Noncardiac Surgery

The risk of a perioperative MI with major noncardiac surgery is only 1–2% in patients over 40 yr. However, the risk of a perioperative MI increases to 3–10% in elderly patients and those with cardiovascular disease *(49)*. In one report, 22 patients who underwent minor orthopedic surgery and 12 patients who underwent lung surgery by median sternotomy had no detectable serum cTnT over 6 d of postoperative serial testing *(48)*. Four of the orthopedic surgery patients showed elevations of CK-MB activity, as did 5 of the lung surgery patients. CK activity was elevated in all of the lung surgery patients and 17 of the orthopedic surgery patients. None of the patients had experienced perioperative MI. These findings were supported in a study of patients undergoing thoracic surgery for lung disease *(50)*. In a large study of 1175 patients undergoing major noncardiac surgery, cTnT and CK-MB had comparable performance for the detection of perioperative MI ($n = 17$, 1.4% of patients) *(51)*. cTnT had a clinical sensitivity of 87% and specificity of 84% for the diagnosis of AMI (cutoff 0.1 ng/mL). A relative risk for AMI of 32.8-fold was associated with an elevated cTnT. Two patients who met the study criteria for the diagnosis of AMI did not have elevated cTnT: one had nonspecific ECG changes and elevated CK and CK-MB following knee surgery, and the other had ECG changes consistent with ischemia, and slightly elevated CK-MB. Neither patient had cardiovascular complications. Among the patients who did not receive the diagnosis of AMI were 17 who suffered major cardiac complications (primarily pulmonary edema). cTnT had a clinical sensitivity of 62% and specificity of 85% for the diagnosis of these major cardiac complications. Elevations were also detected in an additional 148 patients (16%) without AMI or major cardiac complications. However these elevations were significantly correlated with supraventricular tachycardias, chest pain with ECG changes consistent with ischemia, ECG changes without chest pain, and congestive heart failure (CHF). CK-MB elevations were not found in any of the patients with major cardiac complications, and were significantly correlated only with supraventricular tachycardia in the third cohort of patients. cTnT may be superior to CK-MB for detection of myocardial injury in patients undergoing major noncardiac surgery.

Elective Percutaneous Transluminal Coronary Angioplasty (PTCA)

Patients undergoing coronary angioplasty are at risk for myocardial infarction, side-branch occlusion, abrupt vessel closure, and early restenosis. Principal among these is abrupt vessel closure, which occurs in 3–8% of all procedures *(52)*. Cardiac marker measurements are one of the primary tools used to assess myocardial injury associated with PTCA. Measurements of cTnT have been conducted in patients undergoing PTCA. In one study, cTnT > 0.2 ng/mL was found in 3 of 23 PTCA patients, indicating myocardial damage *(53)*. Elevated CK-MB mass was also seen in these three patients and in three additional patients. In a larger study *(54)* of 100 PTCA patients, 41 patients had an increase in cTnT (>0.04 ng/mL above baseline). Eighteen of these also had elevations of CK-MB mass (>5.0 ng/mL above baseline). Postprocedural cTnT elevations were associated with a higher incidence of complex lesion morphology (73% of patients), intracoronary thrombus (29% of patients), abrupt closure (10% of patients), and side-branch occlusion during angioplasty (15% of patients). Similar findings have been reported in studies by others *(55)*. No increase in cTnT concentrations is seen in patients with uncomplicated successful PTCA *(56)*.

Cardiac Surgery

Perioperative myocardial injury is the most common cause of morbidity and mortality following cardiac surgery. The diagnosis of perioperative MI is further complicated by the release of cardiac markers owing to the surgical injury to the heart, producing a higher baseline level of cTnT against which the myocardial injury from AMI must be assessed. During the first 24 h after uncomplicated coronary artery bypass graft (CABG) surgery, baseline levels of cTnT reach approx 1 ng/mL *(57,58)*, although there are some reports of higher baseline levels, up to 3.5 ng/mL *(59)*. It has been suggested that higher baseline levels may be associated with longer aortic crossclamp time, leading to diffuse myocardial damage *(48)*, or with cardiotomy *(58)*. In patients experiencing perioperative MI, cTnT peak concentrations were 2–10 times the baseline *(48,57)*. One study suggested that a single cTnT determination 12 or 24 h postsurgery may be sufficient evidence to confirm the diagnosis of perioperative MI *(58)*.

There has been great interest in the utility of cTnT to assess the effectiveness of cardioprotective procedures *(60)* and drugs *(61)* during cardiac surgery. It has also been reported that cardiac markers, including cTnT, are elevated in shed blood used for autotransfusion in coronary operations *(62)*.

TROPONIN T IN HIGH-RISK UNSTABLE ANGINA (UA) PATIENTS

Non-Q-wave AMI in UA

Patients with the diagnosis of UA are a heterogeneous group with varying extent of coronary artery disease *(63)*. Some of these patients have suffered small non-Q-wave AMIs (or microinfarctions) and are at high short-term risk for AMI or cardiac death *(64–66)*. Similarly, some patients in other

Table 3
Perioperative cTnT Measurement in Patients Undergoing CABG Surgery[a]

Diagnosis	Number of patients with elevated cardiac marker			
	cTnT, >0.2 ng/mL	CK-MB activity, >12 U/L	CK-MB/CK, >6%	CK-MB mass, >6 ng/mL
Stable angina (n = 31)	1 (3.2%)	0	0	0
UA (n = 21)	19 (90.5%)	0	1 (4.8%)	2 (9.5%)

[a]Data from ref. *73*.

diagnostic groups, such as chronic renal failure and polymyositis, are also at high risk for cardiac events.

Troponin T in High-Risk UA Patients

Elevated cTnT in patients with the diagnosis of UA signifies a poor prognosis. This has been well established by numerous studies and by meta-analysis *(67)*. In a large study by the FRISC Study Group *(68)*, the prognostic value of cTnT measurements was assessed in 967 unstable coronary artery disease patients participating in a randomized trial of low-mol weight heparin. cTnT was measured within 24 h of enrollment, and patient outcomes were monitored for 6 mo, starting at day 2. The risk of cardiac events increased with increasing maximal cTnT concentrations, ranging from a relative risk of 4.3% for patients with cTnT < 0.06 ng/mL in the lowest quintile to 17% in the highest quintiles with cTnT ≥ 0.62 ng/mL. In comparison, the incidence of cardiac death or MI was 8.7% in patients with CK-MB mass below the upper reference limit (<6.0 ng/mL). However, 50% of these patients had maximal cTnT ≥ 0.06 ng/mL and were found to have a risk of 13.0% for cardiac death or MI, compared to 4.6% in those with maximal cTnT < 0.06 ng/mL. The risk of subsequent cardiac events (cardiac death, MI, or revascularization) was most pronounced early after the initial event, with approximately

half of the events occurring within the first 6 wk. The diagnosis at enrollment (non-Q-wave AMI or UA) did not add any independent prognostic information. Elevated cTnT in UA is correlated with the severity of coronary artery lesions, as determined by coronary angiography *(69)*.

Troponin T and Intervention in Acute Coronary Syndromes

Treatment of UA patients with thrombolytic agents is not accepted at the present time *(70)*; antithrombotic drugs (aspirin and heparin) are indicated in UA patients, who are often referred for revascularizations (CABG and PTCA) in an attempt to reduce morbidity and mortality *(71)*. In the FRISC trial of dalteparin (low-mol-wt heparin) in patients with unstable coronary artery disease *(72)*, patients with cTnT < 0.1 ng/mL fared equally well, whether they received dalteparin or placebo (4.7 vs 5.7% 40-d mortality, respectively). However, patients with cTnT ≥ 0.1 ng/mL had reduced mortality if they received dalteparin rather than placebo (7.4 vs. 14.2% 40-d mortality, respectively). Troponin T measurements provided an indication of which patients would benefit from dalteparin therapy. In a retrospective study of revascularization intervention, cardiac marker concentrations were measured in 52 patients who had elective CABG surgery (Table 3) *(73)*. Elevated cTnT was found in

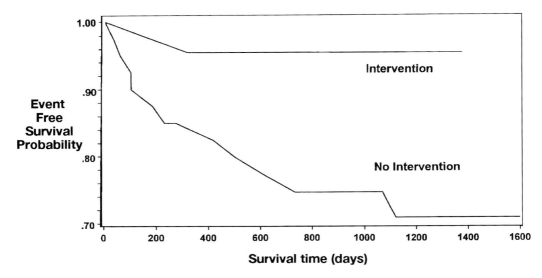

Fig. 5. Kaplan-Meier plot of survival among 62 cTnT-positive (>0.2 ng/mL) UA patients with and without revascularization. Twenty-two patients underwent elective revascularization, but 40 did not. One (4.5%) of the 22 suffered cardiac death during the follow-up period compared to 11 (27.5%) of the nonrevascularized patients. (Used with permission from ref. *74*.)

19 of 21 UA patients prior to surgery, indicating that many of the UA patients who require CABG surgery would have been identified as high-risk patients by cTnT testing prior to surgery. In another study, 183 UA patients were followed for 3 yr after their initial admission and cTnT measurement *(74)*. Initial cTnT levels were ≥0.2 ng/mL in 62 (34%) of patients. Of these, 22 patients underwent elective PTCA or CABG surgery during the follow-up period. Only 1 of these patients died, compared to 11 cardiac deaths among the 40 cTnT-positive UA patients who did not undergo elective revascularization (Fig. 5). The relative risk of death among cTnT-positive UA patients who did not undergo elective revascularization was 7.95. These studies provide the first data on the benefit of therapeutic or revascularization intervention in cTnT-positive UA patients and underscore the high risk that these patients face for adverse outcomes without intervention. In patients who have experienced AMI, a serum cTnT level > 2.8

ng/mL predicts a left ventricular ejection fraction of <40% with a sensitivity of 100% and a specificity of 92% *(75)*. This can be used to identify patients who may benefit from long-term angiotensin-converting enzyme (ACE) inhibitor therapy.

TROPONIN T IN OTHER HIGH-RISK PATIENT POPULATIONS

Chronic Renal Failure (CRF) and Dialysis Patients

Patients with chronic renal disease often present with other underlying disease(s) and multiple organ failure owing to diabetes and hypertension, which contribute to significant cardiovascular disease. Cardiomyopathies unique to renal failure and to diabetes have been described *(76,77)*. However, their etiologies have not been fully delineated. Furthermore, CRF treated with dialysis is associated with accelerated atherosclerosis *(78)*. It has been reported that 79% of ECGs on patients starting dialysis are abnormal *(79)*. Hemodialysis is associated with acute complications (hypotension, sudden death) explained by typical dialysis-induced effects on the heart *(80)*. AMI and cardiovascular disease account for 40–60% of deaths in dialysis patients *(81)*.

False elevations of CK and CK-MB activity in chronic dialysis patients have been reported *(82,83)*. These findings did not vary with alternative dialysis methods or because of the dialysis procedure itself. Elevation of these markers has been attributed to abnormal protein metabolism, muscle wasting, and the inherent lack of quantitation and variable sensitivity of CK-MB activity measurement by the electrophoretic method *(82)*. Measurement of CK-MB mass rather than activity may be more specific in dialysis patients *(84)*. Underlying hypothyroidism *(83)* in CRF patients can lead to delayed clearance of the enzyme from the reticuloendothelial system. Furthermore, endothelial dysfunction has been described in early diabetic nephropathy *(85)* and in dialyzed uremic patients *(86)*. Elevated CK-MB in dialysis patients has been associated with an increased risk for subsequent AMI or angina pectoris *(87)*.

Elevated cTnT *(88,89)* concentrations have been reported in 29–63% of CRF patients, but cTnI is reported to be elevated only rarely in these patients *(90)*. Unfortunately, these cTnI reports may be misleading. Troponin I was detected in many of these CRF patients, but failed to exceed the high clinical cutoffs used in the commercial cTnI assays *(31,89,91,92)*. When lower clinical cutoffs are used, as reported for the detection of microinfarction in high-risk UA patients *(32)*, a higher incidence of abnormal cTnI in CRF patients are reported *(93)*.

Elevated cTnT has been associated with an increased risk for subsequent angina pectoris or death owing to AMI in some hemodialysis patients *(94)*, but this is not a consistent finding *(89)*. It has been speculated that elevated cTnT findings in renal

disease patients may be owing to skeletal troponin T (sTnT) interference resulting from the 3.6% crossreactivity previously noted for the first-generation commercial assay *(90)*. High sTnT concentrations were speculated to be present because of uremic myopathy in CRF. Elevated cTnT in these particular patients could indeed arise from sTnT interference in the ELISA troponin T assay. The interference from sTnT using the first-generation ES 300 assay may occur when total CK exceeds 5000 U/L *(7)*. However, rhabdomyolysis was only rarely found in CRF patients *(95)*. Total CK generally does not correlate with abnormal cTnT findings *(95)*. Furthermore, myoglobin cannot be used as a marker of skeletal muscle injury or disease in these patients because of its renal mode of clearance. sTnT interference in the original ELISA assay was distinguishable from reaction with cTnT because of the nonlinear change in measured cTnT when samples containing sTnT were diluted in series *(96)*. Samples containing cTnT produced a linear change in measure when diluted in series. Skeletal muscle interference did not account for elevated cTnT measured in this study of 116 renal dysfunction patients. However, the frequency and magnitude of cTnT elevations correlated with the severity of disease, as confirmed by others *(97,98)*. In a study of cardiac markers in serum from both juvenile and adult CRF patients *(98)*, elevated serum cTnT was observed in 71% of hemodialysis patients, 57% of peritoneal dialysis patients, and 30% of CRF patients not on dialysis. cTnT concentrations were not affected by hemodialysis, with elevations persisting after treatment. In a study comparing the performance of the original ELISA cTnT assay with the second-generation assay, Enzymun-Test® Troponin T, the magnitude of cTnT concentrations in some hemodialysis patients was reduced *(99)*. The MAb with 12% crossreactivity toward sTnT has been replaced with a cTnT-specific MAb in both Enzymun-Test® and Elecsys® tests. The crossreactivity of these new assays with sTnT is <0.005 and <0.001%, respectively. These results suggest that sTnT interference may have been responsible for elevated cTnT findings in some renal failure patients. cTnT measurements on serum from 20 hemodialysis patients comparing the original ELISA cTnT assay with Enzymun-Test® and Elecsys® Troponin T are shown in Table 4. It can be seen that 4 (20%) of the cTnT measurements using the ELISA cTnT method were falsely elevated (presumably owing to interference from sTnT).

Myopathies

Polymyositis-dermatomyositis (PM-DM) is a chronic inflammatory myopathy of unknown origin that is mediated by autoimmune and cellular events *(100)*. The heart is affected in 50–70% of cases with about 20% of deaths in these patients owing to cardiac causes. The effect of the disease on the heart is similar to the pathological changes seen in the skeletal muscle, involving an inflammatory process with necrosis and fibrosis of the myocardium *(101)*. Cardiac involvement and poor prognosis are usually associated with severe, progressive disease *(100)*. Abnormalities have been reported in ECG, echo, and radionuclide imaging studies *(102)*.

cTnT has been measured in several groups of patients with autoimmune diseases, including patients with PM-DM *(103)*. There were no cTnT increases (≥ 0.25 ng/mL) among 30 normal subjects, 25 rheumatoid arthritis patients, or 28 systemic lupus erythematosus patients. However, high cTnT was found in 8 of 30 randomly selected PM-DM patients. cTnT concentration was not correlated with total CK activity. In one case *(104)* of exacerbated polymyositis with a cTnT concentration of 15 ng/mL at presentation, the ECG was

Table 4
cTnT in Hemodialysis Patients[a]

Patient no.	ELISA cTnT	Enzymun-Test cTnT	Elecsys cTnT
1	0.457	0.517	0.583
2	0.460	0.510	0.571
3	0.121	0.229	0.273
4	0.264	0.348	0.432
5	0.532	0.495	0.655
6	0.909	0.280	0.330
7	1.057	0.853	1.065
8	1.049	1.041	1.186
9	1.235	1.210	1.433
10	0.074	1.752	2.011
11	2.911	1.752	2.011
12	0.153	0.158	0.190
13	0.074	0.140	0.191
14	0.200	0.275	0.368
15	0.574	0.702	0.944
16	0.166	0.028	0.013
17	0.255	0.280	0.350
18	0.665	0.617	0.814
19	0.104	0.182	0.256
20	1.271	0.044	0.079

[a]All results in ng/mL.

normal and Holter monitoring indicated a small number of supraventricular premature contractions, but myocardial [201]TI scintigraphy showed a loss of accumulation in the anterior wall. There was no ischemic pathology, as seen in AMI, but there was clear evidence of focal myocardial necrosis localized in the anterior wall of the cardiac muscle. Subsequent steroid therapy resulted in an improved accumulation loss on [201]TI scintigraphy, and cTnT levels dropped to zero. cTnT measurements are helpful in the management of PM-DM patients.

cTnT has also been studied in children with Duchenne/Becker muscular dystrophies (DMD/BMD). Dilated cardiomyopathy is often seen particularly in the late stages of the disease, and may be the only clinical manifestation of the disease in heterozygous female carriers. Heart failure is the leading cause of death in DMD/ BMD *(105)*. Grossly elevated serum cTnT concentrations have been found in DMD patients using the original BMC commercial assay, as shown in Table 5. However, the frequency and magnitude of abnormal cTnT findings are greatly reduced with the second-generation cTnT assays *(106)*. Interference from sTnT using the first-generation ES 300 assay may occur when total CK exceeds 5000 U/L *(7)*. However, it is not surprising to find evidence of minor myocardial injury in some patients with DMD, similar to cTnT levels seen in patients with end-stage cardiomyopathy *(107)*, given the nature and clinical course of the disease.

It has been suggested that elevated cTnT findings in myopathy patients could be the result of re-expression of a fetal isoform of cTnT during muscle regeneration *(91)*. Because patients with renal disease, PM/DM, and DMD patients are at high risk for cardiac complications, it is not surprising to find abnormal cTnT in serum. Elevated cTnT in these patients should not automatically be dismissed as a false.

Critically Ill Patients

High cTnT and cTnI concentrations have been reported in critically ill patients who had not been diagnosed with a comorbid AMI. In one study, increased cTnT identified 94% of patients with myocardial injury, whereas CK-MB mass identified 69% of these patients *(108)*. The clinical investigation into the cause of abnormal cTnT or CK-MB mass focused on ECG and echo findings. Although the only myocardial injury that was diagnosed was AMI, cardiac injury was plausible in many of the cases cited (e.g., patients with HIV, polymyositis, and CRF). Only myocardial oxygen supply and consumption in the critically ill have been suggested as a cause of myocardial injury in cTnI-positive patients

Table 5
cTnT in Muscular Dystrophy Patients[a]

Patient no.	ELISA cTnT ng/mL	Enzymun cTnT ng/mL	CK U/L
1	0.21	0.06	1001
2	0.24	0.09	460
3	0	0	39
4	0.95	0.11	2970
5	0.14	0.18	565
6	1.39	0.13	2670
7	0	0	133
8	0.14	0.03	1021
9	1.59	0.11	2849
10	7.3	0.23	5280
11	5.7	0.21	3949
12	0.23	0	3984
13	0.11	0.04	669
14	0.84	0.10	2256
15	7.0	0.27	4512
16	4.8	0.29	4080
17	0.01	0.02	100
18	0.13	0.01	655
19	0.95	0.15	1812
20	2.52	0.19	2160

[a]Data from ref. *106.*

(109). However, others have argued that other causes of myocardial injuries can result in the release of cTnT *(110)*.

TROPONIN T AND OTHER MYOCARDIAL INJURIES

Cardiac Contusion and External Defibrillation

Blunt trauma to the chest and closed heart massage can produce cardiac contusions and necrosis in the absence of AMI. Serum cTnT increases similar in magnitude, time to peak, and duration to those seen in cardiac surgery patients have been reported in cardiac contusion patients *(111)*. However, cTnT findings did not correlate with the presence or absence of cardiac complications, such as ST-T-wave changes. The clinical findings on admission, including ECG findings, are still the most practical means of identifying patients in need of specialized care *(112)*.

External defibrillation is also reported *(113)* to result in the release of cTnT and CK-MB, with serum concentrations correlating with defibrillation energy (which reflects duration of resuscitation). The release of cTnT from the combination of closed heart massage (possible cardiac contusion) and external defibrillation in patients with ventricular fibrillation and suspected AMI leads to a higher baseline level of cTnT against which the myocardial injury from AMI must be assessed. An elevated cutoff concentration of 4.0 ng/mL cTnT has been used in these cases rather than 0.1 or 0.2 ng/mL. cTnT was found to be superior (fewer false positives) to CK-MB mass for the detection of AMI in these patients.

Cardiac Transplants

The value of cTnT measurements has been examined for assessing myocardial injury that may occur in potential heart transplant donors, ischemic preservation of the heart, and detection of cardiac allograft rejection *(114–116)*. cTnT is valuable in cardiac donors in assessing the myocardial damage associated with brainstem death for the identification of high-risk donors, whereas CK-MB activity measurements are not helpful *(114)*. Furthermore, elevated donor serum cTnT was associated with a significant increase in the incidence of catecholamine support in the immediate postoperative period. The initial release slopes, but not peak levels of CK-MB mass and cTnT in cardiac allograft recipients correlate with ischemic preservation time and donor age *(115)*.

Acute allograft rejection is the most serious complication in the early course following cardiac transplantation *(117)*. Accelerated coronary artery disease, AMI, and sudden cardiac death are the most serious threats to long-term survival *(118)*. Histo-logical examination of endomyocardial biopsies serves as the standard for the diagnosis of acute rejection. In one study, there were no differences in serum cTnT concentrations in orthotopic heart transplant recipients before biopsy with grades II and III rejection compared to those with grades 0 and I rejection *(119)*. However, in patients who later had important acute rejection episodes, serum cTnT were significantly increased at a median of 13 d prior to the histological evidence of rejection as seen on biopsy. In contrast, others found that increases in cTnT, but not CK-MB activity, showed a gradual and significant rise with increasing degrees of rejection in a rat model *(120)*. Clearly further studies will be necessary to determine whether cTnT in cardiac allograft recipients has prognostic value for severe acute rejection episodes.

Myocarditis

Myocarditis is an inflammatory disease involving the myocardium. Cardiac injury can occur with invasion of the myocytes by the infecting organism, damage by the host's immune system, or with primary injury to vascular cells resulting in coronary microcirculatory endothelial swelling, thrombosis, and small infarctions. cTnT is a more sensitive marker than the CK-MB index for autoimmune myocarditis in humans *(121)*. In one study, 21/25 (84%) of suspected myocarditis patients with elevated cTnT levels also had immunohistochemical evidence of lymphocytic infiltration in endomyocardial biopsies *(122)*. Although all of these studies conclude that high cTnT is a useful and sensitive marker for myocardial cell damage in myocarditis, a negative serum cTnT does not exclude the presence of disease.

Cardiotoxicity

Cardiotoxicity is a well-known side effect of doxorubicin and daunorubicin (anthracycline) therapy for cancers in children that can lead to long-term cardiac impairment *(123)*. Doxorubicin cardiotoxicity studies in a rat model reveal that elevated cTnT in serum is correlated with morphologic alterations of cardiac myocytes, including vacuolization and myofibrillar loss *(124)*. The release of troponin T from cTnT measurements have also been used to monitor cardiotoxicity-associated myocardial necrosis in children receiving anthracycline therapy. Using a cutoff of 0.04 ng/mL, cTnT has been used to identify myocardial necrosis associated with doxorubicin therapy in children *(125)*. Modest elevations in cTnT were observed in 6 of 10 children undergoing treatment, but not CK, CK-MB, or myoglobin, or children who had completed therapy. cTnT has been used to monitor for cardioprotective effects of the ACE inhibitor Cilazapril on doxorubicin cardiotoxicity in a rat model, the effects of fibric acid derivatives on cultured chick myocardial cells, the cardiotoxicity of calcium antagonists and β-adrenergic agonists in tocolysis, and myocardial damage from radiation treatment of breast cancer *(126–129)*. Zidovudine (AZT) has been shown to cause cardiotoxicity in humans and animals *(130)*, with its primary effect on the myocyte mitochondria. This may lead to the detection of elevated cTnT in HIV-positive patients, although these patients may also have abnormal cTnT if they have myocarditis.

TROPONIN T AND SKELETAL MUSCLE INJURY

Physical Training

Release of cardiac markers, such as cTnT, in competitive athletes is of interest because of sudden death cases in asymptomatic individuals *(131)*. Mild exercise in cardiac patients above the ischemic threshold (with release of CK that remains normal) does not appear to result in sufficient injury to cause

the release of cTnT *(119)*, nor does more vigorous exercise with release of CK activity two to five times above normal *(131,132)*. Individuals with yet higher CK activities may have acute exertional rhabdomyolysis *(134)*. Those with CK activity greater than five times the normal limit may have a high cTnT concentration with the first-generation BMC assay, as seen in a marathon runner with a postrace CK activity of 12,360 U/L and cTnT of 0.48 ng/mL. Use of the second-generation cTnT assay, however, did not produce any abnormal cTnT results among those running in the 1995 Boston Marathon *(135)*.

Rhabdomyolysis

Extraordinary CK activities can be seen in some patients with severe rhabdomyolysis. Serious complications can develop in severe rhabdomyolysis, including disseminated intravascular coagulation, myoglobinuric renal failure, and acute cardiomyopathy. Cardiac involvement is not common, but may be seen when rhabdomyolysis is produced by a drug or toxin that acts directly on striated muscle. This has been reported in fluoroacetate poisoning, ethanol-induced rhabdomyolysis, and heroin abuse *(136)*. Abnormal cTnT concentrations have been reported in 19/20 patients with severe rhabdomyolysis using the first-generation cTnT assay *(137)*. cTnI was elevated in only 6/20 patients. AMI was not diagnosed in any patients. However, 3/20 had ischemic ECG changes on admission to the hospital, and both cTnT and cTnI were elevated in these patients. It is not clear whether elevated cTnT in these patients is owing to:

1. Crossreactivity of sTnT *(7)*;
2. The fetal cardiac isoform that is expressed in skeletal muscle during fetal development being re-expressed and released into the blood by regenerating skeletal muscle in these patients; or
3. These patients experiencing undetected myocardial injury.

No elevations of cTnT were found in 219 healthy subjects with exertional rhabdomyolysis (CK activities up to 4500 U/L) prolonged over a 6-mo period *(133)*. Re-expression and release of fetal cTnT was not evident, even after 24–29 wk of repeated injury, regeneration, and repair. Others found cTnT <0.02 ng/mL in 43 marathon runners and 24 rhabdomyolysis patients using the second-generation Enzymun-Test® method for cTnT, which has <0.005% crossreactivity with human sTnT *(8)*. Further studies are needed to determine whether fetal cTnT is re-expressed in regenerating adult skeletal muscle in rhabdomyolysis or degenerative skeletal muscle disease patients. However, studies with the second-generation Enzymun-Test® method for cTnT *(8)* suggest that if fetal cTnT is re-expressed, it may not appear in serum in clinically significant concentrations.

ABBREVIATIONS

ACE, Angiotensin-converting enzyme; AMI, acute myocardial infarction; AZT, azidovudine; BMC, Boehringer Mannheim Corporation; CABG, coronary artery bypass graft; CHF, congestive heart failure; CK, creatine kinase; CRF, chronic renal failure; cTnI, T, cardiac troponins I and T; DMD/BMD, Duchenne/Becker muscular dystrophies; ECG, electrocardiogram; ED, emergency department; ELISA, enzyme-linked immunosorbent assay; FRISC, Fragmin during Instability in Coronary Artery Disease; PM-DM, polymyositis-dermatomyositis; PTCA, percutaneous transluminal angioplasty; PVC, polyvinylchloride; sTnT, skeletal muscle troponin T; TIMI, Thrombolysis In Myocardial Infarction; UA, unstable angina; WHO, World Health Organization.

ACKNOWLEDGMENT

The author gratefully acknowledges the assistance of Stephen D. Cunningham, Boehringer Mannheim Corp., who provided invaluable information and literature searches.

REFERENCES

1. Trahern CA, Brewster-Gere J, Krauth GH, and Binham DA (1978) Clinical assessment of serum myosin light chains in the diagnosis of acute myocardial infarction. Am. J. Cardiol. 41:641–645.
2. Cummins P, McGurk B, and Littler WA (1979) Possible diagnostic use of cardiac specific contractile proteins in assessing cardiac damage [Abstract]. Clin. Sci. 56:30.
3. Katus HA, Remppis A, Looser S, Hallermeier K, Scheffold T, and Kuebler W (1989) Enzyme linked immuno assay of cardiac troponin T for the detection of acute myocardial infarction in patients. J. Mol. Cell. Cardiol. 21:1349–1353.
4. Katus H, Borgya A, Hallermayer K, and Looser S (1995) Specific antibodies against troponin T, their manufacture and use in a reagent for the determination of heart muscle necrosis. European Patent Office EP 0 394 819 B1.
5. Katus HA, Remppis A, Neumann FJ, Scheffold T, Diederick KW, Vinar G, Noe A, Matern G, and Kuebler W (1991) Diagnostic efficiency of troponin T measurements in acute myocardial infarction. Circulation 83:902–912.
6. Katus HA, Looser S, Hallermayer K, Remppis A, Scheffold T, Borgya A, Essig U, and Geuss U (1992) Development and *in vitro* characterization of a new immunoassay for cardiac troponin T. Clin. Chem. 38:386–393.
7. Katus HA, Simon M, Zorn M, Scheffold T, Remppis A, Zehelein J, Grvenig E, and Fiehn W (1993) Cardiac troponin T measurements are highly specific for myocardial damage [Abstract]. J. Am. Coll. Cardiol. 21:88A.
8. Mueller-Bardoff M, Hallermayer K, Schroeder A, Ebert C, Borgya A, Gerhard TW, Remppis A, Zehelein J, and Katos HA (1997) Improved troponin T ELISA specific for the cardiac troponin T isoform. Part I: development, analytical and clinical validation of the assay. Clin. Chem. 43:458–461.

9. Mueller-Bardorff M, Freitag H, Scheffold T, Remppis A, Kubler W, and Katus HA (1995) Development and characterization of a rapid assay for bedside determinations of cardiac troponin T. Circulation 92: 2869–2875.

10. Bialk P, Vogel D, Mayr S, Richter S, and Franken N (1995) Electro-chemiluminescent immunoassay for troponin T using the random-access analyzer Elecsys (Abstract). Clin. Chem. 41:S60.

11. Gerhardt W, Katus HA, Ravkilde J, and Hamm CW (1992) S-troponin T as a marker of ischemic myocardial injury [Letter]. Clin. Chem. 38:1194–1195.

12. Antman E, Grudzien C, and Sacks D (1995) Evaluation of a rapid bedside assay for the detection of serum cardiac troponin T. JAMA 273:1279–1282.

13. Boehringer Mannheim Corporation (1997) CARDIAC T® ultra sensitive rapid assay. Package Insert.

14. Yasuda K, Ishiwata Y, and Ikeda R (1995) Determination of serum biotin levels by HPLC-ECD in patients with hemodialysis therapy [Abstract]. Clin. Chem. 41:S145.

15. Kricka LJ and the HAMA Survey Group (1992) Interlaboratory survey of methods for measuring human anti-mouse antibodies [Letter]. Clin. Chem. 38:172–173.

16. Bakker AJ, Koelemay MJW, Gorgels JPMC, van Vlies B, Smits R, Tijssen JG, and Haagen FD (1994) Troponin T and myoglobin at admission: value of early diagnosis of acute myocardial infarction. Eur. Heart. J. 15:45–53.

17. Wu AH (1994) Cardiac troponin T: biochemical, analytical, and clinical aspects. J. Clin. Immunoassay 17:45–48.

18. World Health Organization, Copenhagen, Regional Office for Europe. Ischemic heart disease registers: report of the fifth working group (1971) WHO Europe 8201(5):27–31.

19. Kruger D, Stierle U, Kerner W, Potratz J, Mitusch R, Schmucker G, Schwabe K, Taubert A, Sheikhzaden A, and Diederich KW (1994) No release of cardiac troponin-T after short-lasting severe myocardial ischemia [Abstract]. Eur. Heart J. 15:221.

20. Lavigne L, Waskiewicz S, Pervaiz G, Fagan G, and Whiteley G (1996) Investigation of serum troponin I heterogeneity and com-plexation to troponin T [Abstract]. Clin. Chem. 42:S312.

21. Feng YJ, Moore RE, and Wu AHB (1997) Identification and analysis of cardiac tro-ponin complexes in blood by gel filtration chromatography [Abstract]. Clin. Chem. 43: 5519.

22. Bakker AJ, Koelemay MJW, Gorgels JPMC, Van Vlies B, Smits RT, Tijssen JG, and Haagen FD (1993) Failure of new biochem-ical markers to exclude acute myocardial infarction at admission. Lancet 242: 1220–1222.

23. Gerhardt W, Katus H, Ravkilde J, Hamm C, Jorgensen PJ, Peheim E, Ljungdahl L, and Lofdahl P (1991) S-Troponin T in suspected ischemic myocardial injury compared with mass and catalytic concentrations of S-creatine kinase isoenzyme MB. Clin. Chem. 37:1405–1411.

24. Gerhardt W, Ljungdahl L, and Herbert AK (1993) Troponin-T and CK MB (mass) in early diagnosis of ischemic myocardial injury. The Helsingborg Study, 1992. Clin. Biochem. 26:231–240.

25. Burlina A, Zaninotto M, Secchiero S, Rubin D, and Accorsi F (1994) Troponin T as a marker of ischemic myocardial injury. Clin. Biochem. 27:113–121.

26. Adams JE III, Schechtman KB, Landt Y, Landenson JA, and Jaffe AS (1994) Com-parable detection of acute myocardial infarc-tion by creatine kinase MB isoenzyme and cardiac troponin I. Clin. Chem. 40:1291–1295.

27. Fitzgerald RL, Fraukel WL, and Herold DA (1996) Comparison of troponin I with other cardiac markers in a VA hospital. Am. J. Clin. Pathol. 106:396–401.

28. Wu AHB, Valdes R Jr, Apple FS, Gornet T, Stone MA, Mayfield-Stokes S, Ingersoll-Stroubos AM, and Wiler B (1994) Cardiac tro-ponin-T immunoassay for diagnosis of acute myocardial infarction and detection of minor myocardial injury. Clin. Chem. 40:900–907.

29. Mair J, Puschendorf B, and Michel G (1994) Clinical significance of cardiac contractile proteins for the diagnosis of myocardial injury. Adv. Clin. Chem. 31:63–98.

30. Bhayana V and Henderson R (1995) Bio-chemical markers of myocardial damage. Clin. Biochem. 28:1–29.

31. Baxter Diagnostics Inc. (1995) Stratus® cardiac troponin-I fluorometric immunoassay. Package Insert Rev7/95:7.

32. Antman EM, Tanasijevic MJ, Thompson B, Schactman M, McCabe CH, Cannon CP, Fischer G, and Braunwald E (1995) Cardiac troponin I on admission predicts death by 42 days in unstable angina and improved survival with an early invasive strategy: results from TIMII III B [abstract]. Circulation 92(suppl.): I–663.

33. Lindahl B, Venge P, and Wallentin L (1995) Early diagnosis and exclusion of acute myocardial infarction using biochemical monitoring. Coronary Artery Disease 6: 321–328.

34. de Winter RJ, Koster RW, Sturk A, and Sanders GT (1995) Value of myoglobin, troponin T, and CK-MB$_{mass}$ in ruling out an acute myocardial infarction in the emergency room. Circulation 92:3401–3407.

35. Ohman EM, Armstrong PW, Christenson RH, Granger CB, Katus HA, Hamm CW, O'Hanesian MA, Wagner GS, Kleiman NS, Harrell FE, Califf RM, and Topol EJ (1996) Risk stratification with admission cardiac troponin T levels in acute myocardial ischemia. N. Engl. J. Med. 335: 1333–1341.

36. Collinson PO, Moseley D, Stubbs PJ, and Carter GD (1993) Troponin T for the differential diagnosis of ischaemic myocardial injury. Ann. Clin. Biochem. 30:11–16.

37. Panteghini M and Pagani F (1994) Diagnostic value of a single measurement of troponin T in serum for suspected acute myocardial infarction [Letter]. Clin. Chem. 40:673,674.

38. Bhayana V, Cohoe S, Pellar TG, Jablonsky G, and Henderson AR (1994) Combination (multiple) testing for myocardial infarction using myoglobin, creatine kinase-2 (mass), and troponin T. Clin. Biochem. 27:395–406.

39. Rentrop KP (1995) Restoration of anterograde flow in acute myocardial infarction: the first 15 years. J. Am. Coll. Cardiol. 25:1S–2S.

40. Burns WB and Davidson CJ (1995) Thrombolysis or primary angioplasty? reviewing the evidence. Emerg. Med. 28:18–33.

41. Klootwijk P, Cobbaert C, Fioretti P, Kint PP, and Simoons ML (1993) Noninvasive assessment of reperfusion and reocclusion after thrombolysis in acute myocardial infarction. Am. J. Cardiol. 72:75G–84G.

42. Mair J, Wagner I, Jakob G, Lechleitner P, Dienstl F, Puschendorf B, and Michel G (1994) Different time courses of cardiac contractile proteins after acute myocardial infarction. Clin. Chim. Acta. 231:47–60.

43. Abe S, Arimaa S, Yamashita T, Miyata M, Okino H, Toda H, Nomoto K, Ueno M, Tahara M, Kigonaga K, Nakao S, and Tanaka H (1994) Early assessment of reperfusion therapy using cardiac troponin T. J. Am. Coll. Cardiol. 23:1382–1389.

44. Apple FS, Voss E, Lund L, Preese L, Berger CR, and Henry TD (1995) Cardiac troponin, CK-MB and myoglobin for the early detection of acute myocardial infarction and monitoring of reperfusion following thrombolytic therapy. Clin. Chim. Acta. 237: 59–66.

45. Sobel BE, Roberts R, and Larson KB (1976) Considerations in the use of biochemical markers of ischemic injury. Circ. Res. 38(Suppl. I):I99–I108.

46. Wagner I, Mair J, Fridrich L, Artner-Dworzak E, Lechleitner P, Morass B, Dienstl F, and Puschendorf B (1994) Cardiac troponin T release in acute myocardial infarction is associated with scintigraphic estimates of myocardial scar. Coronary Artery Disease 4:537–544.

47. Omura T, Teragaki M, Takagii M, Tani T, Nishida Y, Yamagishi H, Yanagi S, Nishikimi T, Yoshiyama M, Toda I, Akioka K, Takeuchi K, and Takeda T (1995) Myocardial infarct size by serum troponin T and myosin light chain 1. Jpn. Circ. J. 59:154–159.

48. Katus HA, Schoeppenthau M, Tanzeem A, Bauer HG, Saggau W, Diederich KW, Hagl S, and Kuebler W (1991) Non-invasive assessment of perioperative myocardial cell damage by circulating cardiac troponin T. Br. Heart J. 65:259–264.

49. Goldman L (1994) Assessment of perioperative cardiac risk. N. Engl. J. Med. 330: 707–708.

50. Yamamoto S, Takagi Y, Gomi K, and Takaba T (1995) Clinical significance of

early-stage breast cancer. J. Clin. Oncol. 13:2582–2584.

130. Hsai J (1994) Cardiovascular consequences of AIDS. In: Cardiology and co-existing disease, Rapaport E, ed., New York, Churchill Livingstone, pp. 349–370.

131. Maron BJ, Pelliccia A, and Spirito P (1995) Cardiac disease in young trained athletes: insights into methods for distinguishing athlete's heart from structural heart disease, with particular emphasis on hypertrophic cardiomyopathy. Circulation 91:1596–1601.

132. Mair J, Wohlfarter T, Koller A, Mayr M, Artner-Dworzak E, and Puschendorf B (1992) Serum cardiac troponin T after extraordinary endurance exercise [Letter]. Lancet 340:1048.

133. Collinson PO, Chandler HA, Stubbs PJ, et al. (1995) Measurement of serum troponin T, creatine kinase MB isoenzyme, and total creatine kinase following arduous physical training. Ann. Clin. Biochem. 32:450–453.

134. Berardi RS and Jetter WW (1987) Acute exertional rhabdomyolysis in a runner with elevated serum cardiac isoenzyme (CK-MB). Penn. Med. 90(4):44–48.

135. Siegel AJ, Sholar M, Yang J, et al. Elevated serum cardiac markers in asymptomatic marathon runners after competition: is the myocardium stunned? Cardiology, in press.

136. Curry SC, Chang D, and Connor D (1980) Drug- and toxin-induced rhabdomyolysis. Ann. Emerg. Med. 18:1068–1084.

137. Lofberg M, Tahtela R, Harkonen M, and Somer H (1995) Myosin heavy-chain fragments and cardiac troponins in the serum in rhabdomyolysis. Arch. Neurol. 52:1210–1214.

Cardiac Troponin I

Fred S. Apple

BIOCHEMISTRY

In striated muscle, the thin filament contains a protein complex containing three polypeptides: troponin C, I, and T, which are involved in calcium regulation. Troponin I (TnI) is the subunit of the troponin complex that inhibits actomyosin ATPase activity. Three isoforms of TnI have been described, a cardiac (cTnI)* and two skeletal muscle (slow twitch [sTnI] and fast twitch [fTnI]) *(1)*. Each of the three cTnI isoforms is encoded by three different genes located on different chromosomes *(2)*. The skeletal isoforms show approx 40% heterogeneity of primary sequence, but the cardiac isoform displays a similar degree of sequence heterogeneity compared to each skeletal isoform. Owing to the presence of an additional 31 amino acids at the N-terminal region, cTnI (24 kDa) is uniquely different than either fTnI or sTnI (19.8 kDa). During human development, both sTnI and cTnI are expressed in the myocardium. At birth, however, as shown in Fig. 1, only cTnI is expressed in the myocardium *(3)*. cTnI has been shown not to be expressed in any type of skeletal muscle, independent of developmental or disease stimuli. Therefore, knowledge that cTnI is 100% tissue-specific for the myocardium makes it an excellent candidate to serve as a biochemical marker for detecting of myocardial injury in serum.

Human cTnI DNA has been isolated, and the amino acid sequence of human cTnI has been confirmed. The gene has been assigned to chromosome 19p13.2–19q13.2 *(4)*. cTnI appears to have a uniform distribution throughout the atrial and ventricular chambers *(5)*. The general relationship between cardiac and skeletal muscle isoforms of TnI is common in several different species, including rabbit, cow, baboon, monkey, and humans *(6)*.

MEASUREMENT

Because only one cardiac isoform is present in the heart and because it contains a unique N-terminal amino acid sequence, the immunochemical reactivity of TnI is less complex than other contractile proteins. Both polyclonal antibodies and monoclonal antibodies (MAb) to human cTnI have been raised that show little to no crossreactivity to sTnI or other proteins.

The first reported immunoassay for human cTnI was reported in 1983 *(7)*. It used sheep and rabbit polyclonal antibodies directed against human or baboon cTnI, with

---

*See p. 240 for list of abbreviations used in this chapter.

From: Cardiac Markers *Edited by: Alan H. B. Wu*
© *Humana Press Inc., Totowa, NJ*

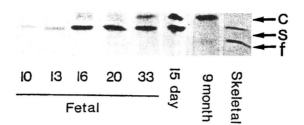

Fig. 1. Expression of TnI isoforms in developing human heart and skeletal muscle. Note transition from expression of sTnI to cTnI between 20 wk fetal development and 9 mo postnatal life (reprinted by permission from ref. *3*).

radioisotopic detection. The level of cross-reactivity against sTnI was minimal up to 1000 ng/mL. The sensitivity of this radioimmunoassay was improved in 1987, detecting down to 10 ng/mL, with <2% cross-reactivity with sTnI *(8)*. However, this assay was never commercialized. The lack of analytical sensitivity to be able to distinguish small changes within the normal reference limits or at critical medical decision limits led to the development and reporting of several specific, nonisotopic enzyme immunoassays using pairs of MAb directed against cTnI. This has allowed low-level detection of cTnI in the circulation that is highly specific for myocardial injury.

Several manufacturers have reported the development of immunoassays for the detection of cTnI, as shown in Table 1. The initial specific MAb-based assay was a double monoclonal "sandwich" enzyme immunoassay *(15)*. The cTnI-specific MAb used in this assay have now been incorporated in the worldwide (FDA-approved) commercially available Dade International (Deerfield, IL) Stratus fluorometric immunoassay. Further, Behring Diagnostics (Westwood, MA) and Beckman Instruments (formerly Sanofi Pasteur Diagnostics, Chaska, MN) have FDA-approved cTnI assays on the Opus Plus/Magnum, and Access systems, respectively. The Opus assay uses two goat anti-cTnI polyclonal antibodies. The Access assay was derived from a one-step immu-noenzymatic assay (IEMA) utilizing a pair of antihuman cTnI MAb *(16)*. A research (5-h) ELISA on a microliter plate utilizing monoclonal anti-cTnI antibodies supplied by Spectral Diagnostics has recently been described *(16)*. Abbott Laboratories (Abbott Park, IL) *(12)*, Bayer Diagnostics (Tarrytown, NY) *(14)*, and Chiron Diagnostics have also described immunoassay systems that are FDA approved. Further, several rapid whole blood devices have been described and or shown by manufacturers for potential bed-side testing (point of care) for cTnI. These systems also include the diversity of multiple analyte measurements in addition to cTnI; First Medical System, FDA approved (Mountain View CA; total CK, myoglobin, CK-MB mass); Biosite Diagnostics, FDA approved (San Diego CA, myoglobin, CK-MB mass); Dade (Deerfield, IL, myoglobin, CK-MB mass) not FDA approved. Further, a rapid, one-step qualitative immunoassay system (positive, negative based on specific cutoffs) was recently FDA approved (Cardiac STATus, Spectral Diagnostics (Toronto, Canada).

Normal ranges, detection limits, and medical decision cutoffs vary between assay systems owing to the lack of standardization and differences in antibody recognition of different cTnI subunit complexes *(17)* for cTnI. Therefore, when comparing published clinical studies, absolute comparisons of cTnI concentrations are difficult. However,

Table 1
Commercial Immunoassays for cTnI Mass Determination
That Utilize Specific anti-TnI-Antibodies

Supplier	Detection	Initial anchor	Ab tag	Detection limit	Reference range	Assay time
Dade-Stratus (9)	Fluorescence	Monoclonal-anti-cTnI glass fiber paper	Monoclonal anti-cTnI-ALP	0.35 ng/mL	≤0.6	10 min
Behring Opus (10)	Fluorescence	Polyclonal-anti-cTnI-	Polyclonal anti-cTnI-ALP	0.50 ng/mL	≤1.9	20 min
Beckman-Access (11)	Chemiluminescence	Monoclonal-anti-cTnI	Monoclonal-anti-cTnI-ALP	0.03 ng/mL	≤0.1	15 min
Abbott-Axsym (12)	Fluorescence	Monoclonal-anti-cTnI-microparticle	Polyclonal-anti-biotin-ALP	0.75 ng/mL	≤2.1 ≤0.8	13 min
Spectral Diagnostics (13)	Colorimetric	Monoclonal-anti-cTnI-qualitative	Polyclonal-anti-cTnI	0.2 ng/mL	—	15 min
Bayer Immuno (14)	Fluorescence	Monoclonal-anti-cTnI-magnetic particles	Polyclonal-anti-cTnI-ALP	0.1 ng/mL	≤0.1	23 min

relative changes for cTnI based on upper reference limits in the numerous clinical studies should allow for comparability of findings for different assay systems used for the measurement of cTnI (*see* Table 1).

CLINICAL UTILITY

Over 20 studies that have utilized several different cTnI immunoassays will be discussed in this section. Since no primary standard is used by the different assay systems, the reader must be aware that absolute concentrations used for medical decision and reference ranges will vary considerably (*see* Table 1). However, comparisons can be made between studies using the different assay systems regarding relative changes related to normal reference limits. This section will discuss studies that have measured cTnI for the detection of AMI, monitoring reperfusion after thrombolytic therapy in AMI, detection of myocardial injury in renal disease, and studies involving skeletal muscle injury with possible concomitant

AMI. Since cTnI is 100% cardiac-specific *(16)*, the studies reviewed in this section will show how cTnI can be used to distinguish elevations of serum CK-MB caused by skeletal muscle injury from those caused by acute myocardial infarction (AMI).

Acute Myocardial Infarction

cTnI has been shown to be a very sensitive and specific marker for AMI *(10,15, 17–20)*. The early release kinetics for cTnI are similar to creatine kinase (CK)-MB, in that it takes 4–8 h to increase above the upper reference limit (Fig. 2). Thus, cTnI does not provide an earlier detection for AMI than CK-MB *(9,21,22)*. The initial cTnI rise is from release of 3–6% cytoplasmic fraction of troponin in the cell following ischemic injury *(18)*. cTnI peaks between 14 and 36 h after onset of AMI and remains elevated 3–7 d after AMI. The mechanism for the lengthy time for elevations of cTnI is most likely owing to the ongoing release of troponin from the 94–97% myofibril-bound fraction *(18)*. This can be

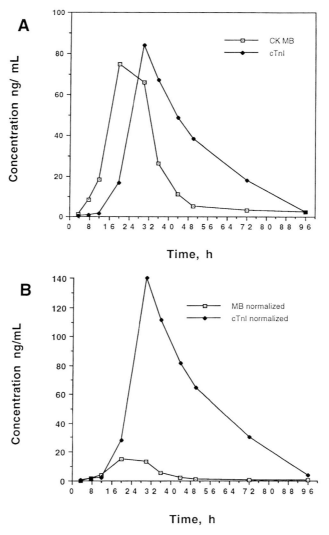

Fig. 2. Serial serum CK-MB and cTnI concentration profiles following AMI **(A)** Cardiac markers are plotted as a function of the upper reference limits = 1 **(B)** Time is from the onset of chest pain.

considered the biological half-life. The ongoing release and clearance thus give the impression that cTnI has a long half-life. However, the true half-life of cTnI is <2 h. Owing to the lengthy time of increase of cTnI following onset of chest pain, it should clinically replace lactate dehydrogenase (LD) isoenzymes in detection of late-presenting AMI patients. Recent studies have demonstrated (Fig. 3) that regardless of whether AMI patients received thrombolytic therapy or not, cTnI was more

sensitive than the LD1/LD2 ratio (cutoffs of either 1.0 or 0.8) for detection of myocardial infarction (MI) up to 7 d after admission *(23,24)*. The very low to undetectable cTnI values in serum from noncardiac-diseased and normal patients, permit the use of very low discrimination values compared to higher values of CK-MB for the determination of myocardial injury. This is because of ongoing release of the low percentage of CK-MB found in skeletal muscle *(25,26)*.

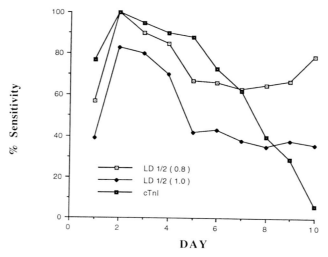

Fig. 3. Comparison of the LD isoenzyme LD1/LD2 ratios vs cTnI following AMI (adapted from ref. *24*).

Several studies have shown that cTnI is comparable to CK-MB for the sensitive detection of AMI during the initial 48 h after AMI. However, diagnostic sensitivities are insufficient for effective, very early diagnosis of AMI 0–4 h post onset of chest pain. Because of the slow release kinetics of cTnI, it takes hours before it increases above the upper reference. It has been hypothesized that the early release of cTnI (<30 kDa) compares to CK-MB (80 kDa), because cTnI is released as the three-subunit I, T, and C complex (80 kDa). The early findings of three different studies that examined large numbers of patients presenting to the hospital to rule in or rule out AMI in chest pain patients were not prospectively performed *(11,15,18)*. The studies all addressed patients either admitted to a coronary care unit (CCU) with MI or with a high probability of MI. As expected, cTnI sensitivity remains >90%, a much longer time compared to CK-MB, owing to the extended appearance rate of cTnI.

Several studies have also demonstrated excellent and improved specificity (> 90%) for cTnI vs CK-MB during the entire post-AMI time period *(9,21)*. As shown in Fig. 4, the overall sensitivity and specificity of AMI

detection are dependent on medical decision cutoff values used for cTnI and the times studied following presentation to ED after onset of chest pain studied *(21)*.

Reperfusion Assessment

Three studies have examined the early and rapid release kinetics of cTnI following successful reperfusion after initiation of thrombolytic therapy in AMI patients *(28–30)*. Since there are many positive benefits of thrombolytic therapy conferred by reperfusion of infarct-related arteries, the use of rapid analytical determinations for early cTnI measurements would serve as an excellent noninvasive assessment. In successfully reperfused AMI patients, cTnI significantly increased 30, 60, and 90 min after thrombolytic therapy compared to baseline and showed significant increases compared to nonreperfused patients at all times (Fig. 5). By utilizing a calculated relative ratio index of reperfusion at 90 min after thrombolytic therapy (cTnI at 90 min divided by cTnI at 0 min baseline), preliminary findings showed a >80% sensitivity for detection of reperfusion *(30)*. Thus, measurement of cTnI may be more sensitive than

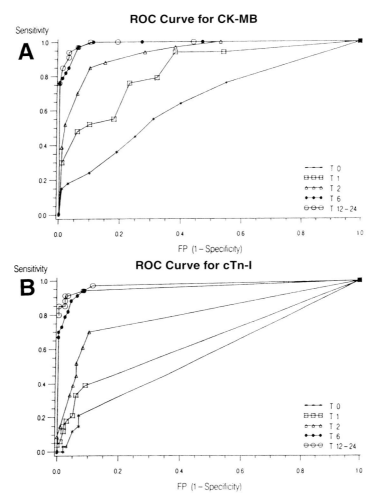

Fig. 4. ROC curves to establish the best discriminator limits for AMI for CK-MB (**A**) and cTnI (**B**) following time (T, h) after presentation to emergency department. Each curve represents a different time period for 35 AMI patients (adapted from ref. *21*).

CK-MB and myoglobin for early detection of reperfusion. Larger population studies will be necessary to confirm these findings before clinical use will be implemented.

Surgery

Several studies have used cTnI measurements following surgical procedures to detect myocardial injury. In 22 patients with angina who underwent uneventful percutaneous transluminal coronary angioplasty (PTCA), no increases in cTnI were found

7–13 h after *(31)*. This supports the view that no substantial myocardial injury occurred in successful PTCA. In 28 patients undergoing coronary artery bypass grafting (CABG), owing to surgical cutting of the myocardium, all patients showed elevation of cTnI *(32)*. However, in four patients with electrocardiogram- (ECG)–documented perioperative AMI, cTnI concentrations were significantly greater at peak, 12, or 24 h. In a study involving patients receiving aortic valve replacements, a positive correlation was found

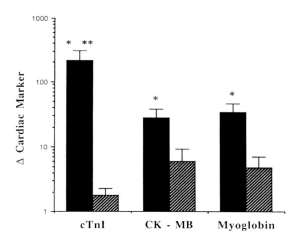

Fig. 5. Relative ratio index increases (plotted on a log scale) for cTnI (ΔcTnI), CK-MB (ΔCK-MB), and myoglobin (Δmyoglobin) 90 min after the initiation of thrombolytic therapy. Group 1 = reperfused patients, solid bars; group 2 = nonreperfused patients, hatched bars. *Significantly ($p < 0.05$) greater than CK-MB and myoglobin within group 1. Error bars represent standard error (reprinted by permission from ref. *30*).

between aortic crossclamping time and cTnI in serum *(33)*. In another study involving 108 patients undergoing noncardiac-related vascular surgery, eight patients experienced new abnormalities in the echocardiogram, which was used to diagnose perioperative MI *(34)*. All eight had increased cTnI (Fig. 6). Of the other 100 without perioperative infarction, 19 had false-positive elevations of CK-MB. In each of these surgical studies, cTnI was found to be a specific and reliable marker of cardiac ischemia during heart and noncardiac surgeries. In contrast, cTnI, cTnT, and CK-MB do not appear to be useful in monitoring cardiac transplant patients for acute rejection, since one study showed no difference in protein levels with grades 2 and 3 rejection vs those with grades 0 and 1 *(35)*.

Occult Myocardial Injury

Numerous studies have determined the incidence of increased cTnI for detection of cardiac injury in several patient groups that have often shown falsely increased CK-MB concentrations. These have included patients with chest trauma, with cocaine-associated

chest pain, in the critically ill intensive care patients, and hypothyroid patients. Patients with cocaine-induced chest pain frequently have abnormal ECG tracings and increases in total CK and CK-MB. In a study of emergency department patients with confirmed cocaine use, results of ECG, CK, and CK-MB (mass assay) were abnormal on 84%, 74%, and 16%, respectively, whereas cTnI (Stratus) and cTnT were normal on all subjects (Fig. 7) *(36)*. In patients with blunt chest trauma, 26 of 37 patients had falsely elevated CK-MB concentrations. cTnI was positive in six of six patients with blunt chest trauma and was falsely positive in only one case (Fig. 8) *(37)*. Among critically ill patients, cTnI was accurate in determining the high incidence (32 of 209 patients) with cardiac injury (a frequently unrecognized [20 of 32 patients] complication) (Fig. 9) *(38)*. Mortality in patients with myocardial injury that was recognized (42%) or unrecognized (40%) was higher than in those without myocardial injury and normal cTnI concentrations (15%). In patients with hypothyroidism, high CK and CK-MB are

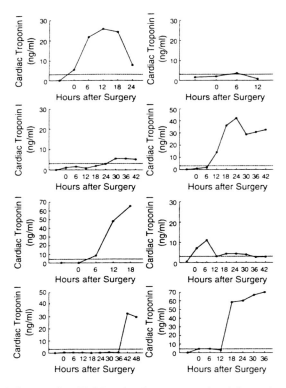

Fig. 6. Time-course of changes in cTnI levels after surgery in eight patients with AMI. Initial elevations were present in six patients on day 1 and in two patients on day 2. The broken lines denote the upper limit of normal values. Preoperative values are indicated by the first symbol in each curve (reprinted by permission from ref. *34*).

frequently observed, because there is reduced clearance of the enzyme *(39)*. Coronary artery disease is a frequent complication of hypothyoridism owing to hypetension and hypercholesterolemia *(40)*. In a study of 52 hypothyroid patients, CK and CK-MB were increased in 64 and 13%, whereas cTnI (Stratus) was normal in all subjects *(41)*. These results suggest that CK and CK-MB are nonspecific when compared to cTnI.

Skeletal Muscle Injury

Several studies involving skeletal muscle injury have examined the use of cTnI to facilitate distinguishing whether increases of CK-MB are owing to myocardial or skeletal muscle injury. In marathoners, all pos-

trace cTnI concentrations were normal, compared to >80% with CK-MB increases *(42,43)*. In acute or chronic skeletal muscle injury or disease patients, the only increases in cTnI were found in ECG and echocardiogram-documented MIs (Fig. 10) *(43)*.

Renal Disease

Demonstration of the cardio-specificity of cTnI for detection of myocardial injury in renal disease patients was first addressed in 1993 *(43)*. Evaluation of 159 patients with chronic renal failure demonstrated a 3.8% false-positive rate for CK-MB mass, with the one patient demonstrating an increased cTnI having an AMI. Since then, several letters to the editor, case papers, and abstracts have evaluated the clinical significance of

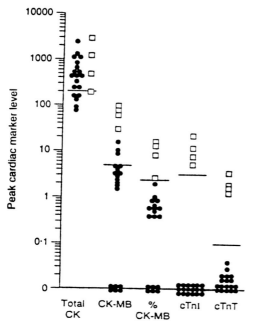

Fig. 7. Graph of peak serum values for total CK activity, CK-MB isoenzyme (CK-MB) concentration, %CK-MB, cTnI concentration, and cTnT concentration in patients admitted with cocaine-induced chest pain (●) and in patients with documented myocardial infarction (□). Horizontal lines indicate the upper reference limit of the respective assay; total CK (200 U/L). CK-MB (5.0 ng/mL), % CK-MB (2-5%), cTnI (3.1 ng/mL), and cTnT (0.1 ng/mL) (reprinted by permission from ref. *36*).

cTnI, cTnT, and CK-MB measurements in patients with renal failure *(44–50)*. A summation of these studies showed that in over 400 chronic renal disease patients evaluated, falsely elevated (no direct evidence of myocardial injury) cardiac marker concentrations were found as follows: first generation cTnT assay in 47% of cases; CK-MB in 10.3% of cases; cTnI in 2.6% of cases *(50)*. However, in two recent studies that compared cTnI with the improved second generation cTnT assay, more comparable false positive findings are reported; 5% cTnI vs 10–15% cTnT. The value of cTnI is further suggested in a study of patients undergoing renal transplantation, where there were no cases of cTnI (Opus) increased either before or after the transplant *(51)*.

The underlying mechanisms for the large number of nonspecific elevations of cTnT and CK-MB in renal disease as well as in the other pathology entities noted above are unclear. Several potential mechanisms can be postulated. First, both CK-MB and cTnT have been shown to be re-expressed in regenerating human and animal skeletal muscle *(50,52,53)*. Thus, expression of cTnT and CK-MB may occur in the skeletal muscle myopathy associated with chronic renal disease *(54)*. Second, an increase in cTnT may be owing to low-level immunoassay cross-reactivity errors from sTnT *(46)*. However this is eliminated using the second generation cTnT-assay. Third, the possibility of minor myocardial injury undetected clinically may be responsible for true-positive increased cTnT or cTnI values. However, for cTnI, its tissue specificity for the heart is unchallenged, with no expression of cTnI in myopathic skeletal muscle from patients diagnosed with muscular dystrophy, polymyositis, and chronic renal disease *(50)*. Finally, it is possible that cTnI is falsely low because of the presence of autoantibodies *(55)*. This rare occurrence is a highly unlikely explanation for the hundreds of samples from patients with dialysis that have been tested for undetectable cTnI.

Unstable Angina

Reports have now described that analysis of cTnI has prognostic value in non-AMI (unstable angina) patients with cardiac disease. Determination of elevated serum cTnI levels at presentation in patients (*n* = 1402) with unstable angina predicted a significantly increased mortality at 42 d and identified improved survival occurred in patients treated with early invasive versus conservative strategy *(56)*. In samples collected from unstable patients (*n* = 106) admitted to a

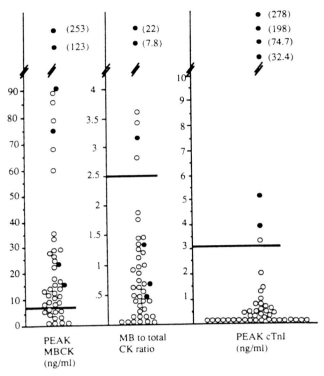

Fig. 8. Peak CK-MB, peak CK-MB to total CK ratio, and peak cTnI values found in patients with blunt chest trauma. Open circles indicate patients without cardiac contusion; solid circles indicate those with contusion. Heavy horizontal lines indicate upper reference limits for each parameter (reprinted by permission from ref. *37*).

CCU over a 3 d period, the presence of minor degrees of myocardial damage was identified by increased cTnI values (*57*). Using as a primary endpoint death or non-fatal AMI at 30 d, increased cTnI concentrations were a significant predicator of adverse short and long term prognosis. CTnI measurements were used for risk stratification in 74 consecutively admitted non-AMI patients with chest pain. Odds ratios showed that poor outcomes were significantly more frequent in the high cTnI group than in the low cTnI group, a significant improvement over CK-MB (*58*). There has only been one study on 33 patients with unstable angina that suggested no value for cTnI (Access) and risk stratification (*59*). Direct comparison studies of cTnI and cTnT in the same patient populations showed no differences in the

prognostic value of these two markers (*50,60,61*). These direct comparisons of cTnI and cTnT in similar patient groups with unstable angina, have preliminary demonstrated similar prognostic value of these two markers with both demonstrating and adverse 30 d prognosis in patients with an increased concentrate. Overall, 20–40% of unstable angina patients have an increased cardiac troponin with a 4–12% incidence of death or nonfatal AMI 30 to 40 deep following presentation.

In summary, these studies show that cTnI is a more tissue-specific marker than CK-MB and cTnT for the detection of myocardial injury, including myocardial infarction. When cTnI is increased, one should "think heart." Increased cTnI levels in patients with little clinical evidence sug-

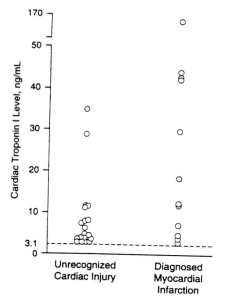

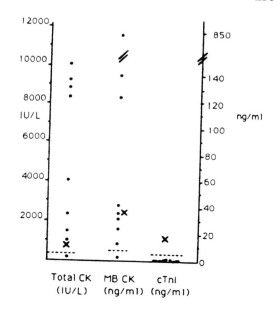

Fig. 9. Peak levels of cTnI in patients with diagnosed myocardial infarction and patients with unrecognized cardiac injury. The mean (SD) level for patients with diagnosed myocardial infarction (32.5 [SD 42.8] ng/mL) was significantly ($p = .009$) different from the levels for patients with unrecognized cardiac injury (8.5 [SD 8.6] ng/mL) (reprinted by permission from ref. *38*).

Fig. 10. Graph of values of total CK, CK-MB, and cTnI in patients with chronic muscle disease ($n = 10$). Values for patients with AMI are indicated by an "X." Dotted lines indicate the upper reference limit of the respective assay; cTnI (3.1 ng/mL), CK-MB (6.7 ng/mL), and total CK (170 U/L) (reprinted by permission from ref. *43*.

gesting myocardial injury should alert the clinician to consider occult cardiac injury or disease, placing patients into a high risk group.

IMPLEMENTATION INTO THE CLINICAL LABORATORY

Because nearly 50% of patients with AMI initially present to emergency departments with nondiagnostic ECGs, serial samples for CK-MB (and total CK) have been the gold standard of testing for the diagnosis of AMI *(62)*. If AMI is suspected, serial measurements made approximately at admission and 3, 6, 9, and 12 h after admission will provide the greatest sensitivity and specificity *(63)*. Single measurements should not be relied on for initial triaging because of the poten-

tial of false-negative results owing to the lag time for rising CK-MB concentrations following the onset of chest pain post-AMI *(63)*. Regarding the implementation of cTnI into the clinical laboratory, a serial ordering pattern similar to CK-MB would be most appropriate for optimal diagnostic accuracy (Table 2). Implementation of cTnI would provide a substantial financial saving to institutions willing to be on the cutting edge. For example, a single cTnI determination would replace CK-MB, total CK, total LD, and LD isoenzyme measurements without sacrificing clinical sensitivity and specificity. CK-MB determinations may only be necessary if and when the clinician observed the cTnI levels to be on the downward slope of the AMI curve and might need to determine whether the CK-MB would distinguish

Table 2
Recommending Test Ordering
Guidelines: Implementation of cTnI

Detection of myocardial infarction
  Common protocol with CK-MB *(63)*
  Proposed using cTnI
    cTnI at admission, and 3, 6, and 9 h after
    admission.
      Total CK, CK-MB mass, % RI: at
      admission, and 3, 6, 9, and 12, h after
      admission.
Detection of reperfusion following
thrombolytic therapy
  Proposed
    cTnI at admission, at time of therapy, and
    60, or 90 min after therapy.
Detection of minor myocardial injury in
unstable angina
  cTnI at admission and 12 h after admission

an early (0–3 d) vs late (>3 d) presenting patient. Total CK would no longer be needed for CK-MB percent calculations. Total LD and LD isoenzymes would not be needed to determine late AMI presentations. Regarding the use of cTnI to attempt to determine the success of reperfusion, levels should be measured at admission, at the time of thrombolytic therapy initiation, and at 60, or 90 min after therapy in an attempt to document the early, rapid rise associated with successful reperfusion (Table 2). Finally, preliminary findings are compelling for the use of cTnI measurement in non-AMI, unstable angina patients for both in-hospital and post-hospitalization risk stratification.

ABBREVIATIONS

AB, Antibody; ALP, alkaline phosphatase; AMI, acute myocardial infarction; CCU, coronary care unit; cTnI, T, cardiac troponins I and T; ECG, electrocardiogram; FDA, Food and Drug Administration; fTnI, fast twitch troponin I; HRP, horse radish peroxidase; kDa, kilodaltons; LD, lactate

dehydrogenase; PTCA, percutaneous transluminal coronary angioplasty; sTnI, skeletal muscle troponin I.

REFERENCES

1. Ebashi S, Wakabayashi T, and Ebashi F (1971) Troponin and its components. Biochem. J. 69:441.
2. Larue C, Defacque-Lacquement H, Calzolari C, Le Nguyen D, and Pau B (1992) New monoclonal antibodies as probes for human cardiac troponin I: epitopic analysis with synthetic-peptides. Mol. Immunol. 29:271.
3. Barton PJR, Bhausar PK, Brand NJ, Chan-Thomas PS, Dabhade N, Farza H, Townsend PJ, and Yacoub MH (1992) Gene expression during cardiac development. Symp. Soc. Exp. Biol. 46:251–264.
4. McGesch C, Barton PJR, and Vallins WJ (1991) The human cardiac troponin I locus: assignment to chromosome 19p13.2–19q13.2. Hum. Genet. 88:101–104.
5. Bhavsar PK, Dhoot GK, Cummings DVE, Butler-Brown GS, Yacoub MH, and Barton PJR (1991) Developmental expression of troponin I isoforms in fetal human heart. FEBS 292:5–8.
6. Larue C (1996) Myocardial proteins, in "Muscle proteins" in Structure of Antigens, Van Regenmortel, MHV, ed., New York, CRC, pp. 183–219.
7. Cummins P and Auckland ML (1983) Cardiac specific radioimmunoassay of troponin I in the diagnosis of acute myocardial infarction. Clin. Sci. 64:42–44.
8. Cummins B, Auckland ML, and Cummins P (1987) Cardiac specific troponin I radioimmunoassay in the diagnosis of acute myocardial infarction. Am. Heart J. 113:1333–1344.
9. Brogan GX, Hollander JE, McCuskey CF, Thode HC, Snow J, Sama A, et al. (1997) Evaluation of a new assay for cardiac troponin I vs creatin kinase MB for the diagnosis of acute myocardial infarction. Acad. Emerg. Med. 4:6–12.
10. Wu AHB, Feng YJ, Contois JH, and Pervaiz S (1996) Comparison of myoglobin, creatine kinase-MB and cardiac troponin I for diagnosis of acute myocardial infarction. Ann. Clin. Lab. Sci. 26:291–300.

11. Larue C, Calzolari C, Bertinchant JP, Leciercq F, Gralleau R, and Pau B (1993) Cardiac specific immunoenzymometric assay of troponin I in the early phase of acute myocardial infarction. Clin. Chem. 39:972–979.

12. Laird DM, Biegalski T, Forsythe C, Gall G, Hansen H, Keller A, and Wilson DH (1997) An automated assay for cardiac troponin I on the Abbott AxSYM analyzer [Abstract]. Clin. Chem. 43:S161.

13. Panteghini M and Bonora R (1997) A rapid bedside immunochromatographic assay for cardiac troponin I evaluated [Abstract]. Clin. Chem. 43:S5157.

14. Doth M, Payne RC, and Morris DL (1997) Development of a quantitative assay for troponin I on the Technicon Immuno I System [Abstract]. Clin. Chem. 43:S158.

15. Bodor GS, Porter S, Landt Y, and Ladenson JH (1992) Development of monoclonal antibodies for the assay of cardiac troponin I and preliminary results in suspected cases of myocardial infarction. Clin. Chem. 38: 2203–2214.

16. Bhayana V, Gougoulias T, Cohoe S, and Henderson AR (1995) Discordance between results for serum troponin T and troponin I in renal disease. Clin. Chem. 41:312–317.

17. Katrukha AG, Bereznikova AV, Esakova KP, Lougren T, Severina MD, Pulkki K, Vuopio-Pulkki, LM and Gusev NB (1997) Troponin I is released in blood stream of patients with acute myocardial infarction not in free form but as complex. Clin. Chem. 43:1379–1385.

18. Adams JE, Schectman KB, Landt Y, Ladenson JH, and Jaffe AS (1994) Comparable detection of acute myocardial infarction by creatine kinase MB isoenzyme and cardiac troponin I. Clin. Chem. 40:1291–1295.

19. Zaninotto M, Altinier S, Lachin M, Carraro P, and Plebani M (1996) Fluoroenzymometric method to measure cardiac troponin I in sera of patients with myocardial infarction. Clin. Chem. 42:1460–1466.

20. Behring Opus manufacturer's package insert for cardiac troponin I immunoassay.

20. Maij J, Genser N, Morandell D, Maier J, Mair P, Lechleitner P, Calzolari C, Larue C, Ambach E, Dienstl F, Pau B, and Puschendorg B (1996) Cardiac troponin I in the diagnosis of myocardial injury and infarction. Clin. Chim. Acta 245:19–38.

21. Tucker JF, Collins RA, Anderson AJ, Hauser J, Kalas J, and Apple FS (1997) Early diagnostic efficiency of cardiac troponin I and cardiac troponin T for acute myocardial infarction. Acad. Emerg. Med. 4:13–21.

22. Bertinchant JP, Larue C, Pernel I, Ledermann B, Fabbro-Peray P, Beck L, Calzolari C, Trinquier S, Nigond J, and Pau B (1996) Release kinetics of serum cardiac troponin I in ischemic myocardial injury. Clin. Biochem. 29:587–594.

23. Jaffe AS, Landt Y, Parvin CA, Abendschein DR, Geltman EM, and Ladenson JH (1996) Comparative sensitivity of cardiac troponin I and lactate dehydrogenase isoenzymes for diagnosis of acute myocardial infarction. Clin. Chem. 42:1770–1776.

24. Martins JT, Li DJ, Baskin LB, Jialal I, and Keffer JH (1996) Comparison of cardiac troponin I and lactate dehydrogenase isoenzymes for the late diagnosis of myocardial injury. Am. J. Clin. Pathol. 106: 705–708.

25. Apple FS, Rogers MA, Sherman WM, Casal DC, and Ivy JL (1985) Creatinine Kinase MB isoenzyme adaptation in stressed human skeletal muscle. J. Appl. Physiol. 59:149–153.

26. Adams J, Abendschein DR, and Jaffe AS (1983) Biochemical markers of myocardial injury: is creatinine kinase the choice for the 1990? Circulation 88:750.

27. Collins R, Tucker J, and Apple FS (1995) Early cardiac injury markers in chest pain patients admitted to the emergency department [Abstract]. Clin. Chem. 41:5234.

28. Tanasijeric MJ, Cannon CP, Wybenga DR, Fischer GA, Grudzien C, Gibson CM, et al. (1997) Myoglobin, creative kinase MB, and cardiac troponin-I to assess reperfusion after thrombolysis for acute myocardial infarction; results from TIMI 10A. Am. Heart J. 134:622–630.

29. Apple FS, Sharkey SW, and Henry TD (1995) Early serum cardiac troponin I and T concentrations after successful thrombolysis for acute myocardial infarction. Clin. Chem. 41:1197–1198.

30. Apple FS, Henry TD, Berger CR, and Landt YA (1996) Early monitoring of serum cardiac troponin I for assessment of coronary reperfusion following thrombolytic therapy. Am. J. Clin. Pathol. 105:6–10.

31. Hunt AC, Chow SL, Chilton DC, Cummins B, and Cummins P (1991) Release of creatine kinase MB and cardiac specific troponin I following percutaneous transluminal coronary angioplasty. Eur. Heart J. 12:600–604.

32. Mair J, Larue C, Mair P, Balogh D, Calzolari C, and Puschendorf B (1994) Use of cardiac troponin I to diagnose perioperative myocardial infarction in coronary artery bypass grafting. Clin. Chem. 40:2066–2070.

33. Etievent JP, Chocron S, Toubin G, Taberlet C, Alwan K, Clement F, Cordier A, Schipman N, and Kantelip JP (1995) Use of cardiac troponin I as a marker of perioperative myocardial ischemia. Ann. Thorac. Surg. 59:1192–1194.

34. Adams JE, Sicard GA, Allen BT, Bridwell KH, Lenke LG, Davila-Roman VG, Bodor GS, Ladenson JH, and Jaffe AS (1994) Diagnosis of perioperative myocardial infarction with measurement of cardiac troponin I. N. Engl. J. Med. 330:670–674.

35. Hossein-Nia M, Holt DW, Anderson JR, and Murday AJ (1996) Cardiac troponin I release in heart transplantation. Ann. Thorac. Surg. 61:275–280.

36. McLaurin M, Apple FS, Henry TD, and Sharkey SW (1996) Cardiac troponin I and T concentrations in patients with cocaine associated chest pain. Ann. Clin. Biochem. 33:1–4.

37. Adams JE, Davila-Roman VG, Bessey PQ, Blake DP, Ladenson JH, and Jaffe AS (1996) Improved detection of cardiac contusion with cardiac troponin I. Am. Heart J. 131:308–312.

38. Guest TM, Ramanthan AV, Tuteur PG, Schechtman KB, Ladenson JH, and Jaffe AS (1995) Myocardial injury in critically ill patients: a frequently unrecognized complication. JAMA 273:1945–1949.

39. Chan KM, Ladenson JH, Pierce GF, and Jaffe AS (1986) Increased creatine kinase MB in the absence of acute myocardial infarction. Clin. Chem. 32:2044–2051.

40. Steinberg AD (1968) Myxedema and coronary artery disease-a comparative autopsy study. Ann. Intern. Med. 68:338–344.

41. Cohen LF, Mohabeer AJ, Keffer JH, and Jialal I (1996) Troponin I in hypothyroidism. Clin. Chem. 42:1494.

42. Mair J, Wohlfarter T, Koler A, Mayr M, Artner-Dworzak E, and Puschendorf B (1992) Serum cardiac troponin T after extraordinary endurance execise. Lancet 340:1048.

43. Adams JE, Bodor GS, Davila-Roman VG, Delinez JA, Apple FS, Ladenson JM, and Jaffe AS (1993) Cardiac troponin I: a marker with high specificity for cardiac injury. Circulation 88:101.

44. McLaurin MD, Apple FS, Herzog CA, and Sharkey SW (1995) Cardiac troponin I, T, and CK-MB in chronic hemodialysis patients. Circulation 92(Suppl.):I80.

45. Katus HA, Haller C, Muller-Bardorff M, Scheffold T, and Remppis A (1994) Cardiac troponin T in end-stage renal disease patients undergoing chronic maintenance hemodialysis. Clin. Chem. 41:1201–1202.

46. Collinson PO, Stubbs PJ, and Rosalki SB (1995) Cardiac troponin T in renal disease. Clin. Chem. 41:1671–1673.

47. Trinquier S, Flecheux O, Bullenger M, and Castex F (1995) Highly specific immunoassay for cardiac troponin I assessed in non-infarct patients with chronic renal failure or severe polytrauma. Clin. Chem. 41: 1675–1676.

48. Li D, Jialal I, and Keffer J (1996) Greater frequency of increased cardiac troponin T than increased cardiac troponin I in patients with chronic renal failure. Clin. Chem. 42:114–115.

49. Li D, Keffer J, Corry K, Vazquez M, and Jialal I (1995) Nonspecific elevation of troponin T levels in patients with chronic renal failure. Clin. Biochem. 28:474–477.

50. McLaurin MD, Apple FS, Voss EM, Herzog CA, and Sharkey SW (1997) Serum cardiac troponin I, cardiac troponin T, and CK MB in dialysis patients without ischemic heart disease: evidence of cardiac troponin T expression in skeletal muscle. Clin. Chem. 43:976–982.

51. Wu AHB, Feng YJ, Roper E, Herbert C, and Schweizer R (1997) Cardiac troponins T and I before and after renal transplantation. Clin. Chem. 43:411,412.

52. Bodor GZ, Porterfield D, Voss E, Kelly J, Smith S, and Apple FS (1995) Cardiac troponin-T composition in normal and regenerating human skeletal muscle. Clin. Chem. 41:148.

53. Sagin L, Gorza L, Ausoni S, and Schiaffino S (1990) Cardiac troponin T in developing,

Table 1
Proposed Methods for Determination of Cardiac MHCs in Human Serum[a]

Source	Principle	Detection limit	Between-run precision (CV)	Remarks
Leger et al. *(15)*	RIA (MAb anti-β-MHC)	15 μg/L	<20.0%	Crossreaction with skeletal HC
Larue et al. *(16)*	IRMA (MAbs anti-β-MHC)	10 μU/L	<8.8%	Crossreaction with skeletal HC
Simeonova et al. *(17)*	ELISA (MAb anti-MHC subfragment 1)	Not reported	Not reported	Crossreaction with skeletal HC
Cardone et al. *(18)*	ELISA (solid-phase MAb antiventricular MHC plus conjugate polyclonal chicken anti-MHC IgY)	10 μg/L	Not reported	Crossreaction with skeletal HC

[a]CV, coefficient of variation; RIA, radioimmunoassay; HC, heavy chain; IRMA, immunoradiometric assay; and ELISA, enzyme-linked immunosorbent assay.

dissociated under certain pH or temperature conditions or in the presence of appropriate chemicals, like 5-5′-dithiobis-(2-nitrobenzoic acid) or edetic acid *(13)*. Lowering the pH of purified myosin preparations to levels simulating the acidosis seen during cell necrosis causes the release of light chains into the supernatant *(14)*. In particular, the maximum dissociation of light chains from heavy chains occurred at pH 6.0 near the pH of severely ischemic cells, which probably represents irreversible cellular damage.

ASSAYS

All assays for cardiac MHCs described in the literature so far show significant cross-reactivity with MHCs from skeletal muscle (Table 1) *(15–18)*. Indeed, the coexpression of cardiac β-MHC isoforms in slow skeletal muscle make it very difficult to develop cardiac specific assays. A competition radioimmunoassay was used first to describe MHC release into serum after acute myocardial infarction (AMI) *(15)*. The fact that three out of seven specific MAb produced by these authors did not detect any myosin in sera of AMI patients was presumably owing to the absence of the corresponding myosin fragments in the serum, and suggested for the first time that only MHC fragments and not the whole molecule are in fact circulating after AMI. An immunoradiometric assay using the same MAb has been described *(16)*, which became the basis for a diagnostic "kit" technique. Because the exact molecular mass of the circulating MHC fragments is not known, MHC concentrations were expressed in μU/L instead of ng/mL (μg/L) *(16)*.

Table 2 shows the values of "cardiac" MHCs in sera from apparently healthy subjects calculated by different authors *(15,18–20)*. Reference values were assay-dependent, and the healthy populations used were small and rather poorly defined. The relatively high MHC concentrations observed in the active subjects were possibly connected to the release of MHC fragments from slow skeletal muscle into serum and to the lack of assay specificity *(21)*.

A variety of immunological assays have been used to detect human cardiac MLCs *(13)*. The first-generation radioimmunoassays using polyclonal antibodies encoun-

Table 2
Serum Cardiac MHC Values Calculated from Measurements on Healthy Subjects[a]

Source	Method	No. of subjects	MHC conc.
Leger et al. *(15)*	RIA	20	Not detected (<15 µg/L) in all subjects
Leger et al. *(19)*	IRMA	52 (sedentary)	52 ± 23 µU/L
		63 (active)	95 ± 31 µU/L
Seregni et al. *(20)*	IRMA	20 (children)	109 ± 71 µU/L
Cardone et al. *(18)*	ELISA	25	264 ± 213 µg/L

[a]Values are mean ± SD. RIA indicates radioimmunoassay; IRMA, immunoradiometric assay; and ELISA, enzyme-linked immunosorbent assay.

tered significant problems of crossreactivity in the differentiation between cardiac and skeletal muscle MLCs *(22–25)*. Such crossreactivity is not surprising because the two types of light chains are highly homologous, and unless antibodies are targeted toward totally unique polypeptide segments (i.e., the amino-terminal portion), crossreactivity is to be expected. More recently, several authors have proposed methodological approaches employing MAb that recognize different epitopes on the light chain molecules to overcome these problems and try to achieve the necessary specificity useful in clinical assays (Table 3) *(26–34)*. Theoretically, MAb in combination with a sandwich technique may lead to a desirable low crossreactivity *(35)*. The use of synthetic peptides from MLC variable regions as immunogens was also proposed to obtain cardiac specific assay systems *(32)*. With regard to light chain type, the MLC 1 determination was widely preferred to MLC 2, since the latter is more labile, even if the MLC 2 measurement has the potential for higher cardiac specificity *(27)*. At present, a fully cardiospecific MLC test is not yet commercially available. Quite recently, a rapid-format monoclonal/polyclonal-based immunochromatographic assay for the detection of cardiac MLC 1 in serum or whole blood was developed that can be performed in approx

10 min with no analytical instrumentation *(36)*. A positive/negative cutoff value of 1.0 µg/L was preliminarily established for clinical use *(37)*.

In general, MLC concentrations are very low in serum from healthy persons (Table 4). However, the reference range varies considerably between different reports *(30,32, 33,36,38)*. This may be owing to a number of factors, such as the calibration of the assay, the selected antibodies, and the detection limit of the method. A standardization of MLC immunoassay is therefore desirable.

CLINICAL UTILITY

MHC in AMI and Infarct Sizing

MHCs are efficiently proteolyzed into fragments as soon as they are liberated from the damaged myocardium. These fragments are detectable in serum from 2–10 d after the onset of AMI. The delay in plasma release is longer than for any other contractile protein studied so far *(38,39)*, which supports the hypothesis that an early releasable cytosolic pool of this protein does not appear to exist. This appearance of MHCs in the bloodstream precludes its use in the early phase of AMI, allowing however for a prolonged retrospective determination of myocardial necrosis. In patients with noncomplex AMI, the time-course is mono-

Table 3
MAb-Based Immoassays for Determination of Cardiac MLCs in Human Serum[a]

Source	Principle	Detection limit, μg/L	Between-run precision, CV	Remarks
Looser et al. *(26)*	ELISA (solid-phase polyclonal antibody plus conjugate MAb anti-MLCs)	1.0	<4.5%	Crossreaction with skeletal LC
Hirayama et al. *(27)*	ELISA (MAb anti-MLC 2)	1.0	<8.2%	High conc. of rheumatoid factor affect test
Uji et al. *(28)*	ELISA (MAb anti-MLC 1)	1.0	<8.7%	Crossreaction with skeletal LC
Katoh et al. *(29)*	IRMA (MAb anti-MLC 1)	1.0	<4.3%	Crossreaction with skeletal LC
Wicks et al. *(30)*	ELISA (solid-phase MAb anti-MLC 1 plus conjugated polyclonal antibody)	0.15	<9.0%	Specificity not reported
Michel et al. *(31)*	ELISA (MAb anti-MLC 1)	0.84	<7.4%	Crossreaction with skeletal LC
Nicol et al. *(32)*	RIA (MAb anti-MLC 1 synthetic peptide P348)	1.0	Not reported	Crossreaction with skeletal LC
Ravkilde et al. *(33)*	ELISA (MAb anti-MLC 1)	0.4	<17.0%	Crossreaction with skeletal LC
Bhayana et al. *(34)*	ELISA (solid-phase MAb anti-MLC 1 plus conjugate polyclonal chicken IgY)	0.5	<5.0%	Crossreaction with skeletal LC

[a]CV, coefficient of variation; ELISA, enzyme-linked immunosorbent assay; LC, light chain; IRMA, immunoradiometric assay; and RIA, radioimmunoassay.

Table 4
Serum Cardiac MLC 1 Values Calculated from Measurements on Healthy Subjects Using Last-Generation Immunoassays[a]

Source	No. of subjects	MLC 1, μg/L
Wicks et al. *(30)*	100	0.13 ± 0.28
Nicol et al. *(32)*	65	Not detected (<1.0 μg/L) in all subjects
Ravkilde et al. *(33)*	190	Not detected (<0.4 μg/L) in 99% of subjects
Styba et al. *(36)*	84	0.37 ± 0.24
Mair et al. *(38)*	79	Not detected (<0.84 μg/L) in all subjects

[a]Values are mean ± SD.

phasic, and on the average, peak concentrations occur 5–6 d after the onset of AMI *(19,39)*. MHC release is slightly influenced by successful thrombolytic therapy *(38,39)*. In patients with reperfusion, peak value occurred just 1 d earlier *(19)*. Considering all these properties, MHCs have been proposed as a suitable marker to quantify the extent of myocardial necrosis noninvasively in humans *(7)*. Differences in serum enzyme kinetics owing to reperfusion alter the known relationship between infarct size and enzyme release. This impacts on the correct estimation of infarct size by the analysis of serum enzyme activities and concentrations, such as for total creatine kinase (CK) and CK-MB *(40)*. These limitations are obviated by using MHCs, which are not influenced significantly by reperfusion, and can therefore be used to assess myocardial damage in patients treated with thrombolysis. In experimental animal models and in AMI patients, the necrosed myocardial mass correlated very closely with the cumulative MHC release *(19)*. MHCs were also a sensitive indicator of myocardial necrosis after cardiac operations *(41)*. In particular, all patients have elevated concentrations of MHCs after cardiovascular surgery, but patients with clinical evidence of perioperative AMI show significantly greater elevations between postoperative d 3 and 12 than those without AMI *(42)*. However, this relatively long time span before the appearance of the MHC fragments in the serum after cardiac surgery precludes the use of MHCs as a tool for earlier detection of perioperative myocardial damage.

In conclusion, measurement of MHC fragments in plasma may be a quantitative indicator of myocardial necrosis *(43)*. In particular, MHC assay enables:

1. Retrospective diagnosis of necrosis;
2. Assessment of infarct size; and
3. Detection of perioperative infarction.

However, the limited cardiospecificity of available MHC assays may hamper the definitive usefulness of this marker in clinical practice.

MLC in AMI

A preliminary study with dogs described the changes of MLCs in serum after experimental AMI *(44)*. The time interval curves of MLCs showed peculiar characteristics that were not observed in serum enzymes studied *(45)*; after coronary occlusion, MLCs rose rapidly, remained elevated for a long period, and their changes in serum were biphasic, allowing both early and late diagnosis of AMI *(46)*.

Increased quantities of MLCs in the sera of patients with AMI were first demonstrated in 1978 *(47)*. Subsequently, this preliminary finding was confirmed and the characteristic biphasic release of this marker after AMI was revealed *(23)*. The initial appearance of MLCs in plasma occurs within 3–6 h after the onset of chest pain, simultaneously with the appearance of the CK-MB isoenzyme, reflecting the loss of the cytosolic unassembled light chain pool. Despite a plasma half-life of 75 min, an elevated plasma concentration persists for as long as 10 d, however, reflecting the ongoing breakdown of MLCs in the infarcted myofilaments, resulting from proteolytic degradation or acid pH dissociation of myosin molecules *(7,13)*. In this period, a peak occurs about 4 d after onset of symptoms (Fig. 3). To investigate the value of MLCs as a marker of necrosis, the mitochondrial isoenzyme of aspartate aminotransferase (mAST) was simultaneously measured *(33)*. mAST is a well-accepted marker of necrosis, inasmuch as mitochondrial enzyme leakage only takes place after substantial disintegration of the cell *(48)*. The maximum value for MLCs and mAST was reached simultaneously, and a clear resemblance existed between the time curves of these markers *(33)*. This similarity suggested that MLCs, like mitochondrial enzymes, can be used as an estimate of myocardial necrosis.

MLC in Infarct Sizing

The use and superiority of structural proteins for estimation of infarct sizing were first demonstrated in an animal model. In a study of 18 dogs, myocardial infarction was induced by ligation of the left anterior descending coronary artery *(49)*. Serial measurements of CK, cytosolic aspartate

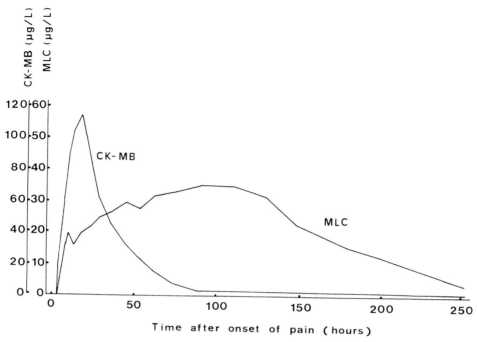

Fig. 3. Typical cardiac MLC and CK-MB mass release in human serum after AMI.

aminotransferase (SAST) and MAST, and MLC 2 were compared against infarct size determined by histologic examination of the left ventriculum after sacrifice. Results showed that measurement of MLC 2 release had the highest correlation to anatomically defined injury (Table 5).

MLCs have been used to distinguish patients with AMI having unfavorable outcomes from those with favorable prognoses *(50)*. The clinical severity and mortality were positively correlated with peak values of MLCs after infarction, and there was a consistently higher correlation between MLC appearance and these clinical variables compared with enzymatic estimates of infarct size *(50)*. In another study, researchers used left ventriculography to conclude that serum MLCs were indicative of infarct size *(24)*. Again, MLCs release correlated well with scintigraphic estimates of myocardial injury *(51)*. In this study, a single MLC measurement on day 6 after

Table 5
Comparison of Cardiac Markers Against Histology for Estimation of Myocardial Infarct Sizing[a]

Marker	Correlation Coefficient
MLC 2, release	0.818
MLC 2, peak	0.683
Total CK, release	0.138
Total CK, peak	0.222
sAST, peak	0.593
mAST, peak	0.492

[a]Data from ref. *49*.

admission yielded useful information on infarct size, without the need for serial blood sampling.

MLC After Thrombolytic Therapy

The effects of thrombolytic therapy on the appearance of MLCs in serum after AMI were also investigated *(52)*. Unlike cytosolic proteins, which showed a more rapid release after thrombolysis, the release of MLCs was not changed significantly by early recanalization of the infarct-related coronary compared with that in nonreperfused AMI. The thrombolytic intervention that alters perfusion of the infarct zone during the initial hours after the onset of pain affected only the release kinetics of the minor fraction of total intracellular MLCs— the cytosolic precursor pool of myosin synthesis—but does not significantly alter the release kinetics of the major MLC pool, i.e., the structurally bound MLCs (13). Later on, other investigators (24,38,39,53) confirmed this MLC characteristic, suggesting the use of the MLC determination as a more accurate estimate of myocardial damage in patients treated with thrombolysis.

MLC in Unstable Angina

MLCs were elevated in about half of the patients with unstable angina (27,54,55), even if, in a comparative study, the MLC assay detected fewer patients at high risk than did troponin T and/or CK-MB mass (33). Elevated concentrations were found only in patients with >75% coronary artery stenosis of at least one of the coronary arteries (54,55). The increase of MLCs correlated with signs of ischemia on the electrocardiogram and with the extent of coronary artery narrowing. Thus, the detection of elevated concentrations of circulating MLCs may enable clinicians to identify subgroups of patients with unstable angina who have more severe coronary artery disease with worse outcomes (56).

MLC in Other Conditions

Recently, two preliminary studies from the same group (57,58) evaluated the use of MLC measurement in the detection of myocardial damage after cardiac surgery. In this relatively small group of patients, MLCs discriminated the actual extent and severity of the myocardial damage better than tro-

ponin T. Measurement of the serum MLC concentrations was also useful in the monitoring of heart transplantation during postoperative period and in the evaluation of heart graft damage during ischemic preservation (59,60).

Increased serum concentrations of cardiac MLCs also were found in subjects with noncardiac disease, such as acute or chronic muscle damage and renal insufficiency (7,13). Elevated MLC values were described in subjects with acute skeletal muscle injury as well as in patients with muscular dystrophy or inflammatory myopathy (33,61–63). In these patients, the levels of MLCs showed positive correlation with other muscular proteins, such as CK and myoglobin, and were useful in evaluating disease severity and treatment response. These elevated results were thought to derive from the crossreaction between cardiac light chains and MLCs of skeletal muscle in the assay method used. On the other hand, since light chains are excreted from the kidney into the urine, serum concentrations of MLCs are influenced by renal function (64).

Conclusion

Evidence suggests that in patients with AMI, cardiac MLCs are continuously released, and therefore may be a very sensitive serum marker to diagnose and quantify myocardial necrosis. Unfortunately, the clinical utility of MLC determination in serum has not yet been widely and rigorously tested because of the lack of a well-established assay for its measurement. Therefore, new rapid and reliable analytic methods are required to evaluate definitively the diagnostic performance of this test.

ABBREVIATIONS

AMI, acute myocardial infarction; m and sAST, mitochondrial and cytosolic aspartate aminotransferase; ATP, adenosine triphosphate; CK, creatine kinase; CV, coefficient of variation; ELISA, enzyme-linked immunosorbent assay; HC, heavy chain; IRMA, immunoradiometric assay; LC, light chain; MAb, monoclonal antibody; MHC, myosin heavy chains; MLC, myosin light chains; RIA, radioimmunoassay.

REFERENCES

1. Murphy RA (1993) Muscle. In: Physiology, 3rd ed., Berne RM and Levy MN, eds., St. Louis, Mosby, pp. 284–287.
2. Matsuoka R, Chambers A, Kimura M, Kanda N, Bruns G, Yoshida M, and Takao A (1988) Molecular cloning and chromosomal localization of a gene coding for human cardiac myosin heavy-chain. Am. J. Med. Genet. 29:369–376.
3. Jaenicke T, Diederich KW, Haas W, Schleich J, Lichter P, Pfordt M, Bach A, and Vosberg HP (1990) The complete sequence of the human beta-myosin heavy chain gene and a comparative analysis of its product. Genomics 8:194–206.
4. Liew CC, Sole MJ, Yamauchi-Takihara K, Kellam B, Anderson DH, Lin L, and Liew JC (1990) Complete sequence and organization of the human cardiac beta-myosin heavy chain gene. Nucleic Acid Res. 18:3647–3651.
5. Matsuoka R, Beisel KW, Furutani M, Arai S, and Takao A (1991) Complete sequence of human cardiac alpha-myosin heavy chain gene and amino acid comparison to other myosins based on structural and functional differences. Am. J. Med. Genet. 41:537–547.
6. Diederich KW, Eisele I, Ried T, Jaenicke T, Lichter P, and Vosberg HP (1989) Isolation and characterization of the complete human betamyosin heavy chain gene. Hum. Genet. 81:214–220.
7. Mair J, Puschendorf B, and Michel G (1994) Clinical significance of cardiac contractile proteins for the diagnosis of myocardial injury. Adv. Clin. Chem. 31:63–98.
8. Seidel U, Bober E, Winter B, Lenz S, Lohse P, and Arnold HH (1987) The complete nucleotide sequences of CDNA clones coding for human myosin light chains 1 and 3. Nucleic Acids Res. 15:4989.
9. Hoffmann E, Shi QW, Floroff M, Mickle DAG, Wu TW, Olley PM, and Jackowski G (1988) Molecular cloning and complete nucleotide sequence of a human ventricular myosin light chain 1. Nucleic Acids Res. 16:2353.
10. Bechet JJ and Houadjeto M (1989) Prediction of the secondary structure of myosin light chains from comparison of homologous sequences: implications for the interaction between myosin heavy and light chains. Biochim. Biophys. Acta. 996: 199–208.
11. Wagner PD and Giniger E (1981) Hydrolysis of ATP and reversible binding of F-actin by myosin heavy chains free of all light chains. Nature 292:560–562.
12. Samarel AM, Ferguson AG, Vander Heide RS, Davison R, and Ganote CE (1986) Release of unassembled rat cardiac myosin light chain 1 following the calcium paradox. Circ. Res. 58:166–171.
13. Panteghini M (1992) Cardiac myosin light chains. Lab. Med. 23:318–322.
14. Smitherman TC, Dycus DW, and Richards EG (1980) Dissociation of myosin light chains and decreased myosin ATPase activity with acidification of synthetic myosin filaments: Possible clues to the fate of myosin in myocardial ischemia and infarction. J. Mol. Cell. Cardiol. 12:149–164.
15. Leger JOC, Bouvagnet P, Pau B, Roncucci R, and Leger JJ (1985) Levels of ventricular myosin fragments in human sera after myocardial infarction, determined with monoclonal antibodies to myosin heavy chains. Eur. J. Clin. Invest. 15:422–429.
16. Larue C, Calzolari C, Leger J, Leger J, and Pau B (1991) Immunoradiometric assay of myosin heavy chain fragments in plasma for investigation of myocardial infarction. Clin. Chem. 37:78–82.
17. Simeonova PP, Kehayov IR, and Kyurkchiev SD (1991) Identification of human ventricular myosin heavy chain fragments with monoclonal antibody 2F4 in human sera after myocardial necrosis. Clin. Chim. Acta. 201:207–222.
18. Cardone B, Skea D, Yang J, and Jackowski G (1994) Development and characterization of monoclonal antibodies to human ventricular myosin heavy chain. Clin. Chem. 40:995.
19. Leger JOC, Larue C, Ming T, Calzolari C, Gautier P, Mouton C, Grolleau R, Louisot P,

Puech P, Peperstraete B, Staroukine M, Telerman M, Pau B, and Leger JJ (1990) Assay of serum cardiac myosin heavy chain fragments in patients with acute myocardial infarction: Determination of infarct size and long-term follow-up. Am. Heart J. 120: 781–790.

20. Seregni E, Luksch R, Crippa F, Bruni GF, and Bombardieri E (1994) Evaluation of serum osteocalcin and myosin in pediatric patients affected by osteosarcoma and rhabdomyosarcoma. Int. J. Biol. Markers 9:260–261.

21. Mair J, Koller A, Artner-Dworzak E, Haid C, Wicke K, Judmaier W, and Puschendorf B (1992) Effects of exercise on plasma myosin heavy chain fragments and MRI of skeletal muscle. J. Appl. Physiol. 72:656–663.

22. Gere JB, Krauth GH, Trahern CA, and Bigham DA (1979) A radioimmunoassay for the measurement of human cardiac myosin light chains. Am. J. Clin. Pathol. 71:309–318.

23. Katus HA, Yasuda T, Gold HK, Leinbach RC, Strauss HW, Waksmonski C, Haber E, and Knaw BA (1984) Diagnosis of acute myocardial infarction by detection of circulating cardiac myosin light chains. Am. J. Cardiol. 54:964–970.

24. Isobe M, Nagai R, Ueda S, Tsuchimochi H, Nakaoka H, Takaku F, Yamaguchi T, Machii K, Nobuyoshi M, and Yazaki Y (1987) Quantitative relationship between left ventricular function and serum cardiac myosin light chain I levels after coronary reperfusion in patients with acute myocardial infarction. Circulation 76:1251–1261.

25. Wang J, Shi Q, Wu TW, Jackowski G, and Mickle DAG (1989) The quantitation of human ventricular myosin light chain 1 in serum after myocardial necrosis and infarction. Clin. Chim. Acta. 181:325–336.

26. Looser S, Hallermayer K, Gerber M, and Katus HA (1988) A new sensitive and specific enzyme immunoassay for human cardiac myosin light chains. Clin. Chem. 34:1273.

27. Hirayama A, Arita M, Takagaki Y, Tsuji A, Kodama K, and Inoue M (1990) Clinical assessment of specific enzyme immunoassay for the human cardiac myosin light chain II (MLC II) with use of monoclonal antibodies. Clin. Biochem. 23:515–522.

28. Uji Y, Sugiuchi H, and Okabe H (1991) Measurement of human ventricular myosin light chain-1 by monoclonal solid-phase enzyme immunoassay in patients with acute myocardial infarction. J. Clin. Lab. Anal. 5:242–246.

29. Katoh H, Sugi M, Chino S, Ishige M, Kuroda M, Fujimoto M, Nagai R, and Yasaki Y (1992) Development of an immunoradiometric assay kit for ventricular myosin light chain I with monoclonal antibodies. Clin. Chem. 38:170–171.

30. Wicks R, Vargas A, Wicks J, and Overdorf L (1992) Development of a solid phase EIA for the quantitation of ventricular myosin light chain 1 in human serum. Clin. Chem. 38:1094.

31. Michel G, Seifert B, and Ritter A (1992) Automated microparticle capture immunoassay for the measurement of human cardiac myosin light chain 1. Clin. Chem. 38:1104.

32. Nicol PD, Matsueda GR, Haber E, and Khaw BA (1993) Synthetic peptide immunogens for the development of a cardiac myosin light chain-1 specific radioimmunoassay. J. Nucl. Med. 34:2144–2151.

33. Ravkilde J, Botker HE, Sogaard P, Selmer J, Rej R, Jorgensen PJ, Horder M, and Thygesen K (1994) Human ventricular myosin light chain isotype 1 as a marker of myocardial injury. Cardiology 84:135–144.

34. Bhayana V, Gougoulias T, Cohoe S, and Henderson AR (1995) Discordance between results for serum troponin T and troponin I in renal disease. Clin. Chem. 41:312–317.

35. Katus HA, Hurrell JG, Matsueda GR, Ehrlich P, Zurawski VR, Khaw BA, and Haber E (1982) Increased specificity in human cardiac-myosin radioimmunoassay utilizing two monoclonal antibodies in a double sandwich assay. Mol. Immunol. 19:451–455.

36. Styba G, Takahashi M, Yang J, Davies E, Youn W, and Jackowski G (1994) Rapid format assay for the detection of cardiac myosin light chain-1 in patients with MI and unstable angina. Clin. Chem. 40:1021.

37. Svanas G, Choi W, Youn W, Leitmann R, Locicero P, Choi YH, Styba G, Kang J, and Jackowski G (1995) Measurement of cardiac myosin light chain 1 in a dry-strip format as an aid in the rapid diagnosis of myocardial injury. Clin. Chem. 41:S61.

38. Mair J, Wagner I, Jakib G, Lechleitner P, Dienstl F, Puschendorf B, and Michel G (1994) Different time courses of cardiac contractile proteins after acute myocardial infarction. Clin. Chim. Acta. 231:47–60.

39. Mair J, Thome-Kromer B, Wagner I, Lechleitner P, Dienstl F, Puschendorf B, and Michel G (1994) Concentration time courses of troponin and myosin subunits after acute myocardial infarction. Coronary Artery Dis. 865–872.

40. Roberts R and Ishikawa Y (1983) Enzymatic estimation of infarct size during reperfusion. Circulation 68(Suppl. I):I183–I189.

41. Triggiani M, Simeone F, Gallorini C, Paolini G, Donatelli F, Paolillo G, Dolci A, and Grossi A (1994) Measurement of cardiac troponin T and myosin to detect perioperative myocardial damage during coronary surgery. Cardiovasc. Surg. 2:441–445.

42. Seguin JR, Saussine M, Ferriere M, Leger JJ, Leger J, Larue C, Calzolari C, Grolleau R, and Chaptal PA (1989) Myosin: A highly sensitive indicator of myocardial necrosis after cardiac operations. J. Thorac. Cardiovasc. Surg. 98:397–401.

43. Leger JJ (1993) Plasma myosin, a marker of necrosis: An update and future trends. Arch. Mal. Coeur 86:29–32.

44. Nagai R, Ueda S, and Yazaki Y (1980) Radioimmunoassay of cardiac myosin light chain II in the serum following experimental myocardial infarction. Adv. Myocardiol. 2:415–420.

45. Nagai R, Chiu CC, Yamaoki K, Ueda S, Iwasaki Y, Ohkubo A, and Yasaki Y (1983) Serial changes in cytosolic, mitochondrial, and lyosomal enzymes and cardiac myosin light chain II in plasma following coronary ligation in conscious closed-chest dogs. Adv. Myocardiol. 4:473–478.

46. Nagai R and Yazaki Y (1981) Assessment of myocardial infarct size by serial changes in serum cardiac myosin light chain II in dogs. Jpn. Circ. J. 45:661–666.

47. Trahern CA, Gere JB, Krauth GH, and Bigham DA (1978) Clinical assessment of serum myosin light chains in the diagnosis of acute myocardial infarction. Am. J. Cardiol. 41:641–645.

48. Panteghini M (1990) Asparate aminotransferase isoenzymes. Clin. Biochem. 23:311–319.

49. Nagai R, Chiu CC, Yamaoki K, Ohuchi Y, Ueda S, Imataka K, and Yazaki Y (1983) Evaluation of methods for estimating infarct size by myosin LC2: comparison with cardiac enzymes. Am. J. Physiol. 245: H413–H419.

50. Katus HA, Diederich KW, Uellner M, Remppis A, Schuler G, and Kubler W (1988) Myosin light chains release in acute myocardial infarction: non-invasive estimation of infarct size. Cardiovasc. Res. 22: 456–463.

51. Mair J, Wagner I, Fridrich L, Lechleitner P, Dienstl F, Puschendorf B, and Michel G (1994) Cardiac myosin light chain-1 release in acute myocardial infarction is associated with scintigraphic estimates of myocardial scar. Clin. Chim. Acta. 229:153–159.

52. Katus HA, Diederich KW, Schwarz F, Uellner M, Scheffold T, and Kubler W (1987) Influence of reperfusion on serum concentrations of cytosolic creatine kinase and structural myosin light chains in acute myocardial infarction. Am. Cardiol. 60:440–445.

53. Yoshida H, Mochizuki M, Sakata K, Takezawa M, Matsumoto Y, Yoshimura M, Mori N, Yokoyama S, Hoshino T, and Kaburagi T (1992) Circulating myosin light chain I levels after coronary reperfusion: a comparison with myocardial necrosis evaluated from single photon emission computed tomography with pyrophosphate. Ann. Nucl. Med. 6:43–49.

54. Hoberg E, Katus HA, Diederich KW, and Kubler W (1987) Myoglobin, creatine kinase-B isoenzyme, and myosin light chain release in patients with unstable angina pectoris. Eur. Heart J. 8:989–994.

55. Katus HA, Diederich KW, Hoberg E, and Kubler W (1988) Circulating cardiac myosin light chains in patients with angina at rest: Identification of a high risk subgroup. J. Am. Coll. Cardiol. 11:487–493.

56. Ravkilde J, Nissen H, Horder M, and Thygesen K (1995) Independent prognostic value of serum creatine kinase isoenzyme MB mass, cardiac troponin T and myosin light chain levels in suspected acute myocardial infarction. J. Am. Coll. Cardiol. 25: 574–581.

57. Uchino T, Belboul A, Liu B, el-Gatit A, and Roberts D (1993) Detection of perioperative

myocardial structural damage by the estimation of cardiac myosin light chain I. J. Cardiovasc. Surg. 34:517–522.

58. Uchino T, Belboul A, Roberts D, and Jagenburg R (1994) Measurement of myosin light chain I and troponin T as markers of myocardial damage after cardiac surgery. J. Cardiovasc. Surg. 35:201–206.

59. Uchino T, Belboul A, el-Gatit A, Roberts D, Berglin E, and William-Olsson G (1994) Assessment of myocardial damage by circulating cardiac myosin light chain I after heart transplantation. J. Heart Lung Transplant 13:418–423.

60. Kawauchi M, Gundry SR, Beierle F, de Begona JA, and Bailey LL (1993) Myosin light chain efflux after heart transplantation in infants and children and its correlation with ischemic preservation time. J. Thorac. Cardiavasc. Surg. 106:458–462.

61. Saitoh M, Miyakoda H, Kitamura H, Kasagi S, and Takamura H (1990) Clinical significance of serum cardiac myosin light chain 1 in patients with muscular dystrophy. Rinsho Shinkeigaku 30:835–839.

62. Fukunaga H, Higuchi I, Usuki F, Moritoyo T, and Okubo R (1992) Clinical significance of serum cardiac myosin light chain 1 in patients with Duchenne muscular dystrophy. No To Shinkei 44:131–135.

63. Mader R, Nicol PD, Turley ii, Bilbao J, and Keystone EC (1994) Inflammatory myopathy—early diagnosis and management by serum myosin light chains measurements. Isr. J. Med. Sci. 30:902–904.

64. Nakai K, Nakai K, Itoh C, Kikuchi M, Nakamura S, Kamata J, et al. (1992) Increased serum levels of human cardiac myosin light chain 1 in patients with renal failure. Rinsho Byori 40:529–534.

Part IV
Future Assay and Format

16

Point-of-Care Testing for Cardiac Markers

Robert H. Christenson

CRITERIA FOR POINT-OF-CARE (POC)* TESTING

Clinical pathology responsibility has evolved into a spectrum of testing ranging from: direct patient and POC monitoring → near patient testing in a satellite laboratory → specimen transport and measurement in an in-house centralized laboratory → referral of esoteric testing to outside institutions. The "wavelength" of a specific analyte in this spectrum is driven by a balance between the urgency with which the results are needed for patient care utilization, the availability of appropriate technology, and cost. However, unlike nature where the spectral wavelength is a static characteristic, the performance site of various analytes can evolve with acquisition of knowledge and technology development.

POC testing considered in this chapter will be operatively defined as assays that may be performed either directly on the patient, at the bedside, or at "near-patient" satellite locations. Also, the technologies available all lend themselves to performance in a centralized area designed for rapid response. Table 1 lists criteria for POC testing of cardiac markers.

The evolution of POC testing is best exemplified by glucose. Originally accurate, precise, and reliable measurements were only available in the central laboratory. However, because real-time glucose measurements were critically needed for clinical decisions regarding triage, monitoring, and treatment adjustments, there was development of the highly accurate and precise POC or "bedside" monitors that are presently available. POC glucose testing must now be considered a "standard of care," because the technology is readily available and immediate treatment decisions (e.g., insulin dosaging) are frequently guided by the data. Also, POC glucose testing is available at a reasonable cost owing to competition from multiple vendors.

The fundamental issue with POC testing is that caregivers in triage, treatment, and patient monitoring areas will base time-sensitive decisions on the results. Cardiac marker testing has evolved from labor-intensive rather esoteric assays that were offered once per day, e.g., Monday through Friday, to systems with turnaround as soon as 10–15 min once the front-end work of transport, centrifugation, serum separation,

---

*See pp. 277–278 for list of abbreviations used in this chapter.

From: Cardiac Markers   Edited by: Alan H. B. Wu
© Humana Press Inc., Totowa, NJ

**Table 1
Criteria for POC Testing
of Cardiac Markers**

A strategy for specimen collection and transfer
    that minimizes risk of infectious disease
Rapid turnaround time
Low volume, preferably whole-blood sample
Direct application of a noncritical volume or
    placement of sample directly into instrument
Disposable device or minimal maintenance
    required
Minimal technical expertise required
Positive identification and specimen tracking
    strategy that eliminates specimen
    identification errors
Simple "goof proof" strategy for recording
    collection time and result reporting
Simple strategy for calibration and QC
Transferability of data to the Laboratory
    Information System (LIS) and/or Hospital
    Information System (HIS)
Agreement of results with accepted "Gold
    Standard" assays
Affordable cost

and instrument setup is completed. The next step forward is to provide cardiac marker assays in real-time or POC, and combine the information into strategies for more rapid, standardized decision making. In any case, the practice of batching these assays, even multiple times per day, will become an anachronism.

TRENDS AND LIMITATIONS
FOR POC TESTING OF CARDIAC
MARKERS

POC testing of myocardial injury markers may evolve into a standard of care for workup of acute cardiac ischemia. Although there has been some controversy regarding need for real-time testing *(1)*, justification of cardiac marker data in real time has been driven by utilization of these data in patient decisions *(2,3)*. There is a clear need for better-defined strategies that integrate the electrocardiogram (ECG), clinical symptoms, biochemical markers, and other technologies for care of cardiac patients. A model for achieving this integration has been implemented in many institutions through establishment of areas that focus on care of patients suspected of having acute cardiac ischemia. These areas are found mainly in the emergency department (ED) and are termed "Chest Pain Evaluation Centers" (CPECs). The National Heart Attack Alert Program, an initiative of NIH's National Heart Lung and Blood Institute, has recently published document no. 93-3278, which endorses rapid identification and treatment of acute myocardial infarction (AMI) patients in ED areas, such as CPECs. The number of CPECs has increased rapidly over the past years, and there seems to be no question that this trend will continue owing to increasing economic pressures, competition between institutions, and a changing standard of medical care *(2,4–6)*.

The role of POC cardiac marker testing must be evidence-based; real-time or POC testing for cardiac markers may not be appropriate for all aspects of care in the context of cardiac ischemia *(1,2)*. Specifically, clinical and economic considerations may never warrant POC testing for the initial assessment of suspected AMI in patients for whom ECG changes are diagnostic of myocardial necrosis.

Thrombolytic Therapy in AMI

POC cardiac marker testing in patients with diagnostic ECG changes or new left bundle branch block is unwarranted, because the presumptive diagnosis of AMI is made based on the ECG, and the patient is likely a candidate for thrombolytic therapy *(4)*. Benefit from thrombolytic therapy is time-sensitive *(7)*, and therefore, biochemical marker testing or any other action that potentiates treatment delay must be shown to be essential to care of these patients. If, however, future studies indicate that use of biochemical markers for immediate risk stratification and guiding treatment decisions is prudent or that broadening the use of thrombolytics can improve outcome in AMI patients for whom the ECG is nondiagnostic, there may be an essential role for POC cardiac marker testing owing to the time-sensitive nature of "opening the artery" *(8)*.

Diagnosis of AMI in Nondiagnostic ECG Patients

Although the ECG is a vital component of assessment and care for the AMI patient, it is important to note that only 24–60% of AMI patients show diagnostic ECG on admission *(9)*. For the remaining ~50% of AMI patients with nondiagnostic ECG, biochemical markers are vital for assessment, particularly considering that the largest source of malpractice dollars for ED physicians is misdiagnosis of AMI *(10)*. Real-time cardiac marker data have been shown to improve diagnostic accuracy and decision making in the CPEC environment as well as facilitating progression through AMI assessment protocols *(3,6,11–15)*. One of the most important of these studies involved the performance of creatine kinase (CK)-MB$_{mass}$ in over 1000 patients, all of whom had nondiagnostic ECG *(14)*. In these patients, the diagnostic sensitivity was 100%, and the diagnostic specificity exceeded 98%, using a strategy that included 0, 3-, 6-, and 9-h sampling after presentation *(14)*.

Risk Stratification

A number of outcome studies indicate that all acute cardiac ischemia patients in whom there is biochemical evidence of minor myocardial necrosis, regardless of their eventual diagnosis, are at increased risk for an adverse outcome *(16)*. Data indicated that

testing for cardiac troponin T (cTnT) *(17–20)* and/or possibly cardiac troponin I (cTnI) *(21,22)* may be appropriate for triage and perhaps decisions relating to interventions, such as cardiac catheterization *(23,24)*. Development of a rapid assay for cTnT *(25,26)* and work toward development of a POC cTnI assay has been prompted by the association of results of markers with risk stratification.

Noninvasive Assessment of Reperfusion After Thrombolytic Therapy

Establishing full thrombolysis in myocardial infarction ([TIMI] 3) patency to the infarct-related artery is important for outcome in the AMI patient *(27)*, yet thrombolytic therapy is successful in achieving TIMI 3 patency in only 60–70% of patients *(8)*. Strategies that include biochemical markers may be a useful tool for assisting clinicians in determining patients for whom patency in the infarct-related artery remains suboptimal, and who may benefit from immediate, alternative intervention. Although at present there is not a precedence for the use and interpretation of biochemical markers of reperfusion, the sampling of CK-MB and myoglobin at baseline (before thrombolytic therapy), and at 60 and 90 min after thrombolytic therapy shows promise *(28,29)*. Rapid and POC testing may be important for this application, because turnaround time is vital if therapy has not been successful, and alternate patient care strategies must be considered in the early phase to "open the artery."

Assessing Infarct Artery Reocclusion and Reinfarction

Reocclusion occurs in a substantial proportion, up to 10–20%, of AMI patients *(30,31)*. Use of biochemical markers for indicating that further myocardial cell necrosis has occurred during the postinfarction phase is an integral part of monitoring the AMI patient. The rapid turnaround that POC measurement of biochemical markers could develop into an important component of care for these patients because the interventional options are time-sensitive.

REGULATORY ASPECTS OF POC TESTING

The POC concept is entirely rational, because it is aimed at providing caregivers with cardiac marker data for real-time use along with the patient's clinical symptoms, the ECG, and other technologies, so that decisions can be reached earlier. In practice, however, there are a number of issues that must be resolved at an institutional level prior to POC implementation. One of the most important and difficult of these issues involves development of an institutional strategy for assuring quality and compliance with all relevant regulatory requirements.

Regulatory requirements for POC testing are mandated by a number of agencies including the Health Care Financing Administration (HCFA), under its "Clinical Laboratory Improvement Act of 1988" (CLIA) regulations, the Joint Commission on Accreditation of Healthcare Organizations (JCAHO), the College of American Pathologists' (CAP) Accreditation Program, and also any additional requirements imposed by local or state government, as is the case with Washington, Florida, New York, and California. CLIA requirements will be included here because they represent the minimum standards for all POC testing in the US. An important caveat: POC testing for cardiac markers or any other analytes should **not** be initiated until any additional requirements imposed by accrediting organizations or state agencies have been investigated. A comprehensive explanation of CLIA requirements, as well as those of the

CAP and JCAHO is available in a recent article *(32)*.

Two CLIA issues must be addressed in the conceptual stage of implementing POC testing. The first issue involves making the institutional decision of who will hold the CLIA certificate that is mandated by HCFA regulation for any in vitro testing. In general, POC testing is either covered by the CLIA certificate held in the central laboratory or individual testing sites may obtain their own CLIA certificate(s). In any case, the individual listed on the CLIA certificate bears the responsibility for assuring compliance with regulations. The second CLIA issue involves the complexity of the testing to be performed. By way of background, CLIA espouses the philosophy of "testing site neutrality," meaning that the same regulatory rules must be followed regardless of the location where the testing is performed. The complexity of testing performed at any site is assigned, based on the technical difficulty of the measurement technology, into the following four categories:

1. Waived;
2. Physician-performed microscopy (not relevant for POC testing);
3. Moderately complex; or
4. Highly complex (not generally relevant for POC testing).

Because the assignment of complexity is technology-based, assays for the same analyte, but measured by different methods can fall into separate categories.

Most believe that the cardinal rule for POC testing is "simpler is better," provided that the performance and other characteristics of the simpler assay is acceptable. Thus, of the four CLIA categories, POC testing implemented should be classified as waived in all cases possible to maximize the flexibility of staffing and facilitate regulatory activities; performance of moderately complex testing is feasible, but has more strin-

Table 2
CLIA 1988 Requirements for Quality Assurance

Requirement	Federal register number	Brief description and comments
Patient test management	493.1703	Entire order process comprised of test order to recording result with interpretation
QC assessment	493.1705	Comprised of seven items[a]
Proficiency testing	493.1707	Participate and perform successfully in CLIA-approved program for regulated analytes[b]
Comparison of test results	493.1709	Minimum twice per year comparison of all analytes performed at more than one location and same CLIA license
Relation of Pt information to test values	493.1711	Must have separate reference intervals for different patient groups, if relevant
Personnel assessment	493.1713	Training and competency testing at specified intervals
Communications	493.1715	Adequate means of communication with users
Complaint investigation	493.1717	Complaint log with documentation of responses to issues
QA review with staff	493.1719	Documented review of QA issues with staff
QA records	493.1721	Documentation of minutes, communications, temperatures, reagents, and so forth

[a]Follow manufacturer's instructions, have a procedure manual, calibrate or check calibration at least every 6 mo, run two levels of QC, follow specified control procedures, perform/document remedial actions, document QC activities, and retain records.
[b]Comparison data if CLIA certificate is held in central lab.

gent requirements. Unfortunately, no POC tests for cardiac markers are classified as waived at present, so the focus of this discussion will be on the moderately complex category.

Personnel criteria for POC and other testing requires designation of four positions: director, clinical consultant, technical consultant, and testing personnel. All four positions may be held by the same individual, provided that educational requirements are met. The minimum education for moderate complexity testing requires that the director and technical consultant hold a Bachelor's degree, the clinical consultant have a doctoral (MD or PhD) degree, and all testing personnel must have a high school diploma. All persons performing POC testing must be appropriately trained and their competency

tested, with documentation twice in their first year, and then once per year thereafter.

Global quality assurance activities required by CLIA for any POC or laboratory testing are listed in Table 2. These responsibilities are further articulated in ref. *(32)*. Again the laboratory director, i.e., the individual listed on the CLIA certificate, has the responsibility for assuring that all global regulations listed in Table 2, in addition to any local regulations, are performed and documented appropriately.

Development of a strategy for compliance with regulatory issues tends to be among the most challenging issues for any POC testing, with cardiac markers being no exception. Communication and cooperation among the central laboratory, clinical areas, and administration are important (and probably essential) for successful implementation and ongoing utilization.

UTILIZATION OF POC CARDIAC MARKERS

Unfortunately the "holy grail" of cardiac markers showing early release, 100% cardiac specificity, a substantial lifetime in circulation, and so forth, has not yet been discovered. In the opinion of many, this situation leads to a panel approach to utilization of markers for the laboratory-assisted care of the patient with acute cardiac ischemia, including AMI diagnosis, risk stratification, assessment of reinfarction, and reperfusion assessment. The constituents of this cardiac panel should include a marker that increases rapidly after cardiac injury. Myoglobin must be considered for this role, because its rise may be as early as 1 h after myocardial injury (*see* Chapter 6). Myoglobin, however, is found in abundant amounts in both cardiac and skeletal tissue, and therefore is not the ideal cardiac marker. To complement myoglobin, a cardiac panel should include a highly tissue-specific marker, even at the sacrifice of the marker being elevated in blood later after myocardial necrosis. A leading candidate for this role has been CK-MB, largely because it has been considered the "gold standard" for diagnosis of AMI (*33*). Measurement of total CK concentration for calculation of a relative index is also advocated (*see* Chapter 9). However, cTnT and cTnI must be considered the markers for the future, because they are more cardiac-specific than CK-MB (*see* Chapters 13 and 14). Cardiac cTnI and, in particular, cTnT are elevated longer after myocardial necrosis, so they may serve an additional application of detecting myocardial necrosis over the previous 4–5 d (for cTnI) to 7–10 d (for cTnT) before presentation (*see* Chapters 12–14). Knowledge of recent myocardial necrosis that may be beyond the "window" of CK-MB elevation could have important implications regarding triage, risk stratification, and patient disposition.

Serial Sampling

A rise and fall of CK-MB in the first 8–12 h after onset of symptoms is nearly pathognomonic for AMI (*34*). A similar rise and fall is also observed for both cTnT and cTnI, and for this reason, a single measurement is inadequate and serial specimen collections are necessary to document myocardial necrosis. As cited earlier, a strategy for CK-MB collections at 0, 3, 6, 9 (*14*), and in some hospitals 12 h, is rapidly becoming a standard in the CPEC environment. Also, promising data have suggested that the negative predictive value of myoglobin be useful for decreasing the serial sampling time to perhaps 3 h (*14,35*). It is important to note, however, that strategies that include myoglobin are intended for more rapid progression of the patient through established CPEC protocols, not strictly for ruling out myocardial necrosis.

Strategies for monitoring reperfusion after thrombolytic therapy may require availability of a panel of cardiac markers at multiple time-points as well (*28,29*). Assessing reinfarction or extension will also require serial sampling to detect an increasing trend in cardiac markers.

Quantitative or Qualitative Results?

Quantitative assays are an obvious requirement for monitoring the rise and fall of cardiac markers, and therefore, assays for POC application intended for AMI monitoring need to yield a quantitative, numerical result with good precision and high accuracy. In the case of CK, this quantitative requirement is further justified because the relative index, usually represented by (CK-MB/total CK × 100%), is part of the diagnostic criteria in many institutions (*see* Chapter 9). Applications, such as monitoring the success of thrombolytic therapy, indicating reinfarction, or an infarction extension, are also based on quantitative rather than qualitative or semiquantitative assays. On the other hand, applications such as AMI triage or risk stratification may not have a strict requirement for a quantitative result if the analytes are not normally present in circulation.

SPECIFIC POC ASSAYS FOR CARDIAC MARKERS

Hybritech ICON

The CK-MB ICON system, manufactured by Hybritech Inc., San Diego, CA, is comprised of an ICON cylinder, associated reagents, and the ICON Reader shown in Fig. 1A. The ICON system was among the first technologies that allowed true near-patient POC testing for quantitative CK-MB$_{mass}$. The system uses a two-site "sandwich" immunoassay format and was cleared by the FDA in the mid-1980s.

The CK-MB ICON system requires a serum specimen and various steps for determination, as outlined in Fig. 2. Technically, the ICON cylinder has a permeable membrane that both provides the solid phase for the immunoassay reaction and modulates sample flow. The capture part of the sandwich immunoassay is based on an antibody with high affinity for the B-subunit of CK-MB that is immobilized in circular orientation on the ICON's membrane (*see* Fig. 1B). Flow through the membrane is optimized such that after any CK-MB in the sample is captured by the immobilized antibody, all other serum contents pass through to the absorptive inner portion of the cylinder. For CK-MB detection, an anti-M-subunit antibody conjugated to horseradish peroxidase binds to the exposed M-subunit of CK-MB captured from the patient sample. Substrate for the horseradish peroxidase is then added, which allows visualization of up to four "spots," two for the sample and one each for high and low calibrators, as indicated in Fig. 1B. The intensity of each spot is directly proportional to CK-MB$_{mass}$ concentration; the ICON cylinder is placed into the reader, which compares the intensity of sample spots with the calibrators for quantitation. Because calibrators and duplicate testing of samples are implicit with each ICON membrane, software in the reader can conduct various quality control (QC)/quality assurance system checks, such as verifying that the CK-MB and calibrator "spots" are developed fully, the results of duplicate sample measurement are in appropriate agreement, and so forth.

There has been substantial experience with the CK-MB ICON from both analytical and clinical perspectives. The analytical characteristics of the ICON system have been described, including definition of the assay's sensitivity of <2 ng/mL (36). Although each institution must establish criteria appropriate for their patient population, a quantitative cutoff of 7 ng/mL is commonly used for indicating myocardial injury with the ICON system. Diagnostic performance of several technologies for CK-MB measurement were compared in a Chest Pain Center environment, concluding that the CK-MB ICON demonstrated better performance characteristics compared to any of the other technologies tested (3).

Several other studies assessing clinical utilization of the CK-MB ICON in the context of AMI have been performed in the ED (13,14). Availability of CK-MB ICON technology has played a large role in documenting that real-time CK-MB data are useful for clinical decision making (3). CK-MB ICON technology has also been used for the noninvasive assessment of reperfusion status where serial CK-MB measurements were combined with clinical indicators (28). The model yielded an area under the Receiver Operator Characteristic curve for predicting successful reperfusion of 0.86 (28).

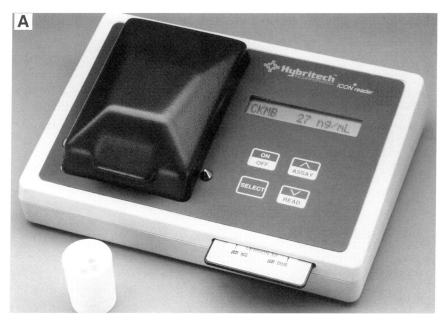

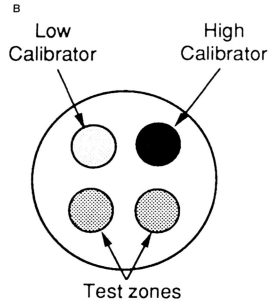

Fig. 1. (A) CK-MB ICON system from Hybritech Inc. **(B)** ICON membrane with four spots, duplicate for the sample and a high and low control.

The CK-MB ICON has a turnaround time of 15–20 min, and although it is appropriate for near-patient POC utilization, this device is less well suited for measurement outside a laboratory environment because the system requires a serum sample, multiple precision pipeting steps, and multiple wash and reagent steps as indicated in Fig. 2.

cTnT Rapid Assay

The cTnT Rapid Assay is a single-step "sandwich" immunoassay manufactured by

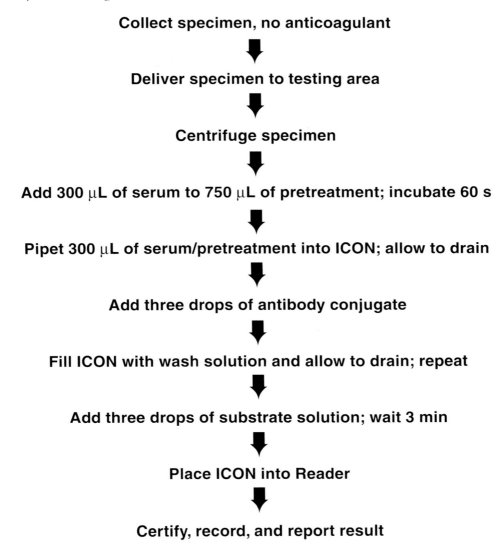

Fig. 2. Testing outline for quantitative CK-MB measurement with the ICON system (courtesy Hybritech Inc., San Diego, CA).

Boehringer Mannheim Corporation (BMC), Indianapolis, IN that utilizes between 135 and 165 µL of either EDTA or heparinized whole blood, or EDTA plasma *(37)*. As indicated in the diagram of the cTnT Rapid Assay in Fig. 3, the cTnT Rapid Assay result is qualitative, i.e., it yields a "positive" or "negative" response. The original 1st generation cTnT Rapid Assay was cleared by the FDA in 1995 and had a cutoff of 0.2 ng/mL *(25,26)*. A 2nd generation Rapid Assay is now available that has a more sensitive cutoff of 0.08 ng/mL.

The cTnT Rapid Assay procedure is outlined in Fig. 4. After whole blood or plasma is dispensed into the sample well, the sample dissolves a buffer and solulubrizes an adsorbed cocktail of two monoclonal antibodies. The sample then diffuses to a portion of the device containing a "fleece" material, where the cellular constituents are separated from the plasma phase. As shown in Fig. 3A, one of the

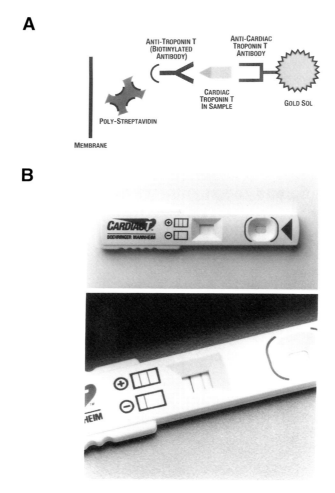

Fig. 3. (A) Components of the sandwich immunoassay used in the cTnT Rapid Assay. **(B)** cTnT Rapid Assay manufactured by BMC, showing a qualitative positive result.

cTnT antibodies is biotinylated (BT); the second antibody is gold-labeled (Au) and binds to a different region of any cTnT molecules to form the immunoassay "sandwich." The (BT-antibody/cTnT/antibody-Au) complexes migrate to the read zone where the BT "tail" of the complex is captured by streptavidin immobilized in a line formation. The Au label on captured complexes forms a red-colored line that is interpreted visually. The control line (Fig. 3B) verifies the integrity of each device. If the control line fails to develop, the test must be repeated using a separate Rapid Assay device. The cTnT Rapid Assay utilizes the same two MAb as the quantitative Cardiac T, ELISA method, also manufactured by BMC. It is of note that falsely increased cTnT measurements have been reported in patients with skeletal muscle disease *(38)* 1st generation Rapid Assay, presumably because of the 12% crossreactivity of the labeled cTnT antibody with skeletal muscle TnT. With the 2nd generation Rapid Assay, however, the capture and label of antibodies are both specific for the cardiac isoform so this issue appears to be eliminated.

Collect EDTA Specimen

Withdraw ~0.5 mL of Whole Blood with Syringe From Tube

Dispense 0.135 to 0.165 mL of Sample into Sample Well

Result is Fully Developed at 20 min (see legend note)

Interpret, Certify, Record, and Report Results

Fig. 4. Rapid assay procedure outline for qualitative measurement of cTnT system (courtesy BMC). *Note:* The 2nd generation Rapid Assay requires only 15 min for full development.

With regard to QC, each testing site must at a minimum run "cTnT-positive" and "cTnT-negative" liquid controls with each new lot of devices, even though a control is included in each device to assure proper technical performance. Of course, it is critical to verify that this strategy is in compliance with local QC/QA regulations.

Studies have examined utilization of the cTnT Rapid Assay device for diagnosis of AMI *(16,39)*. The Rapid Assay's diagnostic performance during the first 4–8 h after presentation showed sensitivities of 86 and 100% with specificities of 86–100 and 85%, respectively, in published studies *(16,39)*. In addition to assessment of AMI, cTnT measurements have also been documented being as useful for risk stratification, as discussed in Chapter 2. Although to date no studies have thoroughly addressed utilization of the Rapid Assay for risk stratification, such a study has been presented in abstract form *(40)*.

The second-generation assay will allow more sensitive detection of myocardial necrosis and may be particularly useful for risk stratification applications.

STATus Myoglobin and CK-MB Device

Figure 5 shows the device and analytical concept for the STATus system from Spectral Diagnostics Inc., Toronto, Canada; this device was cleared by the FDA in 1995. Methodology is based on two-site (sandwich) immunoassay technology, and the device is designed to provide qualitative results for a testing panel that includes both myoglobin and $CK-MB_{mass}$. A second device for qualitative measurement of cTnI was FDA cleared in 1997 and is available for use. Devices that include other markers, such as human ventricular myosin light chains, have been evaluated for release in the near future.

The testing flow for the STATus system is displayed in Fig. 6. With whole blood, a seven-drop sample (precise volume not critical) collected with heparin as anticoagulant is placed into the collection membrane; with serum or plasma samples are simply applied. After initial separation of plasma from the cellular material, the myoglobin, CK-MB or cTnI in the sample reacts with dye-labeled

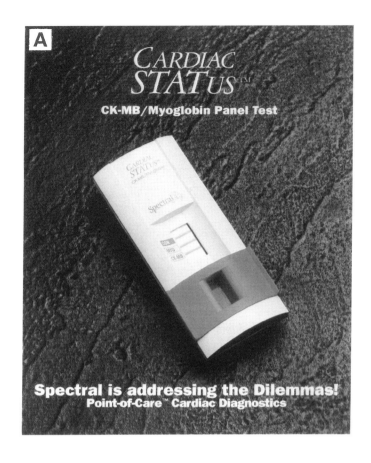

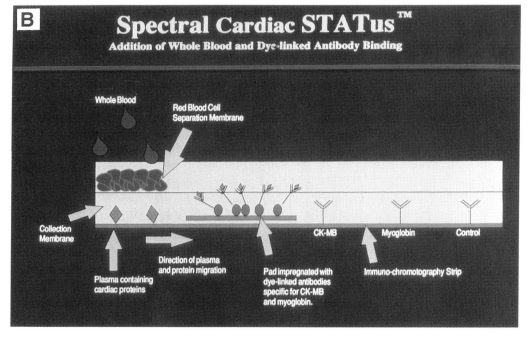

270

Collect Heparinized Specimen

Withdraw ~1 mL through Stopper with Porex Device

Apply 7 Drops from Porex Device Onto Sample Area; Wait 3 min

Remove and Dispose of Application Clip

Apply 4 Drops of Developer on Sample Area; Wait 15 min

Interpret, Certify, Record, and Report Results

Fig. 6. Procedure outline for qualitative measurement of a CK-MB/myoglobin panel with the STATus System (courtesy Spectral Diagnostics Inc.).

antibodies that are analyte-specific. The (dye-labeled antibody/analyte) complexes migrate by immunochromatography to the detection zone, where capture antibodies directed at different epitopes of myoglobin, CK-MB or cTnI are immobilized at different positions, each in line formation (*see* Fig. 5B). For the CK-MB and myoglobin device, the immobilized capture antibodies specifically bind the complex containing either myoglobin or CK-MB; in this way, two lines are visually apparent for positive samples; one line represents the (dye-labeled antibody/myoglobin/capture antibody) complex and the other represents (dye-labeled antibody/CK-MB/capture antibody). A third control line is also visually apparent in the detection zone to help assure proper performance of the device (*see* Fig. 5A). A similar

strategy is used for the cTnI device; however, two lines are present for a positive test, one for cTnI and one for the control.

The cutoff, i.e., concentration at which a definite band appears, is 100 ng/mL for myoglobin and has been determined to be 5 ng/mL for CK-MB and ~1.0 ng/mL for cTnI (similar to Dade stratus cutoff of 1.5 ng/mL). Studies have examined utilization of both the FDA-cleared device for CK-MB and myoglobin (*41*), and the cTnI device (*42*) in the context of triage for AMI and acute cardiac ischemia.

The STATus system has been classified as moderately complex under CLIA regulations. Performance of positive and negative control specimens is necessary with each shipment of reagents. It is important to note that confirmation of any positive CK-MB,

---

Fig. 5. (*opposite page*) (**A**) STATus Device, from Spectral Diagnostics, showing qualitative positive CK-MB and myoglobin results. (**B**) Experimental design of the STATus device.

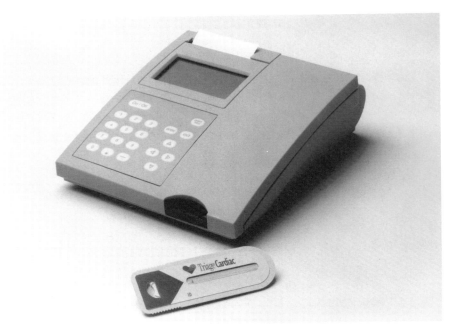

Fig. 7. The Triage® Meter and Triage® Cardiac Panel, showing the instrument and immunoassay cartridge (courtesy Biosite Diagnostics).

myoglobin, or cTnI results by a quantitative laboratory assay is not required.

Biosite Diagnostics Inc.

A prototype of the Triage® Cardiac system, manufactured by Biosite Diagnostics, San Diego, CA, is displayed in Fig. 7. This system provides measurement of a fixed cardiac marker panel consisting of myoglobin, CK-MB, and cTnI, each quantified simultaneously in respective one-step "sandwich" immunoassays with fluorescence detection. The sample requirement for the Triage® Cardiac system is a single, six-drop aliquot of heparinized whole blood; the precise volume of the drops is not critical.

The analytic system consists of two basic components. The first component is a wafer-shaped test panel, about 3 × 1 in in size, that contains all of the reagents necessary for the myoglobin, cTnI, and CK-MB immunoassays in addition to two positive controls. Test panels are stable at room temperature for a

minimum of 6 mo, and each is labeled with a bar code specifying lot number, expiration date, and other critical information. After sample dosing, the cartridge is placed into the "keyed" slot of the second component: the Triage® Meter. The reader is approximately the size of telephone and contains the hardware for fluorescence detection of the cartridge's immunoassay reactions as well as software enabling quantification. The Triage® Meter also has a printer and an LED display for results, specimen identification, time of analysis, and so on. Calibration of the system is accomplished electronically by use of a code chip that is lot-specific and is included with each shipment of cartridges. The code chip is plugged into the appropriate port on the meter, whereupon it downloads performance and documentation data, such as lot number, expiration date, values for internal control checks, and relevant fluorescent signal information for each assay. The Triage® Meter can be interfaced with a host computer through a

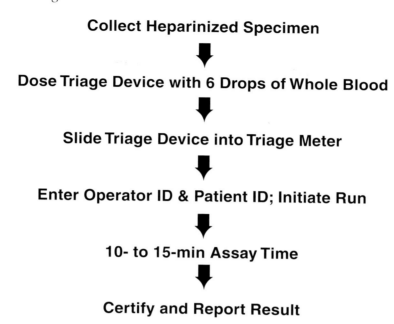

Collect Heparinized Specimen

Dose Triage Device with 6 Drops of Whole Blood

Slide Triage Device into Triage Meter

Enter Operator ID & Patient ID; Initiate Run

10- to 15-min Assay Time

Certify and Report Result

Fig. 8. Testing outline for the Triage® Cardiac System intended for quantitative measurement of a myoglobin, CK-MB, and cTnI panel (courtesy Biosite Diagnostics).

RS232 port, and has a keypad for entry of operator ID and patient information.

The measurement protocol for the Triage® Meter is outlined in Fig. 8. After dosing the cartridge with six drops of whole blood, the plasma and cellular phases are separated when the sample is filtered. The plasma phase is delivered to areas on the cartridge containing immunoassay reagents specific for myoglobin, cTnI, or CK-MB measurement. Two internal fluorescence controls are also activated during this process for analytic QC of the system. When the dosed cartridge is placed into the Triage® Meter, its bar code is scanned to verify that all lot-specific information has been downloaded from the EPROM and is valid for measurement. After an incubation time, the fluorescence signal of the two analytic controls is measured to verify performance of the system; the signal for each cardiac marker is compared to its specific analytical curve allowing quantitative measurement. The entire assay requires about 10 min.

From a regulatory perspective, the system's internal controls are sufficient to satisfy daily quality control according to the Survey Procedures and Interpretive Guidelines for Laboratories and Laboratory Services—Appendix C. Therefore, users have the latitude of designing QC frequency through the software resident in the Triage® Meter. If QC has not been performed within the prescribed period, the system manager may enable a lockout feature or allow control performance to be overridden with documentation on the report. The system's software will store and analyze QC data with rules that are flexible to user definition. CLIA classification of the Triage® Cardiac System will most probably be moderately complex.

The Alpha Dx System

The Alpha Dx System from First Medical Inc., Mountain View, CA uses an EDTA whole blood sample to measure quantitatively a panel of cardiac markers comprised of myoglobin, cTnI, CK, and CK-MB$_{mass}$,

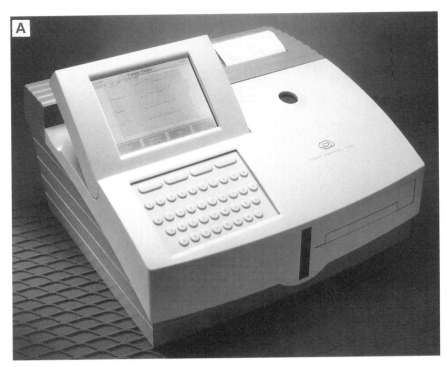

Fig. 9. (A) The Alpha Dx system from First Medical Inc.

all by sandwich immunoassay technology with fluorescence detection. The Alpha Dx system includes two components: an instrument that is the size of a small fax machine, shown in Fig. 9A, and analytical disks that contain the immunoassay reagents necessary for measurement of each analyte, displayed in Fig. 9B.

The Alpha Dx instrument has an alphanumeric keyboard, LCD, bar code reader, floppy disk drive, interface port, and safe-T-coupler (blood tube holder). Patient information, operator ID, reagent lot number, and related information can be entered into the system manually through the keyboard, or with the bar code system. The instrument also allows selection of special features, including QC trending on the LCD and display of temporal patient results. The interface port allows communication with various laboratory and hospital information (computer) systems.

The outline for assay performance is shown in Fig. 10. A whole-blood sample collected in a standard EDTA blood tube is inverted and placed into the instrument's Safe-T-Coupler (blood tube holder). Direct sampling is accomplished by firmly pressing the tube such that the needle at the bottom of the Safe-T-Coupler pierces the blood tube's top. The needle is connected to a flexible plastic tubing assembly with a filter at its end. On operator activation, a peristaltic pump acts on the flexible tubing, causing sample to be withdrawn from the blood tube and through the filter assembly to remove microclots. The sample metering device allows a precise volume of filtered sample to be delivered into the sample chamber on the analytical disk shown in Fig. 9B.

The analytical disk is actually a rotor that is divided into three zones; two of these zones have wells for "on-board" high and low con-

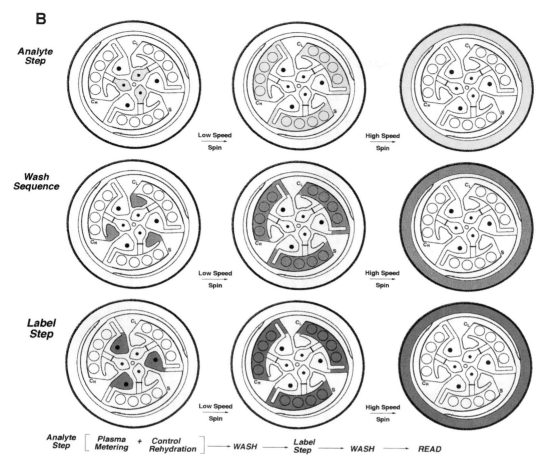

B

Analyte Step — Low Speed Spin — High Speed Spin

Wash Sequence — Low Speed Spin — High Speed Spin

Label Step — Low Speed Spin — High Speed Spin

Analyte Step [Plasma Metering + Control Rehydration] → WASH → Label Step → WASH → READ

Fig. 9. *(continued)* **(B)** Diagram of the system disk that contains the immunoassay components of the CONSULT system.

trols; the third zone contains the sample chamber. Simultaneous with sample delivery, the high and low controls are reconstituted, and there is a short incubation period, during which time fluorescein labeled antibodies specific for myoglobin, cTnI, CK, and CK-MB react to form antibody-fluorescein/analyte complexes. After incubation, the disk is spun at low speed, causing the Ab-fluorescein/analyte complex in the sample and controls to channel to an area with four "divots," each containing an immobilized capture antibody specific for either myoglobin, cTnI, CK, or CK-MB (*see* Fig. 9B). Antibody-fluorescein/analyte complexes are captured by the divot's immobi-

lized antibodies forming the (fluorescein-antibody/analyte/capture-Ab) immunoassay sandwich. Wash solution is then aliquoted into the disk, which is then spun at high speed to remove the fluid matrix of the sample and control to the waste ring at the outside of the disk. The fluorescent label (Cy5-anti-fluorescein-Dextran) is then reconstituted and transferred centrifugally into the reaction zone, where it binds to the fluorescein-antibody/analyte/capture-Ab complex. Centrifugal separation and washing remove unbound Cy5 label. The fluorescence signal of each divot is read multiple times, to improve precision, and compared to a standard curve for quantification. The

Collect EDTA Specimen

⬇

Insert Collection Tube into Safe-T-Coupler

⬇

Place Safe-T-Coupler into Instrument

⬇

Place Appropriate Test Disk in Instrument

⬇

Enter Operator ID; Press "Run"

⬇

18-min Assay Time

⬇

Certify and Report Result

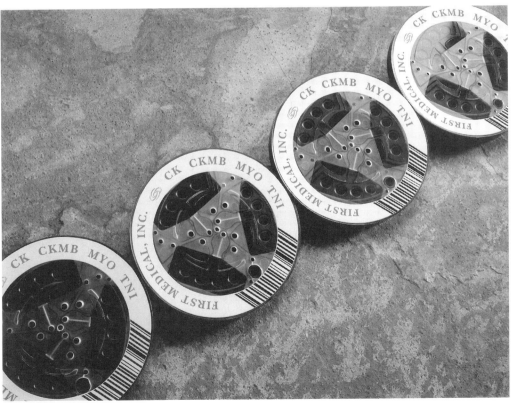

Fig. 10. Testing outline for the CONSULT System intended for quantitative measurement of a myoglobin, CK, CK-MB, and cTnI panel (courtesy First Medical Inc.).

hematocrit of the sample is determined and an algorithm converts the whole blood result to a serum equivalent value.

The Alpha Dx system has demonstrated precision between 4 and 9% for the myoglobin, cTnI, CK, and CK-MB analytes as well as good analytical sensitivity and agreement between 91 and 99% with accepted methods. It is of note that the CK measurement in the Alpha Dx system is actually a "mass" measurement rather than the activity, as has been conventional. The Alpha Dx system will probably be classified as moderately complex.

ECONOMIC ISSUES FOR POC IMPLEMENTATION

In a global sense, economic and clinical considerations are ultimately linked by the following question: Does availability of POC testing for cardiac markers affect outcome of patients with (or suspected of having) acute cardiac ischemia? Economic outcome from availability of cardiac marker results may represent a reduced length of stay or more rapid transfer of a patient to a stepdown unit. Clinical outcome represents the decrease in morbidity and mortality that may occur owing to earlier intervention based on earlier knowledge of cardiac marker results. More properly designed studies providing appropriate evidence are needed.

In addition to regulatory concerns regarding POC testing, cost is frequently a major issue. Ideally, of course, POC testing would be less expensive than testing in a centralized location. In reality, however, achieving both simplicity and cost parody with the central laboratory is difficult. Thus, POC testing for cardiac markers will almost certainly be more costly than centralized testing, and implementation decisions must be based on practice guidelines at individual institutions.

For cost evaluation of POC testing, it is critical to achieve a "normalized" cost for POC testing so that a direct comparison with performance in the centralized lab is possible. The cost components of POC testing include reagents, labor, oversight of the program, and institutional overhead. In addition, reagent costs for patient testing, expense for QC materials, the testing reagents required to perform QC testing, and any sample collection device. An effective means of calculating cost is to develop a "map" or flow diagram of the process that includes all steps in the testing process from sample collection through result reporting and documentation. Labor must include the cost for technical performance, the cost for employee benefits, and also time required to track employee competency, collate QC results, development of training materials, training, and other oversight activities necessary for appropriate patient care and to comply with regulatory requirements. Institutional overhead may vary from region to region depending on local labor costs for support personnel, the cost of space for the testing, taxes, utilities, and administrative costs. Calculating costs for institutional overhead is often complicated and inexact, so that this quantity is usually expressed as a percent of overall cost.

Potential lost revenue based on the individual institution's method of measuring activity and charge capture are also issues. Reimbursement for POC testing is complicated to determine. For in-patients who are covered under "Diagnosis Related Groups" (DRGs) or patients covered by capitated insurance programs, specific reimbursement for POC or any other testing cannot always be expected. For other patients, it may be possible to seek reimbursement by using appropriate current procedural terminology (CPT) based billing codes.

ABBREVIATIONS

AMI, acute myocardial infarction; BMC, Boehringer Mannheim Corporation; BT, biotinylated; CAP, College of American Pathologists; CK creatine kinase; CLIA, Clinical Laboratory Improvement Act; CPECs, chest pain evaluation centers; CPT, current procedural terminology; cTnI and T, cardiac troponins I and T; ECG, electrocardiogram; EDTA, ethylenediaminetetraacetic acid; ELISA, enzyme-linked immunosorbent assay; EPROM, erasable programmable read only memory; FDA, Food and Drug Administration; HCFA, Health Care Finance Administration; ID, identification; JCAHO, Joint Commission on Accreditation of Healthcare Organizations; LCD, liquid crystal display; NIH, National Institutes of Health; POC, point-of-care; QC, quality control; TIMI, thrombolysis in myocardial infarction.

REFERENCES

1. Jaffe AS (1993) More rapid biochemical diagnosis of myocardial infarction: Necessary? Prudent? Cost effective? [Editorial] Clin. Chem. 39:1567–1569.
2. Newby LK, Gibler WB, Ohman EM, and Christenson RH (1995) Biochemical markers in suspected acute myocardial infarction: the need for early assessment [Editorial]. Clin. Chem. 41:1263–1265.
3. Young G, Hedges JR, Gibler WB, Green TR, and Swanson RJ (1990) Do CK-MB results affect chest pain decision making in the Emergency department? Ann. Emerg. Med. 19:1218–1219.
4. Emergency department: Rapid identification and treatment of patients with acute myocardial infarction. Ann. Emerg. Med. 23: 311–329, 1994.
5. Bahr RD (1995) The changing paradigm of acute heart attack prevention in the emergency department: A futuristic viewpoint. [Editorial] Ann. Emerg. Med. 25:95–96.
6. Sayre MR and Gibler WB (1996) New approaches to ruling out acute ischemic coronary syndrome in the emergency department. Ann. Emerg. Med. 27:1–7.
7. Gruppo Italiano per lo Studio dell nell'Infarto Miocardico (GISSI) (1986) Effectiveness of intravenous thrombolytic treatment in acute myocardial infarction. Lancet 1:397–402.
8. The GUSTO angiographic investigators (1993) The effects of tissue plasminogen activator, streptokinase, or both on coronary-artery patency, ventricular function, and survival after acute myocardial infarction. N. Engl. J. Med. 329:1615–1622.
9. Fesmire FM, Wharton DR, and Calhoun FB (1995) Instability of ST segments in the early stages of acute myocardial infarction in patients undergoing continuous 12-lead ECG monitoring. Am. J. Emerg. Med. 13:158–163.
10. Rusnak RA, Stair TO, Hansen K, and Fastow JS (1989) Litigation against the emergency physician: Common features in cases of missed myocardial infarction. Ann. Emerg. Med. 18:1029–1034.
11. Tucker JF, Collins RA, Anderson AJ, Hess M, Farley I, Hagemann DA, Harkins HJ, and Zwicke D (1994) Value of serial myoglobin levels in early diagnosis of patients admitted for acute myocardial infarction. Ann. Emer. Med. 24:704–708.
12. Brogan GX, Friedman S, McCuskey C, Cooling DS, Burrutti L, Thode HC, and Bock JL (1994) Evaluation of a rapid immunoassay for serum myoglobin versus CK-MB for ruling out acute myocardial infarction in emergency department. Ann. Emer. Med. 24:665–671.
13. Hedges JR, Rouan GW, Toltis R, Goldstein-Wayne B, and Stein EA (1987) Use of cardiac enzymes identifies patients with acute myocardial infarction otherwise unrecognized in the emergency department. Ann. Emer. Med. 16:248–252.
14. Gibler WB, Runyon JP, Levy RC, Sayre MR, Kacich R, Hattemer CR, Hamilton C, Gerlach JW, and Walsh RA (1995) A rapid diagnostic and treatment center for patients with chest pain in the emergency department. Ann. Emerg. Med. 25:1–8.
15. Levitt MA, Promes SB, Bullock S, Disano M, Young GP, Gee G, and Pearslee D (1996) Combined cardiac marker approach with adjunct two-dimensional echocardiography to diagnose acute myocardial infarction in the emergency department. Ann. Emerg. Med. 27:1–7.
16. Antman EM, Grudzien C, and Sacks DB (1995) Evaluation of a rapid bedside assay for detection of serum cardiac troponin T. JAMA 273:1279–1282.

17. Wu AHB and Lane PL (1995) Metaanalysis in Clinical Chemistry: validation of cardiac troponin T as a marker for ischemic heart diseases. Clin. Chem. 41:1228–1233.

18. Alonsozana GL and Christenson RH (1996) The case for cardiac troponin T: A marker for effective risk stratification of patients with acute cardiac ischemia. Clin. Chem. 42: 803–808.

19. Lindahl B, Venge P, and Wallentin L (1996) Relation between troponin T and the risk of cardiac events in unstable angina. Circulation 96:1651–1657.

20. Ohman EM, Armstrong PW, Christenson RH, Granger CB, Katus H, Hamm CW, O'Hanesian MA, Lee KL, Wagner GS, Kleiman NS, Harrell FE Jr, Califf RM, and Topol EJ, for the GUSTO-IIa Investigators (1996) Risk stratification with admission cardiac troponin T levels in acute myocardial ischemic. N. Engl. J. Med. 335:1333–1341.

21. Wu AHB, Feng YJ, and Contois JH (1996) Prognostic value of cardiac troponin I in patients with chest pain [Letter]. Clin. Chem. 42:651–652.

22. Antman EM, Tanasijevic MJ, Thompson B, Schactman M, McCabe CH, Cannon CP, Fischer GA, Fung AY, Thompson C, Wybenga D, and Braunwald E (1996) Cardiac-specific troponin I levels to predict the risk of mortality in patients with acute coronary syndromes. N. Engl. J. Med. 335:1342–1349.

23. Wu AHB, Abbas SA, Green S, Pearsall P, Dhakam S, Azar R, Onoroski M, Senaie A, McKay R, and Waters D (1995) The prognostic value of cardiac troponin T in patients with unstable angina. Am. J. Cardiol. 76: 970–972.

24. Stubbs P, Collinson P, Moseley D, Greenwood T, and Noble M (1996) Prognostic significance of admission troponin T concentrations in patients with myocardial infarction. Circulation 94:1291–1297.

25. Muller-Bardorff M, Freitag H, Scheffold T, Remppis A, Kubler W, and Hatus HA (1995) Development and characterization of a rapid assay for bedside determinations of cardiac troponin T. Circulation 92:2869–2875.

26. Christenson RH, Fitzgerald RL, Ochs L, Rozenberg M, Frankel WL, Herold DA, Duh SH, Alonsozana GL, and Jacobs E (1997) Characteristics of a 20-minute whole blood rapid assay for cardiac troponin T. Clin. Biochem. 30:27–33.

27. Anderson JL, Karagounis LA, Becker LC, Sorensen SG, and Menlove RL (1993) TIMI perfusion grade 3 but not grade II results in improved outcome after thrombolytic therapy. Circulation 87;1542–1550.

28. Ohman EM, Christenson RH, Califf RM, George BS, Samaha JK, Kereiakes DJ, Worley SJ, Wall TC, Berrios R, Sigmon KN, Lee KL, and Topol EJ (1993) Noninvasive detection of reperfusion after thrombolysis based on serum creatine kinase MB changes and clinical variables. Am. Heart J. 126: 819–826.

29. Christenson RH, Ohman EM, Topol EJ, O'Hanesian MA, Sigmon KN, Duh SH, Kereiakes D, Worley SJ, George BS, Alonsozana Wall TC, and Califf RM (1997) Combining myoglobin, creatine kinase-MB and clinical variables for assessing coronary reperfusion after thrombolytic therapy. Circulation 96:1776–1782.

30. Buda AJ, MacDonald IL, Dubbin JD, Orr SA, and Strauss HD (1983) Myocardial infarct extension: prevalence, clinical significance, and problems in diagnosis. Am. Heart J. 105:744–749.

31. Weisman HF and Healy B (1987) Myocardial infarct expansion, infarct extension, reinfarction and pathophysiological concepts. Prog. Cardiovasc. Dis. 30:73–110.

32. Ehrmeyer SS and Laessig RH (1995) Regulatory requirements (CLIA '88, JCAHO, CAP) for decentralized testing. Am. J. Clin. Pathol. 104(suppl 1): S40–S49.

33. Lee TH, Rouan GW, Weisberg MC, Brand DA, Cook EF, Acampora D, and Goldman L (1987) Sensitivity of routine clinical criteria for diagnosing myocardial infarction within 24 hours of hospitalization. Ann. Intern. Med. 106:181–186.

34. Lott JA and Stang JM (1989) Differential diagnosis of patients with abnormal serum creatine kinase isoenzymes. Clin. Lab. Med. 9:627–642.

35. de Winter RJ, Koster RW, Sturk A, and Sanders GT (1995) Value of myoglobin, troponin T and CK-MB$_{mass}$ in ruling out an acute myocardial infarction in the emergency room. Circulation 92:3401–3407.

36. Piran U, Kohn DW, Uretsky LS, Bernier D, Barlow EK, Kiswander CZ, and Stastny M (1987) Immunochemiluminometric assay of creatine kinase MB with a monoclonal antibody to the MB isoenzyme. Clin. Chem. 33:1517–1520.

37. Collinson PO, Thomas S, Siu L, Vasudeva P, Stubbs PJ, and Canepa-Anson R (1995) Rapid troponin T measurement in whole blood for detection of myocardial damage. Ann. Clin. Biochem. 32:454–458.

38. Katus HA, Looser S, Hallermayer K, Remppis A, Scheffold T, Borgya A, Essig U, and Geub U (1992) Development and *in vitro* characterization of a new immunoassay of cardiac troponin T. Clin. Chem. 38:386–393.

39. Mach F, Lovis C, Chevrolet JC, Urban P, Unger PF, Bouillie M, and Gaspoz JM (1995) Rapid bedside whole blood cardiospecific troponin T immunoassay for the diagnosis of acute myocardial infarction. Am. J. Cardiol. 75:842–845.

40. Goldmawn BU, Hamm CW, Schneider JC, Geschen M, and Melnertz T (1997) The value of bedside troponin T testing in the emergency room for risk stratification in patients with chest pain after discharge from hospital. J. Am. Coll. Cardiol. 27(Suppl):359A.

41. Brogan GX, Bock J, Hollander J, McCuskey C, Khan S, Thode H, Broderick J, Henry M, Dinowitz S, Katz K, and Valentine S (1996) Evaluation of cardiac STATus creatine kinase-MB/myoglobin device for rapidly ruling out acute myocardial infarction [Abstract]. Acad. Emerg. Med. 3:106.

42. Murthi P, Young GP, Levitt A, and Gawad Y (1996) Serial use of rapid qualitative multimarker bedside immunoassays for the detection of cardiac ischemia in ED patients with chest pain and possible acute myocardial infarction [Abstract]. Acad. Emerg. Med. 3:107.

17

New Biochemical Markers for Heart Diseases

Alan H. B. Wu and Robert G. McCord

INTRODUCTION

The practice of cardiology continues to evolve with a better understanding of the pathophysiology of coronary artery diseases and the development of new therapeutic modalities. Although many groups, such as the American Heart Association, have been successful in making the general public better aware of risk factors, the incidence of coronary artery disease (CAD)* continues to be very high, because the average age of the population in Western countries continues to increase. As such, there are new demands being placed on the in vitro diagnostics (IVDs) industry to improve the performance of existing cardiac markers and to develop novel markers for new cardiac disease indications.

In the clinical laboratory, advancement of new technologies must be balanced with cost-effective delivery. If new services do not improve patient outcomes or reduce costs, it will be very difficult for clinical laboratorians to justify the implementation of these new tests. Important clinical outcome measures include hospital lengths of stay (LOS), morbidity, mortality, and an assessment of the quality of life (1,2). The evaluation of costs cannot be restricted to individual laboratory costs alone. For example, new tests that produced a higher degree of diagnostic accuracy might lead to a reduction in hospital LOS, which would far outweigh the additional laboratory costs for providing that service. If a new test led to better treatment or avoidance of side effects or complications, substantial cost savings would be realized, even if this occurred in a small minority of cases. Clearly, multidisciplinary cost outcome studies will be required with implementation of new test procedures or services. The areas of active research in new cardiac markers are described in the subsequent sections of this chapter. Today, the IVD's greatest effort has been in the development of tests for early AMI diagnosis. One strategy is to find a test that is earlier and more specific than myoglobin. Another is to find markers that are designed to be used in combination with myoglobin to make the latter more cardiac-specific.

EARLY DIAGNOSIS OF CORONARY ARTERY ISCHEMIA

Need for Early Diagnosis

The need for early diagnosis of AMI has been clearly demonstrated in large clinical

---

*See p. 290 for list of abbreviations used in this chapter.

From: Cardiac Markers   Edited by: Alan H. B. Wu
© Humana Press Inc., Totowa, NJ

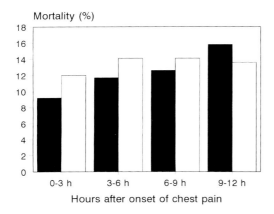

Fig. 1. The in-hospital mortality rate of the GISSI streptokinase trial *(3)*.

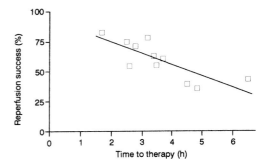

Fig. 2. Reported incidence of reperfusion success vs time from symptoms onset to treatment with IV streptokinase therapy following AMI *(8)*.

trials involving thrombolytic therapy *(3–5)*. For example, in the Italian iv streptokinase study, the mortality of AMI patients treated within 3 h of chest pain was substantially better than AMI patients (Fig. 1) *(3)*. It has been estimated that each hour delay in receiving thrombolytic therapy results in a loss of 21 lives/1000 within 30 d *(6)*. In terms of reperfusion success, earlier treatment relative to the onset of chest pain is associated with a higher success rate (Fig. 2) *(7)*. Because of the increased incidence of bleeding for treated patients relative to placebo *(8)*, the diagnosis of AMI must also be definitive (i.e., a minimal number of false-positive results) *(8)*. Currently, thrombolytic therapy is only given to AMI patients with ST-segment elevations on the electrocardiogram (ECG) *(9)*. However, this strategy may change if high-risk patients with unstable angina (UA) can be identified. Irrespective of how thrombolytics are used now or in the future, early markers for ruling out AMI are needed for the effective triage of patients from the emergency department. Each hour of delay in the triaging equates directly with increased hospital costs.

Assays for myoglobin and CK-MB isoforms provide an early indication for AMI relative to CK-MB and cardiac troponin

(10,11), although there are some studies that question the early utility of these tests *(12–14)*. Myoglobin is not specific toward cardiac injury, and CK-MB isoforms currently require high-voltage electrophoresis to perform. Neither assay consistently produces abnormal results during the first 3 h after AMI onset. As the result of these shortcomings, there is an ongoing search to find new cardiac markers that can provide earlier and more definitive indications of AMI.

Strategies for New Markers Based on the Pathophysiology of Acute Coronary Syndromes

All traditional markers of AMI have focused on the measurement of a specific protein or enzyme that is released after the onset of irreversible damage. In general, smaller proteins appear in blood before larger ones, because they can more easily pass from the interstitial space to the general circulation. Myoglobin has been used as an early marker because of its small size (17 kDa) relative to CK-MB (84 kDa) and lactate dehydrogenase (134 kDa). Markers that are found at high concentrations within the cytoplasm (e.g., myoglobin) are also better candidates than nuclear or mitochondrial proteins (e.g., mitochondrial aspartate aminotransferase), since they must pass through an extra set of membranes, or contractile proteins (cTnT or cTnI),

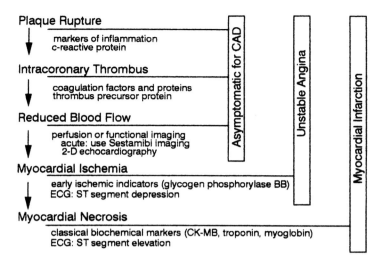

Fig. 3. Role of proposed new cardiac markers for early AMI diagnosis in relation to the pathophysiology of acute coronary syndromes.

Table 1
Summary of New Biochemical Markers for Cardiac Diseases

Marker	Pathophysiologic and/or biochemical role	Size[a]	Clinical utility
C-reactive protein	Acute phase protein	115–140	Marker of inflammation
Thrombus precursor protein	Protein preceding formation of insoluble fibrin formation	>300	Early detection of thrombosis
P-selectin	Platelet activation	140	Detection of platelet aggregation
Glycogen phosphorylase	BB ischemia-induced glycogenolysis	188	Early marker of ischemia
Fatty acid binding protein	Fatty acid protein carrier	15	AMI rule out
α-actin	Striated muscle contraction	43	Heart injury
Brain natriuretic peptide	Natriuresis factor function	4, 10	Sensitive marker for left ventricular

[a]In kilodaltons.

since they require degradation of the actin-myosin unit. Markers of cellular necrosis cannot consistently detect the presence of AMI during the first 3 h of onset, because for most patients, substantial irreversible injury has only just begun. Therefore, a laboratory test that detects AMI earlier than myoglobin must be sensitive to pathophysiologic events that occur during the reversible phase of the disease. Figure 3 reviews some of these events and the biochemical indicators of these

events. Because UA and AMI share a common pathophysiology, a very early serum marker will not likely be successful in differentiating between these two clinical diseases. Nevertheless, both diseases require clinical workups in a hospital setting. If iv thrombolytic therapy becomes important in the treatment of UA patients, a distinction between Q-wave and non-Q-wave (UA) will not be as important. Table 1 summarizes the new markers discussed in this chapter.

EXPERIMENTAL MARKERS FOR EARLY DIAGNOSIS

Markers of Inflammation

As shown in Fig. 3, acute coronary syndromes are associated with inflammation and release of acute-phase proteins, such as C-reactive protein (CRP), amyloid protein A, total sialic acid, and others. Prior to the development of AMI, these acute-phase proteins may be released into the circulation and be used to determine the presence of an acute coronary event. CRP has been used for many years as a marker of inflammation. It may also be possible, therefore, that increased serum levels of inflammatory proteins signify presence of some "initiating" event (infection, trauma, and so forth) that triggers the acute CAD process. CRP has a molecular weight between 115 and 140 kDa, migrates in the γ-region following serum protein electrophoresis, and is typically measured using rate nephelometric or turbidimetric methods *(15)*. The normal range in adults is 6.8–820 µg/dL. Abnormal concentrations in blood are observed in any condition of stress, such as trauma, infection, inflammation, surgery, or neoplasia. CRP concentrations are increased in patients with AMI and may correlate with infarct size when thrombolytic therapy is not given *(16)*. In an experimental model of injury, CRP was increased after elective percutaneous transluminal coronary angioplasty (PTCA) relative to baseline levels, whereas no increase was observed in control patients (i.e., those undergoing coronary angiography) *(17)*.

The major interest in CRP has been in the short- and long-term risk stratification of patients with CAD. In patients with stable angina, CRP along with fibrinogen, von Willebrand factor antigen, and tissue plasminogen activator antigen were correlated to AMI and coronary death within 2 yr *(18)*. In patients with UA, high concentrations of CRP and amyloid protein A were correlated to an increased incidence of AMI or coronary death (35%), when compared to UA patients with normal results (0% incidence) *(19)*. Later studies showed that only CRP and not amyloid A was associated with risk of coronary events *(20)*. In patients with AMI, higher CRP results were found in those AMI patients who developed acute heart failure *(21)* and cardiac rupture *(22)*, compared to AMI patients who had no complications. Although highly nonspecific, CRP can be useful to indicate the presence of acute coronary syndromes and to differentiate it from stable forms of CAD. Moreover, in a recent study, risk of AMI and stroke can be reduced with salicylate use, which may act by reducing inflammation, as demonstrated by a decrease in plasma CPR concentrations *(23)*.

Similar findings have been reported for fibrinogen, another acute-phase protein *(24)*. Plasma fibrinogen levels exceeding 300 mg/dL were associated with bad cardiac outcomes at 42 d from the initial presentation. Fibrinogen has been implicated more as a long-term risk assessment marker, similar to cholesterol.

Markers of Thrombus Formation

Thrombus Precursor Protein™ (TpP)

As discussed in Chapters 2 and 3, thrombus plays a pivotal role in coronary artery disease *(25)*. Plasma markers that indicate the presence of active clot formation can provide valuable information in the differential diagnosis of chest pain. A diagnosis of AMI might effectively be ruled out if there is no evidence of active thrombosis. As shown in Fig. 4, insoluble fibrin forms from fibrinogen under the action of thrombin (Factor IIa) *(26)*. Two pairs of peptides are released in this process. In the presence of Factor XIIIa, soluble fibrin undergoes crosslinking to form insoluble fibrin polymers. During fibrinolysis, plasmin degrades

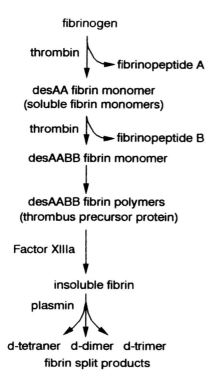

fibrinogen

thrombin ⟍
→ fibrinopeptide A

desAA fibrin monomer
(soluble fibrin monomers)

thrombin ⟍
→ fibrinopeptide B

desAABB fibrin monomer

desAABB fibrin polymers
(thrombus precursor protein)

Factor XIIIa

insoluble fibrin

plasmin

d-tetraner   d-dimer   d-trimer
fibrin split products

Fig. 4. Conversion of fibrinogen to insoluble fibrin monomers and insoluble fibrin polymers. (Adapted from ref. *28.*)

fibrin to peptides known collectively as fibrin degradation (or split) products. One of these products includes the complex known as D-dimer, which can be assayed directly.

Recently, two new tests have been developed that measure precursor proteins of fibrin: desAA fibrin with cleavage of fibrinopeptide A (known as soluble fibrin monomers) and desAABB fibrin with cleavage of fibrinopeptide B (fibrin soluble polymers, commercially known as thrombus precursor protein, TpP™, American Biogenetic Sciences, Inc., Boston, MA). Studies have suggested that monoclonal antibodies (MAb) to soluble fibrin polymers react with both desAA and desAABB fibrin, as well as select fibrin degradation products *(27,28)*. There have been no studies to date on the usefulness of soluble fibrin monomers in AMI. For TpP, the immediate precursor to

soluble fibrin, a preliminary AMI study demonstrated that this protein is increased in 21 patients with AMI who present within the first 6 h of chest pain *(29)*. The concentration of traditional biochemical markers, such as CK-MB, were normal in many of these patients. After admission, TpP concentrations in subsequent collections showed a dramatic decline in values. This decrease in TpP is thought to be owing to the effect of in vivo heparin therapy given to these AMI patients *(30)*.

In patients where active thrombosis has been ruled out, results of TpP are within the normal range of 0–6 μg/mL. The TpP test, however, is necessarily nonspecific, since active clot formation can occur in a variety of other diseases, such as deep vein thrombosis, pulmonary emboli, and cerebral vascular accident. The clinical presentations of patients with any of these disorders may be sufficiently different such that positive results produced by TpP in these disorders might not add significant ambiguity to the interpretation of data. It may also be possible that irrespective of the in vivo site, evidence of active thrombus may warrant admission and further evaluation. This protocol would be particularly warranted if therapeutic intervention for thrombotic diseases demonstrated a reduction in the appropriate outcome measures.

Because thrombus formation is also a major cause of UA, abnormal results for TpP and other markers of thrombin activity would be expected in this disease as well. In a preliminary study of 18 UA patients, 15 were within the normal range *(29)*. In the remaining three with high values, a progression to AMI was noted. In a separate study, serum fibrinopeptide A concentration was increased in 50% of 150 patients with UA *(31)*. Kaplan-Meier survival curves showed fibrinopeptide A might be useful for risk-stratify patients for cardiac death, Q-wave, and non-Q-wave AMI. If the specificity of coagulation markers can be thoroughly documented, it may be very useful in clinical practice for evaluation of patients with CAD.

P-Selectin

The activation and aggregation of platelets constitute another important step in the formation of insoluble clots. The first step in the process is adhesion of platelets to the vessel wall. There it can be activated by agonists, such as thrombin, adenosine diphosphate (ADP), or arachidonic acid (30). Fibrinogen binds to the platelet through glycoprotein IIb/IIIa receptors located on each cell. This enables binding of other circulating platelets to form aggregates. A protein known as GMP-140 or P-selectin is translocated to the activated platelet surface, where it functions to promote leukocyte adhesion and consolidation of the thrombotic plug (32–34). Release of P-selectin from the α-granules of platelets and Weibel-Palade bodies of endothelial cells into the circulation is an indicator of platelet activation and is associated with acute thrombotic disease states (35).

The evaluation of soluble P-selectin into blood of CAD patients has been reported in a few clinical studies. In patients with UA, high levels of P-selectin have been reported within 1 h after onset of symptoms (36). In contrast, normal levels were observed in patients with stable angina, even after they were put on a treadmill and stressed to the point of ST-segment depression on ECG. Following AMI, P-selectin is also increased for the first 3 d of hospitalization (37). For AMI patients acutely treated with PTCA, platelet-bound P-selectin levels transiently decrease immediately after the procedure (4–8 h), but return to high levels on the following days (38). It has been suggested that the initial decline is owing to sequestration of highly adhesive platelets, followed by platelet activation caused by exposure of the endothelial tissue produced

by the angioplasty procedure itself. P-selectin can be useful in understanding the pathophysiologic role of platelets in acute coronary syndromes. It may also be useful for therapeutic strategies involving new antiplatelet drugs. For early AMI diagnosis, the role of P-selectin is currently being investigated.

Functional Imaging

The occlusion of a coronary artery will lead to a disruption in the perfusion of myocardial tissue. This condition can be detected through the use of noninvasive perfusion imaging techniques, such as single-photon emission computed tomography (SPECT) following injection of ^{201}thallium or ^{99m}technetium (sestamibi and tetrosfosmin) (39). The technical details of radionuclide ventriculography are beyond the scope of this volume. Discussion of clinical data is included in this chapter because ventriculography can provide an early indication of CAD, and results will likely complement the use of serum cardiac markers.

In the clinical setting of chest pain with a negative or nondiagnostic ECG, acute myocardial imaging has been successful when radionuclides are injected while the patient is experiencing chest pain. In a study of 45 ED patients, ^{99m}technetium sestamibi tomography provided a sensitivity and specificity of 96 and 79%, respectively (40), for detection of CAD. Corresponding values for 12-lead ECG were 35 and 74%. In another study, nuclear imaging results compared favorably against regional wall abnormalities as assessed by echocardiography. Both the sensitivity (100% vs 42%) and specificity (93% vs 80%) were improved (41). When sestamibi was used to stratify short-term risk of adverse events, positive scans provided a relative risk ratio of 13.9-fold compared to patients with normal scans (42).

In the presence of equivocal ECG results, radionuclide ventriculography can detect the presence of CAD at a time when cardiac markers are still within the normal range *(43)*. Use of sestimibi is superior to thallium scanning, because it does not require a cyclotron for generation of nuclides, and imaging can be performed 1–2 h after injection of sestimibi, a time when patients are more likely to be clinically stable. Although these preliminary results are promising, the use of these techniques in acute chest pain is experimental. Moreover, the cost of the procedure, estimated at $600/case *(42)*, must be considered. Many centers do not have nuclear imaging centers, or do not offer services on a 24-h basis.

Markers of Early Myocardial Ischemia

The total occlusion of a coronary artery by a thrombus will result in anoxia in myocardial areas that are distal to the site of the lesion. Lack of oxygen delivery inhibits the production of ATP by the mitochondria. In order to survive, myocytes must conserve vital ATP stores by inhibiting unnecessary biological functions, such as the maintenance of ionic gradients (via the ATP-dependent membrane pump), and anaerobically producing as much ATP as possible from glucose, proteins, and fatty acids *(44)*. Initially, the ischemic injury is reversible, i.e., if blood flow is restored to the jeopardized areas, no permanent damage will occur. If coronary artery reperfusion does not occur, irreversible injury will begin, as signified by the release of macromolecules, such as enzymes and proteins. The period of ischemic reversibility is likely to vary from person to person, but it is believed to begin between 1 and 3 h after the onset of symptoms *(44)*.

If proteins and enzymes that participate in these "compensatory" biochemical mechanisms are released into the blood during ischemia, they may be useful as early markers of AMI. Glycogen phosphorylase (GP) catalyzes the degradation of glycogen in the sarcoplasmic reticulum (SR) and provides the necessary substrates for glycolysis. GP is a dimeric enzyme with a relative large molecular weight of 188 kDa. It consists of three isoenzymes: BB found in the brain and heart, MM found in skeletal muscles, and LL found in the liver *(45)*. It has been suggested that after glycogenolysis has occurred in an ischemic tissue, GP is released from the SR to the cytoplasm. If the permeability of the cell membrane is compromised by ischemia, GP would appear in the circulation owing to the large concentration gradient of myocytes relative to blood.

An immunoassay for GP-BB has been developed and evaluated in patients with CAD. In a study of 48 patients admitted for angina, results of GP-BB were compared to CK-MB mass, cTnT, and myoglobin *(46)*. In the absence of transient ST-T-segment alterations on ECG, blood concentrations for these markers were largely in the normal range. However, in 18 patients with ST-T-abnormalities, GP-BB was increased in 16 patients (88%), as compared to 2 (11%), 3 (17%), and 5 (28%) patients for myoglobin, cTnT, and CK-MB, respectively. In a comparison of these markers for AMI, GP-BB was the most sensitive marker during the first 2–4 h after onset of chest pain *(45,47)*. In AMI patients treated with thrombolytic therapy, GP-BB returned to normal levels before CK and CK-MB. GP-BB has also been studied as a marker of myocardial injury following bypass surgery *(48)*. Commercial assays for GP-BB are being developed (Pace Medical Diagnostics Corp., Toronto) and await evaluation by clinical trials.

Other Protein Markers of Myocardial Necrosis

Because myoglobin is not specific for myocardial damage, other small-mol-wt proteins have been examined as potential early markers. Heart fatty acid binding protein (FABP) is part of a family of at least six different low-mole-wt proteins (14–15 kDa) that functions as a carrier for long-chain fatty acids. It is found within the cytoplasm and plays an important role in lipid metabolism *(49)*. Because of its low molecular weight, FABP is freely filtered by the glomerulus, and is rapidly cleared from the circulation. Urine concentration of FABP appear within 2 h after injury *(50)*. In patients with renal failure, FABP increases owing to impaired clearance.

The heart type isoenzyme is distinct from the forms found in the liver and intestines. However, like myoglobin, FABP is also found in significant quantities in skeletal muscles. When FABP is used alone as a marker for AMI, it may have no advantage over myoglobin with respect to specificity and sensitivity for early diagnosis. On the other hand, a testing strategy whereby the ratio of myoglobin to FABP is calculated may provide additional diagnostic information over use of one marker alone. Studies of purified organs and tissues have shown that the heart type isoenzyme of FABP is found in very high concentrations in the myocardium (0.46 mg/g wet wt of the left ventricle *[50]*). This reflects the important role of energy production and fatty acid metabolism in the heart. Myoglobin is found in high concentrations within the skeletal muscles. Thus, a calculation of the ratio of these two proteins can be used to determine the source of elevations of these markers in blood after injury. Table 2 illustrates this relationship *(51)*. In heart tissue, a low ratio is observed, whereas skeletal muscles have high values. After AMI, there is an elevation of both myoglobin and FABP, which is accompanied by a low myoglobin/FABP ratio, reflecting the expected myocardial distribution of these proteins. On the other hand, high results and a high ratio after aortic surgery are owing to release from skeletal muscles produced by the surgery itself. Fol-

Table 2
Results of Myoglobin/FABP Ratio in Various Tissues and Blood after Various Events[a]

Tissue/Event	Ratio	SD
Heart	4.5	1.0
Skeletal Muscles	47	8.0
Blood, AMI no thrombolytic therapy	6.2	1.0
Blood, AMI, thrombolytic therapy	4.4	1.4
Blood, after aortic surgery	45	22
Blood, after cardiac surgery		
0.5 h	11.3	4.7
8 h	6.7	3.7
24 h	32.1	13.6

[a]Adapted from ref. *51*.

lowing cardiac surgery, a previous report showed that the initial injury is from the heart, and is followed by release of proteins from the skeletal musculature *(52)*. Using the myoglobin/FABP ratio, data from Table 2 are consistent with this pattern.

The use of FABP in AMI has been demonstrated in several clinical studies. In a study of 10 AMI patients, FABP was increased in all admission samples (range 1.5–14 h after onset of chest pain), whereas CK-MB activity was within the normal range *(53)*. In another study, the clinical sensitivity for FABP and CK-MB was 91.4% and 20%, respectively, for samples collected within 0–3 h *(54)*. Neither of these two studies compared results against myoglobin or assessed the value of the myoglobin/FABP ratio. Presumably, such studies are forthcoming.

OTHER BIOCHEMICAL MARKERS

α-Actin

The structural proteins that have been extensively studied in blood of patients with CAD include cTnT and cTnI, and myosin light and heavy chains. Many believe that cTnT and cTnI will become the new "gold standard" for the definitive diagnosis of AMI because of their high cardiac specificity. In contrast, skeletal muscle myosin chains crossreact with antibodies for the cardiac forms, and these tests will likely be more useful for infarct sizing.

Actin is another structural protein of the thin filament. It has a molecular weight of 43 kDa and makes up more than 20% of the total cell protein pool. The α-actin is present at a ratio that is seven times higher than troponin or myosin *(55)*. As such, if immunoassays can be developed with high analytical sensitivity and specificity, actin may be a more sensitive marker for minor myocardial injury.

In a study of UA, actin was elevated in 19 of 29 patients. Using an immunoblot technique, the highest circulation concentration was 40 µg/mL *(55)*, considerably higher than troponin or myosin. Unfortunately, the sensitivity of this technique was not described. Thus, it is difficult to determine the magnitude of increase relative to normal or baseline levels. The clinical sensitivity of α-actin in AMI was 95% among 70 patients *(56)*. The highest actin concentration was reported at 112 µg/mL. Actin was detected as early as 1 h after the onset of chest pain and remains positive for up to 170 h. Actin was also observed in patients with silent ischemia and in patients with noninsulin-dependent diabetes mellitus *(57)*. Since troponin and CK-MB were not reported in this study, it is difficult to determine if actin detects a lower degree of injury. It is too early to tell if and how actin might be used in patients with CAD. The key issue for actin will be the clinical specificity of the assay.

Brain Natriuretic Peptide

Most of the discussion on new biochemical markers has focused on the use of the tests for ischemic heart disease. Another important area is in the evaluation of left ventricular function in patients with congestive heart failure (CHF). CHF is produced by chronic heart disease, such as diluted cardiomyopathy, valvular disease, and ischemic heart disease. It affects some 2 million Americans today with an average morality rate of 10% after 1 yr and 50% after 5 yr *(58)*. It is expected to rise with the aging of the population. The disease is classified by a variety of schemes, such as that described by the New York Heart Association (NYHA) *(see* Chapter 1). The NYHA classification is made on clinical grounds. Definitive assessment of heart failure is determined by echocardiography, with measurement of the ejection fraction (EJ). Values between 35 and 40% are associated with heart failure *(59)*, although there are a large number of CHF patients that have an EJ of 50% or more *(60)*.

Recently, biochemical markers have been used to assess CHF. Atrial (ANP) and brain natriuretic peptides (BNP) are important hormones for regulation of fluid volume, sodium balance, and blood pressure. ANP is a 28 amino acid peptide that is secreted from the atria of the heart *(61)*. BNP is a 32 amino acid peptide that originates from the brain and ventricles of the heart. There are two forms that are found in plasma of patients with heart failure (molecular weights of 4 and 10 kDa). The high-mol-wt form is found in the highest concentration in blood *(62)*. Another structurally related hormone is C-type natriuretic peptide (CNP), a 17 amino acid hormone that does not have natriuretic action.

In blood of CHF patients, the concentrations of ANP and BNP are significantly abnormal, as the result of increased synthesis by the heart. The degree of increase has been linked to the severity of CHF. Figure 5 shows the results of BNP as a function of degree, as classified by the NYHA system *(63)*. Although there is significant overlap between groups, there is a stepwise increase of BNP as the severity increases from normal

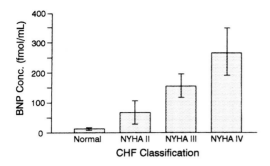

Fig. 5. Results of BNP in different NYHA classification of CHF. Standard deviation given in arrow bars. (Adapted from ref. *59.*)

or stage I–V. The overlap of results is not surprising considering the subjective nature of the NYHA classification. It is presumed that increases in ANP and BNP in CHF are owing to the degree of overload of the atria and ventricles, respectively *(63).* Synthesis of ANP from the ventricles has also been reported *(64).*

When results were compared to ejection fraction (EF), a significant negative linear correlation was produced (i.e., the higher the BNP, the lower the EF). This correlation was observed for dilated cardiomyopathy, but not mitral valve stenosis *(65).* Following AMI, ANP and BNP are both increased in blood *(66).* ANP levels are highest at admission and decline thereafter. BNP undergoes a biphasic release pattern. These hormones appear to reflect the degree of left ventricular dysfunction following the ischemic injury because of the functional role they play in the disease process. There has been no discussion to date on the use of these markers for early AMI detection, since patients with chronic failure may also have abnormal baseline concentrations.

Other Miscellaneous Markers

In a recent review, other very novel markers for myocardial injury were discussed, including protein $S100a_0$, a calcium binding protein, annexin, a phospholipid binding

protein, enolase $\alpha\beta$ isoenzyme, a glycolytic enzyme, and phosphoglyceric acid mutase isoenzyme MB, another glycolytic enzyme *(67).* The performance of these markers has been examined in preliminary studies of patients with UA, AMI, and AMI rule-out. None of these markers are specific to myocardial injury, nor are they released any earlier than existing markers, such as myoglobin and CK-MB isoforms. It is therefore doubtful that that immunoassays for any of these proteins will reach the stage of commercialization.

ABBREVIATIONS

AMI, acute myocardial infarction; ANP, BNP, CNP, atrial, brain and C-type natriuretic peptide; CAD, coronary artery disease; CHF, congestive heart failure; CRP, C-reactive protein; cTnT, cTnI, cardiac troponin T and I; EJ, ejection fraction; FABP, fatty acid binding protein; GISSI, Gruppo Italiano per lo Studio della Streptochinasi nell'Infarcto miocardico; GP, glycogen phosphorylase; iv, intravenous; IVD, in vitro diagnostics; kDA, kilodaltons; LOS, lengths of stay; NYHA, New York Heart Association; PTCA, percutaneous transluminal coronary angioplasty: SPECT, single-photon emission computed tomography; SR, sarcoplasmic reticulum; TpP, thrombus precursor protein; UA, unstable angina.

REFERENCES

1. Ash AS (1993) Outcomes analysis and the practice of medicine. Hosp. Practice 28(10): 10–11.
2. Testa MA and Simonson DC (1996) Assessment of quality-of-life outcomes. N. Engl. J. Med. 334:835–840.
3. The GISSI Study Group (1986) Effectiveness of intravenous thrombolytic treatment in acute myocardial infarction. Lancet 1:397–402.
4. The ISAM Study Group. A prospective trial of intravenous streptokinase in acute myocardial infarction. N. Engl. J. Med. 314:1465–1471.

5. The Thrombolysis in Myocardial Infarction (TIMI) Study Group (1985) The thrombolysis in myocardial infarction (TIMI) trial. N. Engl. J. Med. 312:932–936

6. Rawles J (1996) Magnitude of benefit from earlier thrombolytic treatment in acute myocardial infarction: new evidence from Grampian region early anistreplase trial (GREAT). Br. Med. J. 312:212–216.

7. Sherry S (1987) Recombinant tissue plasminogen activator (rt-PA): is it the thrombolytic agent of choice for an evolving acute myocardial infarction? Am. J. Cardiol. 59: 984–989.

8. Schreiber T (1987) Review of clinical studies of thrombolytic agents in acute myocardial infarction. Am. J. Med. 83:(Suppl. 2A): 20–25.

9. Ryan TJ, Anderson JL, Antman EM, Braniff BA, Brooks NH, Califf RM, Hillis D, Hiratzka LF, Rapaport E, Riegel BJ, Russell RO, Smith EE, and Weaver WD (1996) ACC/AHA guidelines for the management of patients with acute myocardial infarction: a report of the American College of Cardiology/American Heart Assocation Task Force on Practice Guidelines (Committee on Management of Acute Myocardial Infarction). J. Am. Coll. Cardiol. 28:1328–1419.

10. van Blerk M, Maes V, Huyghens L, Derde MP, Meert R, and Gorus FK (1992) Analytical and clinical evaluation of creatine kinase MB mass assay by IMx: comparison with MB isoenzyme activity and serum myoglobin for early diagnosis of myocardial infarction. Clin. Chem. 38:2380–2386.

11. Puleo PR, Guadagno PA, and Roberts R (1990) Early diagnosis of acute myocardial infarction based on an assay for subforms of creatine kinase-MB. Circulation 82: 759–764.

12. Mair J, Morandell D, Genser N, Lechleitner P, Dienstl F, and Puschendorf B (1995) Equivalent early sensitivities of myoglobin, creatine kinase MB mass, creatine kinase iosoform ration, and cardiac troponins I and T for acute myocardial infarction. Clin. Chem. 41:1266–1272.

13. Bhayana V, Cohoe S, and Henderson AR (1995) Evaluation of the Cardio Rep for creatine kinase isoforms analysis. Clin. Chem. 41:S184.

14. Laurino J, Bender EW, Kessimian N, Chang J, Pelletier T, and Usatequi M (1996) Comparative sensitivities and specificities of the mass measurements of CK-MB2, CK-MB, and myoglobin for diagnosing acute myocardial infarction. Clin. Chem. 42: 1454–1459.

15. Silverman LM and Christenson RH (1994) Amino acids and proteins. In: Tietz textbook of clinical chemistry, 2nd ed., Burtis CA and Ashwood ER, eds., Philadelphia, Saunders, 713,714.

16. Pietila K, Harmoinen A, Hermens W, Simoons ML, Van de Werf F, and Verstraete M (1993) Serum C-reactive protein and infarct size in myocardial infarct patients with a closed versus an open infarct-related coronary artery after thrombolytic therapy. Eur. Heart J. 14:915–919.

17. Azar RR, Seecharran B, Feng YJ, Giri S, Wu AH, Kiernan F, McKay R, and Waters DD (1996) Coronary angioplasty induces a systemic inflammatory response. Circulation 94:I559–1560.

18. Thompson SG, Kienast J, Pyke SD, Haverkate F, and van de Loo JC (1995) Hemostatic factors and risk of myocardial infarction or sudded death in patients with angina pectoris. European Concernted Action on Thrombosis and Disabilities Angina Pectoris Study Group. N. Engl. J. Med. 332:635–641.

19. Liuzzo G, Biasucci LM, Gallimore JR, Grillo RL, Rebuzzi AG, Pepys MB, and Maseri A (1994) The prognostic value of C-reactive protein and serum amyloid A protein in severe unstable angina. N. Engl. J. Med. 331:417–424.

20. Haverkate F, Thompson SG, Pyke SDM, Gallimore JR, and Pepys MB (1997) Production of C-reactive protein and risk of coronary events in stable and unstable angina. Lancet 349:462–466.

21. Kazmierczak M, Sobieska M, Biktorowicz K, and Wysocki H (1995) Changes of acute phase proteins glycosylation profile as a possible prognostic marker in myocardial infarction. Int. J. Cardiol. 49:201–207.

22. Ueda S, Ikeda U, Yamamoto K, Takahashi M, Nishinaga M, Nago N, and Shimada K (1996) C-reactive protein as a predictor of cardiac rupture after acute myocardial infarction. Am. Heart J. 131:857–860.

23. Ridker PM, Cashman M, Stampter MJ, Tracy RP, and Hennekins CH (1997) Inflammation, aspirin, and the risk of cardiovascular disease in apparently healthy men. N. Engl. J. Med. 336:973–979.

24. Becker RC, Cannon CP, Bovill EG, Tracy RP, Thompson B, Katterud GL, Randall A, and Braunwald B (1996) Prognostic value of plasma fibrinogen concentration in patients with unstable angina and non-Q-wave myocardial infarction (TIMI IIIB trial). Am. J. Cardiol. 78:142–147.

25. Ambrose JA (1996) Thrombosis in ischemic heart disease. Arch. Intern. Med. 156:1382–1394.

26. Wieding JU and Husias C (1992) Determination of soluble fibrin: a comparison of 4 different methods. Thromb. Res. 65:745–756.

27. Dempfle LE, Dollman M, Lill H, Puzzovio D, Dessauer A, and Heene DL (1995) Binding of a new monoclonal antibody against N-terminal heptapeptide of fibrin alpha-chain to fibrin polymerization site "A": effect of fibrinogen and figrinogen derivatives, and pretreatment of samples with NaSCN. Blood Coagulation and Fibrinolysis 4:79–86.

28. Mosesson MW (1992) The roles of fibrinogen and fibrin in hemostasis and thrombosis. Semin. Haematol 29:177–188.

29. Carville DGM, Dimitrijevic N, Walsh M, Digirolamo T, Brill EM, Drew N, and Gargan PE (1996) Thrombus precursor protein (TpP): marker of thrombosis early in the pathogenesis of myocardial infarction. Clin. Chem. 42:1537–1541.

30. (1997) A blood test for detection of intravascular thrombosis. Measurement of thrombus precursor protein. South Bend, IN, American Biogenetic Sciences.

31. Ardissino D, Merlini PA, Gamba G, Barberis P, Demicheli G, Testa S, Colombi E, Poli A, Fetiveau R, and Montemartini C (1996) Circulation 93:1634–1639.

32. Ushiyama S, Laue TM, Moore KL, Erickson HP, and McEver RP (1993) Structural and functional characteristics of monomeric soluble P-selectin and comparison with membrane P-selectin. J. Biol. Chem. 268:15,229–15,237.

33. George JN, Pickett EB, Saucerman S, McEver RP, Kunicki TJ, Kieffer N, and Newman PJ (1986) Platelet surface glycoproteins. Studies on resting and activated platelets and platelet membrane microparticles in normal subjects and observations in patients during adult respiratory distress syndrome and cardiac surgery. J. Clin. Invest. 78:340–348.

34. McEver RP (1990) The clinical significance of platelet membrane glycoproteins. Hematol. Oncol. Clin. North Am. 4:87–105.

35. Nurden AT, Bihour C, Macchi L, Lacaze D, Durrieu C, Besse P, Dachary J, and Hourdille P (1993) Platelet activation in thrombotic disorders. Nouv. Rev. Fr. Hematol. 3:67–71.

36. Ikeda H, Takajo Y, Ichiki K, Ueno T, Maki S, Noda T, Sugi K, and Imaizumi T (1995) Increased soluble form of p-selectin in patients with unstable angina. Circulation 92:1693–1696.

37. Ikeda H, Nakayama H, Oda T, Kuwano K, Muraishi A, Sugi K, Koga Y, and Toshima H (1994) Soluble form of P-selectin in patients with acute myocardial infarction. Coronary Artery Dis. 5:515–518.

38. Gawaz M, Neumann FJ, Ott I, Schiessler A, and Schomig A (1995) Platelet function in acute myocardial infarction treated with direct angioplasty. Circulation 93:229–237.

39. Morris S, Wu AHB, and Heller GV (1996) New diagnostic approaches to patients with acute chest pain: role of cardiac imaging and biochemical markers. Curr. Opinion Cardiol. 11:386–393.

40. Bilodeau L, Theroux P, Gregoire J, Gagnon D, and Arsenault A (1991) Technetium-99m sestamibi tomography in patients with spontaneous chest pain: correlations with clinical, electrocardiographic and angiographic findings. J. Am. Coll. Cardiol. 18:1684–1691.

41. Varetto T, Cantalupi D, Cerruti A, Compagnoni-Pesenti M, Leone G, and Orlandi C (1990) Tc99m sestamibi and 2D-echo imaging for rule-out of acute ischemia in patients with chest pain and non-diagnostic ECG [Abstract]. Circulation 94 (Suppl.):I367.

42. Hilton TC, Thompson RC, Williams HJ, Saylors R, Fulmer H, and Stowers SA (1994) Technetium-99m sestamibi myocardial perfusion imaging in the emergency room evaluation of chest pain. J. Am. Coll. Cardiol. 23:1016–1022.

43. Morris S, Wu A, Ahlberg AW, Feng YJ, Piriz JM, Shehata A, and Heller GV (1996) Correlation of acute technetium-99m SPECT myocardial perfusion imaging and cardiac serum markers in patients with spontaneous angina [Abstract]. J. Nuclear Med. 37:58.

44. Hearse J (1979) Cellular damage during myocardial ischaemia: metabolic changes leading to enzyme leakage. In: Enzymes in Cardiology: Diagnosis and Research, Hearse DJ and de Leiris J, eds., Chichester, UK, Wiley, pp. 1–19.

45. Rabitzsch G, Mair J, Lechleitner P, Noll F, Hofmann U, Kraus EG, Dienstl F, and Puschendorf B (1995) Immunoenzymometric assay of human glycogen phosphorylase isoenzyme BB in diagnosis of ischemic myocardial injury. Clin. Chem. 41:966–978.

46. Mair J, Puschendorf B, Smidt J, Lechleitner P, Dienstl F, Noll F, Kraus EG, and Rabitzsch G (1994) Early release of glycogen phosphorylase in patients with unstable angina and transient ST-T alterations. Br. Heart J. 72:125–127.

47. Rabitzsch G, Mair J, Leichleitner P, Noll F, Hofmann U, Krause EG, Dienstl F, and Putschedorf B (1993) Isoenzyme BB of glycogen phosphorylase b and myocardial infarction. Lancet 341:1032–1033.

48. Mair D, Mair J, Kraus EG, Balogh D, Puschendorf B, and Rabitzsch G (1994) Glycogen phosphorylase isoenzyme BB mass release after coronary artery bypass grafting. Eur. J. Clin. Chem. Clin. Biochem. 32:543–547.

49. Roos W, Eymann E, Symannek M, Duppenthaler J, Wodzig KWH, Pelsers M, and Glatz JFC (1995) Monoclonal antibodies to human heart fatty-acid binding protein. J. Immunol. Meth. 183:149–153.

50. Yoshimoto K, Tanaka T, Somiya K, Tsuji R, Okamoto F, Kawamura K, Ohkaru Y, Asayama K, and Ishii H (1995) Human heart-type cytoplasmic fatty acid-binding protein as an indicator of acute myocardial infarction. Heart Vessels 10:304–309.

51. van Nieuwenhoben FA, Kleine AH, Wodzig KWH, Hermens WT, Kragten HA, Maessen JG, Punt CD, van Dieijen MP, van der Vusse GJ, and Glatz JFC (1995) Discrimination between myocardial and skeletal muscle injury by assessment of the plasma ratio of myoglobin over fatty acid-binding protein. Circulation 92:2848–2854.

52. Willems GM, Van der Veen FH, Huysmans HA, Flameng W, De Meyere R, Van der Laarse A, Van der Vusse GJ, and Hermens WT (1985) Enzymatic assessment of myocardial necrosis after cardiac surgery: differentiation from skeletal muscle damage, hemolysis, and liver injury. Am. Heart J. 109:1243–1252.

53. Tanaka T, Hirota Y, Sohmiya KI, Nizhimura S, and Kawamura K (1991) Serum and urine human heart fatty acid-binding protein in acute myocardial infarction. Clin. Biochem. 24:195–201.

54. Tsuji R, Tanaka T, Sohmiya K, Hirata Y, Yoshimoto K, Kinoshita K, Kushaka Y, Kawamara K, Morita H, Abe S, and Tanaka H (1993) Human heart-type cytoplasmic fatty acid-binding protein in serum and urine during hyperacute myocardial infarction. Int. J. Cardiol. 41:209–217.

55. Aranega AE, Reina A, Velez C, Alvarez L, Melguizo C, and Arange A (1993) Circulating alpha-actin in angina pectoris. J. Mol. Cell. Cardiol. 25:15–22.

56. Aranega AE, Reina A, Muros MA, Alvarez L, Prados J, and Aranega A (1993) Circulation α-actin protein in acute myocardial infarction. Int. J. Cardiol. 38:49–55.

57. Prados J, Melguizo C, Aranega AE, Escobar-Jimenez F, Cobo V, Gonzales R, and Aranega A (1995) Circulating alpha-actin in angina pectoris. Int. J. Cardiol. 51:127–130.

58. Konstam MA, Dracup K, Baker DW, Bottorff MB, Brooks NH, Daceg RA, et al. (1994) Heart Failure: evaluation and care of patients with left-ventriculay systolic dysfunction. Clinical Practice Guideline, No. 11. US Department of Health and Human Services Public Health Service, Rockville, MD, June.

59. Marantz PR, Tobin JN, Wassertheil-Smoller S, Steingart RM, Wexler JP, Budner N, Lense L, and Wachspress J (1988) The relationship between left-ventricular systolic function and congestive heart failure diagnosed by clinical criteria. Circulation 77:607–612.

60. Dougherty AH, Naccarelli GV, Gray EL, Hicks CH, and Goldstein RA (1984) Con-

gestive heart failure with normal systolic function. Am. J. Cardiol. 54:778–782.

61. Wei CM, Heublein DM, Perrella MA, Lerman A, Rodeheffer RJ, McGregor CGA, Edwards WD, Schaff HV, and Burnett JC (1993) Natriuretic peptide system in human heart failure. Circulation 88:1004–1009.

62. Yandle TG, Richards AM, Gilbert A, Fisher S, Holmes S, and Espiner EA (1993) Assay of brain natriuretic peptide (BNP) in human plasma: evidence for high molecular weight BNP as a major plasma component in heart failure. J. Clin. Endocrinol. Metab. 76: 832–838.

63. Mukoyama M, Nakao K, Hosoda K, Suga SI, Saito Y, Ogawa Y, Shirakami G, Jougasaki M, Obata K, Yasue H, Kambayashi Y, Inouye K, and Imura H (1991) Brain natriuretic peptide as a novel cardiac hormone in humans. Evidence for an exquisite dual natriuretic peptide system, atrial natriuretic peptide and brain natriuretic peptide. J. Clin. Invest. 87:1402–1412.

64. Saito Y, Nakao K, Arai H, Nishimura K, Okumara K, Obata K, Takemura G, Fujiwara H, Sugaware A, Yamada T, Itoh H, Mukogama M, Hosoda K, Kawai C, Ban T, Yasue H, and Imura H (1993) Augmented expression of atrial natriuretic polypeptide gene in ventricle of human failing heart. J. Clin. Invest. 83:298–305.

65. Ungerer M, Bohm M, Elce JS, Erdmann E, and Lohse MJ (1993) Altered expression of β-adrenergic receptor kinase and β_1-adrenergic receptors in the failing human heart. Circulation 87:454–463.

66. Morita E, Yasue H, Yoshimura M, Ogawa H, Jougasaki M, Matsumura T, Mukoyama M, and Nakao K (1993) Increased plasma levels of brain natriureti peptide in patients with acute myocardial infarction. Circulation 88: 82–91.

67. Mair J (1997) Progress in myocardial damage detection: new biochemical markers for clinicians. Crit. Rev. Clin. Lab. Sci. 34:1–66.

Index

About the Editor

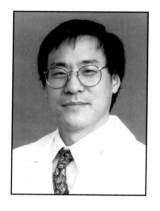

Dr. Alan Wu received his Ph.D. in Analytical Chemistry from the University of Illinois and served a Post-doctoral Fellowship in chemistry at the Hartford Hospital in Connecticut. He is currently the Director of Clinical Chemistry and Toxicology of the Department of Pathology at Hartford Hospital and a Professor of Laboratory Medicine at the University of Connecticut. Board certified in clinical and toxicological chemistry, Dr. Wu is has devoted much of his recent research effort to the study and development of new cardiac markers, and lectures regularly on this topic at international scientific conferences. He has won the American Association of Clinical Chemistry's Outstanding Speaker Award in 1986, 1993, 1996, and 1997. Dr. Wu has authored 113 abstracts, published 134 articles, letters, and reviews, has contributed 20 book chapters, and has co-edited two other books prior to publishing *Cardiac Markers* with Humana Press.